The *Liberty Paradox*

The
Liberty
Paradox

Living with the
Responsibilities of Freedom

DAVID KINLEY

JOHNS HOPKINS UNIVERSITY PRESS
Baltimore

© 2024 David Kinley
All rights reserved. Published 2024
Printed in the United States of America on acid-free paper
2 4 6 8 9 7 5 3 1

Johns Hopkins University Press
2715 North Charles Street
Baltimore, Maryland 21218
www.press.jhu.edu

Library of Congress Cataloging-in-Publication Data

Names: Kinley, David (Lecturer in law), author.
Title: The liberty paradox : living with the responsibilities of freedom /
David Kinley.
Description: Baltimore : Johns Hopkins University Press, 2024. |
Includes bibliographical references and index.
Identifiers: LCCN 2023005905 | ISBN 9781421447957 (hardcover) |
ISBN 9781421447964 (ebook)
Subjects: LCSH: Liberty.
Classification: LCC JC585 .K547 2024 | DDC 323.44—dc23/eng/20230303
LC record available at https://lccn.loc.gov/2023005905

A catalog record for this book is available from the British Library.

*Special discounts are available for bulk purchases of this book. For more information, please
contact Special Sales at specialsales@jh.edu.*

To the memory of Tom Campbell,

who knew a thing or two about freedom and responsibility

And for Suzanne,

who just might read this one

When men yield up the privilege of thinking,

the last shadow of liberty quits the horizon.

—*Thomas Paine*

Contents

The *Liberty Paradox*

Prologue

As I was wrestling with a draft of this book in early 2020, the first murmurings of a new flu-like virus were emerging out of China. As the COVID-19 calamity gathered force inside China and then erupted across an unprepared rest of the world in the months that followed,[1] it quickly dominated every aspect of our lives in ways that were as incredible as they were (for most of us) unpredictable. So pervasive has the pandemic been and so grave its consequences for our daily lives that it seemed to me inevitable it would also dominate this book. And in a way it has. Not in the sense that this is now a book focused on COVID-19, nor even a book that pivots toward viewing freedom through the lens of living with pestilence, but rather in the sense that the compromises COVID-19 has forced us all to make—be it wearing masks, restricting our travel, or getting vaccinated—help validate the book's core argument that in the reality of our entangled lives, freedom is *always* conditional. You might wholly or broadly accept these compromises, or you might resist or rail against them, but whichever the case, conditions of some kind or other constitute an essential part of what freedom is. That is the paradox of liberty.

As we all, to varying degrees, live in the company of others, so our individual freedoms are necessarily a communal affair. This is the very nature of liberty, taking *and* giving. The eternal vigilance ascribed as the price of freedom refers to your keen attention and mine to the nature and boundaries of our respective freedoms insofar as they overlap or clash. Liberty is not and cannot viably be a license to take and not to give; to do as one pleases irrespective of others. Such claims to "freedom without limits," as are increasingly made by so-called libertarians,[2] are not only doomed to fail in any societal setting, but they also gravely misrepresent what liberty is about.

In these circumstances, therefore, the overarching concern of the book is to rehabilitate the notion of liberty by countering such myopic demands and showing what responsibility means in the context of freedom as we experience it today. How, in other words, do we live with the idea of liberty in practice as we negotiate the content of freedom and its boundaries for ourselves and one another in the everyday realms of our lives? Whether in normal, unremarkable times or in times of extraordinary upheaval, the need to recognize and work with the "liberty paradox" remains the same. The global upheaval caused by a pandemic, therefore, does not alter my argument but rather underlines it. COVID-19's impact has been to highlight—in garish technicolor—the contention that responsibilities are not only unavoidable but also elemental to the establishment and preservation of freedom. Freedom, both personal and societal, is a long game, hard fought and at times exhausting, and the enduring challenge is how to set the rules and play by them in ways fair to everyone.

I take on this task by explaining why we need to face up to the liberty paradox and by exploring how we live with it across a broad spectrum of concerns that occupy our daily lives. I use myriad examples to stress specific points about how we try (and sometimes fail) to balance freedoms and responsibilities across the key domains of our health, death, wealth and work, our voice and the voices of others, our pursuit of happiness, our love lives, and our collective and individual security, and whether and how much we trust and respect our leaders, as well as one another, to negotiate the balance justly and wisely. These are not, of course, the only domains of quotidian concern, but I do believe them to be important ones that are, undeniably, large and present for all of us at some time or other and to varying degrees, depending on our circumstances.[3]

And while the lessons of COVID-19 certainly help fortify what I say about the benefits and burdens of living with the responsibilities of freedom, I don't spell out these lessons in all the places they might apply, though I dare say you will see points of relevance drawing from your own knowledge and experiences as you read through the book. This is not to downplay the significance of a pandemic but to place it in the context of the struggle for freedom that has preoccupied human civilizations from their earliest days, a struggle that will continue to do so long after this coronavirus is relegated to just another contagion we have learned to live with.

Introduction
Tea with a Dictator

It was a moment of chilling clarity. It stopped me dead in my tracks when the meaning of what he said sank in. He had spoken so quietly, with a smile on his face and looking directly into my eyes, all totally at odds with the intent of his words. "You must remember, Mr. Kinley, that it is my head on the block, not yours." This was Tin Hlaing, a colonel in the Myanmar military and Minister of Home Affairs. It was 2002, Myanmar was ruled by a brutal military dictatorship, and we were sitting at a small rickety table on the patio of a Yangon hotel, having afternoon tea. I was there to lead a small team of international lawyers providing human rights training to public servants, many of whom were employed in the colonel's ministry. Myanmar was almost completely ostracized by the rest of the world at the time, and so our Australian government–backed initiative was controversial, both inside and outside Myanmar.

Tin Hlaing had been a key broker on the Myanmar side of this deal, which he knew very well was not popular within the junta.[1] He was at risk being seen to reach out to the West at all, but doing so on the topic of human rights was especially eyebrow raising. What had led to our conversation over tea was our team's use of Amnesty International and United Nations publications on Myanmar as reading material for the public servants we were training. Credible, well-researched, and publicly available (outside Myanmar), these documents were highly critical of the government's "continuing pattern of gross and systematic violations of human rights."[2] For each training session, the papers were carefully counted out and back and then locked away, so concerned were our hosts that the material might make it out of the classroom. What Tin Hlaing was telling me, therefore, was that while I might be enjoying the freedom to use these publications, it came with responsibilities. Most especially, that I accept the necessity of restricting access to the materials lest their inflammatory contents reach the eyes or ears of his less tolerant colleagues. Contrary though that might be to my liberal, professorial sensibilities, he was telling me that was nothing compared to what he stood to lose.

As inside all autocracies, there are some good guys (or less bad guys); Tin Hlaing was one of those in Myanmar's recent dark past. He did indeed survive the regime in a physical sense but suffered a "social death," being stripped of his ministerial position and military rank and retreating to a Buddhist monastery for a time. The reformatory path he trod, however, eventually led to Myanmar's coming in from the cold in 2012 (before relapsing following the military coup in February 2021), and today he lives quietly in semi-retirement and runs a charitable foundation established in his wife's honor.

Then and now, I regard this little episode as one of life's tipping points.[3] A sharp reminder of the tenuousness of freedom, how hedged and compromised it can be and yet, to the extent that it does exist, precious nonetheless. It also brought home to me that using freedom—however broad or limited its scope—is never carefree. There are consequences, impacts that may often be beneficial or neutral but that can also be detrimental and even dangerous. Freedom holders, its users and advocates, must always bear this in mind, no matter how zealously they guard it.

Freedom's Questions

Freedom is indeed the catchcry of our time. We covet it and claim it as our right. We fight for it and many have died in its name. Above all we argue about it. Endlessly. Freedom to do what? Where to do it and when? Freedom for whom and how much? For in the reality of our messy lives, freedom has limits and responsibilities, boundaries that separate my freedom from yours, and both of ours from everyone else's.

We are all individuals living in the presence of others. We don't live alone in the true meaning of the word; we all live in societies, big or small, intimate or disparate. The same freedoms we demand for ourselves, therefore, will be demanded by our neighbors, with the unavoidable prospect that some will clash. Freedom, necessarily, comes with responsibilities. Both must be managed, and their balance negotiated between relevant parties either directly or through social means. Here, governments and lawmakers play a role. By setting some boundaries, issuing rules to guide our deliberations over others, and sometimes—when serious conflicts do arise—by mediating between disputing parties, they are supposed to represent our individual and collective interests openly and fairly. It is our responsibility to make sure they do so. But that is not our only responsibility, and not even necessarily the most important one.

For within these broadly defined confines, our personal freedoms and our responsibilities to others are continuously refined through the fluidity of our interpersonal relations and social settings. Individual freedom in the absolute sense is a *non*sense.[4] But do we really understand this? Do we accept that our own freedoms might be restricted to protect the rights of others (and theirs limited to protect ours), as well as to preserve the interests of us all as a whole? Or do we sidestep the inconvenient claims of others and furtively (or frankly) resent it when our freedoms are restricted? Has freedom made a rod for its own back by appearing to promise more than it can deliver?

I have spent a lifetime pondering such questions. Whether personally or professionally, implicitly or explicitly, they've always been present. For nearly forty years I've worked in human rights—in parliaments and assemblies, courtrooms and jailhouses, on the streets, in lecture halls and libraries, in broken homes, dingy offices, and stately boardrooms. And alongside (or against) a host of organizations—governments, corporations, nongovernmental organization (NGOs), aid agencies, and international bodies such as the UN, the World Bank, and the EU, as well as universities and some truly remarkable activists, refugees, lawyers, entrepreneurs, great thinkers, and "ordinary" people. It has taken me across the globe, from Europe and the Americas, to Africa, South and Southeast Asia, and the Pacific islands (both big, like Australia, and small, like Kiribati). Together these experiences have provided me with a wealth of understanding of what freedom can do to promote human rights and improve lives, and to crush both, when it is unfairly denied or brutally quashed.

One might perhaps expect no less of someone occupying a university chair in human rights law, but of course that is only my day job. What propelled me toward such an occupation had as much to do with personal experiences and inclinations as it did with intellectual interest and professional ambition. What freedom means in practice, when two sides have such apparently implacable opinions on the matter that they fight a guerrilla war over the question for thirty years in the streets of your childhood and adolescence, unavoidably and profoundly shapes one's own opinions on freedom and much else besides. I was born in Belfast, Northern Ireland, and raised there during some of the worst years of the Troubles in the 1970s and '80s. While my upbringing was fortunate despite eight years in an Irish boarding school (itself a *Lord of the Flies*–style lesson in negotiating freedom), you could not avoid the effects of the violence, either physically or psychologically.

This book's journey into freedom and responsibility, therefore, is also something of a reflection on my own long, winding path in and around the subject. As such, the book is peppered with accounts of my personal encounters with tough questions about freedom and its limits. From bombs in Belfast and tea with Burmese dictators, to whispered conversations with human rights advocates in China, and louder lectures from bankers about making money; to a former Viet Cong soldier's unlikely love story forged during battle; to the crippling poverty of brick kiln workers in Nepal; to how an Iraqi translator nearly caused an international incident trying to save the blushes of an Australian judge; and the bravery of activists opposing the suffocating expansion of palm oil corporations in Indonesia. Lessons in French slang learned from deciphering the freedom protests scrawled on the vests of the *gilets jaunes* in Paris, what Aung San Suu Kyi's dog did to her copy of the Myanmar constitution, how to get law students to think seriously about free speech, and an uncomfortably private confession of unrequited thespian aspirations are also tales told throughout the book. Even my mother's ordinary life of extraordinary dedication gets an airing, precisely because it is a story of freedom-crimping selflessness shared by millions like her.

But the book is more than a ragbag collection of personal and professional memoirs. I draw extensively on decades of my research in the field, as well as on the research, experiences, and contemplations of many others—writers, philosophers, policy wonks, and data nerds—to create a series of storytelling doorways through which to engage with the big ideas inside. I hope that, together, these narratives provide both context and insight into the various ways we negotiate the boundaries between freedom and responsibility across our lives today. I hope also that they give us cause to reflect on what we need to do to make the negotiated outcomes fairer and more sustainable. In so doing, however, I am conscious of the dangers of epistemic trespass. I am not a professional philosopher or a political scientist, still less an economist, ethicist, or psychologist, yet I must engage with all these fields and others when considering the nature of freedom. Such breadth is often, unavoidably, the lot of a human rights lawyer who nonetheless brings their own perspectives, experiences, and disciplinary rigor to any topic, which, in the present case, I would characterize as a jurisprudentially pragmatic approach to the dynamic between individual rights and social order. Inevitably, I will disappoint purists in one or all of the above disciplines, but as my goal is to reach beyond and across boundaries to better explain liberty's past, present, and future in terms meaningful to general readers rather than (only) specialists, I hope that greater breadth will be considered a fair exchange for any shortfalls in depth.

Liberty's Answers

Of all the messages I'm trying to convey in the book, the most important is simple. It is that freedom's limits are both essential and desirable. What this means in practice, however, is where the difficulties lie. To this end, I invite you to join me on an exploration of how well we go about deciding where to draw these limits, by highlighting who wins and who loses. I show why it is so important that we embrace the responsibilities of freedom as individuals in the ways we conduct our own lives, and together in the ways we build and organize the societies we live in. I conclude by urging us all to reestablish respect and trust between one another in matters of liberty, while at the same time reasserting our demands that governments respect the trust we invest in them. The real-time consequences of the COVID-19 pandemic have shown us grounds for both hope and despair about what good stocks of social trust can achieve and what their absence or inadequacy can destroy.

That there is a word for acknowledging the fundamental necessity of these limits and for shouldering these responsibilities constitutes the fulcrum upon which my argument turns. The word as properly understood has fallen into disuse, overtaken in more recent times by the apparently irresistible appeal of the word "freedom" itself. That word is "liberty."[5]

Liberty denotes freedom within borders, even if, to some, that seems paradoxical. It incorporates the duties that necessarily accompany any exercise of individual freedom in social, political, or economic settings, if we are to preserve everybody's freedom and not just those of the privileged or powerful. These duties rest on all our shoulders, including, and especially, those of our leaders and institutions of government. For if history has taught us anything about the fortunes of liberty, it is that people's freedom is never more in danger than when those in authority spurn the responsibilities they owe to the societies they live in, by supposing or asserting that their freedoms are more important than those of others. Liberty bestows on no one a mandate to do what they please.

In the pages that follow, I chronicle the remarkable history of liberty and the vital role it has played in the evolution of our modern world. I dissect liberty's twin-like relationship with the notion of freedom and explain how and why the one has come to displace the other, and with what consequences. Most of all, I argue for the rehabilitation of the idea of liberty, that freedom is conditional and that those conditions are matters of contestation and perpetual debate. As freedom's rights holders, we are also its duty bearers. Defining liberty is not a one-way street protecting your freedoms or mine, come what may. It is instead more like a roundabout whereby we must first contemplate alternative or competing freedom claims coming from different directions, and then shoulder the burden of deciding who gets priority and why. Liberty, in other words, requires us to work for our freedom.

Living with Liberty Every Day

As a passionate defense of liberty, the book seeks to unravel what freedom really means in practice by examining the role it plays in the most significant domains of our lives: from the ways we work and play, through the levels of health and safety we enjoy, our use (and abuse) of wealth, what personal, philosophical, or religious convictions we hold and how we express them, to how we love and die. And I've sought to employ vivid and telling examples of freedom's peculiarities, problems, and possibilities in the everyday settings of these domains to illustrate how its borders are negotiated and its responsibilities defined.

Threaded through lines of personal and professional narrative, these examples range far and wide. Some focus on fear. Such as the swift and overwhelming dread that pandemics like the previous century's Spanish flu and this century's COVID-19 exert over almost every aspect of daily life and death. Or the more gradual foreboding that our wholesale surrender of personal data online has already so shrunken our capacity to act freely that the choices we make are in fact profoundly manipulated by others. The bitter disputes in many countries over proposals that vaccinations should be made compulsory in order to protect the health of the community despite the objections of individuals. Free speech debates over restrictions on hate speech and sedition (what the Chinese government calls a lack of "ideological firmness"), or how to respond to offensive jokes or fake news. And the disturbingly surreal arguments over whether restrictions on the ownership and use of firearms in the United States safeguards or endangers lives.

Other examples rely on the sobering results of evidence-based research. Such as findings that freedom is nearly always relative and circumstantial, as shown by multiple studies revealing the poor to be just as happy as the rich, and often more so. The scarcely understood implications for our freedoms inside (and outside) the workplace of predictions that nearly half of all jobs consist of activities that can and will be significantly automated in the coming decade.[6] And how education triumphed over prejudice in Ireland, once one of the world's most theocratic states, in decriminalizing blasphemy and abortion and legalizing same-sex marriage (while at the same time banning smoking in pubs), all in little more than a decade.

Reflections on the many ways freedom and responsibility play out across our everyday lives invite a raft of existential questions. Are we free to work, make money, and spend it as we please? Will a high-tech gig economy increase or decrease our levels of privacy and personal freedom? Can wealth buy freedom? Should it? Why are there any restrictions at all on our pursuit of happiness? Surely we should be free to love whomever or whatever and however we want? Ought we be compelled to be healthy, at least to some degree, or should we be free to endanger our health however we choose? And if we can be forced to respect the health of others in a pandemic, should the same apply when the pandemic has passed? Why can't we decide the manner of our death and when and where it happens? What about our opinions and beliefs: can't we hide, express, or practice them without interference? Is it necessary to trade some freedoms for more security? And if so, whose freedoms and whose security?

These are some of life's most pressing questions and ones that, daily, in one way or another we are all trying to answer. This is the art of living with liberty, of navigating freedom within limits, whether too many and too rigid, or not enough and too weak. It is the imperative of taking seriously freedom's responsibilities. The book investigates the techniques we employ in trying to answer these and other liberty-related questions, while highlighting the old and new challenges we face along the way and suggesting how we can best overcome them.

Perspectives matter greatly in this quest. Those on the Left of politics often (though, interestingly, not always) have different views on where to draw freedom's boundaries from those on the Right. Whether the freedoms in question are being mainly or wholly exercised in private or public significantly influences their scope. The extent to which the facts of climate change should restrict our present freedoms in order to preserve the future environment and future generations is both pressing and moot. The elemental psychological question of whether any of us truly exercises a "free will" also bears on our individual perceptions of freedom and its constraints. As does the equally abstruse question of how far we must alter our understanding and expectations of freedom as technological advances in machine learning and artificial intelligence increasingly affect all aspects of our lives.

Throughout this book, I traverse all these points of view as together we journey through liberty's deservedly illustrious past to its underappreciated present and onward to an uncertain future.

By showing how thoroughly misplaced its current neglect is, I mount what I hope you'll believe is a compelling argument for the restoration of liberty's paradox as the guiding principle by which we can best define our freedoms today, defend their borders tomorrow, and share the benefits they generate in the days to come.

PART I
Understanding Liberty

In which the scene is set by defining liberty in terms of freedom *and* responsibility, and by surveying the historical antecedents, theoretical landscape, and practical implications of the relationship.

1

From "Liberty Dogs" to "Freedom Fries"

The liberty of man, in society, is to be under no other legislative
power, but that established by consent in the Commonwealth.
—John Locke

Celebrating Liberty

A few years before he began work on the famous tower to which
his name is now attached, Frenchman Gustave Eiffel's exceptional
engineering skills were put to the test on another project of monumental significance. In the winter of 1879, he was hired to construct the iron framework on which the sculptor Frédéric Auguste
Bartholdi would mount a 46-meter-high copper statue of a Roman goddess. It must have been a remarkable sight as, over the
next three years, the statue rose out of the workshop to dominate
the skyline of Paris's Plaine-Monceau. Paris, however, was not its
intended location. Because it was the world's first major monument built in kit form, and because it was a gift from the people
of France to the people of the United States, the entire structure
was dismantled and shipped across the Atlantic. After reaching
New York, the piece was duly reassembled and over the summer
of 1886 erected on a massive stone pedestal built by American
masons on a small island off the southwestern tip of Manhattan.
The Roman goddess was Libertas, and the statue was inscribed

with the words "La Liberté éclairant le monde" (Liberty enlightens the world). It was and is the Statue of Liberty.

As a joint project between two nations marking their respective centenaries of freedom from monarchical rule (Gustave's eponymous tower unveiled in Paris three years later, in 1889, was intended to honor that very event in France), the term "liberty" resonated deeply. Further, coming just two decades after an enervating civil war fought over slavery in the United States—the outcome of which had been an additional reason why the French were so keen to recognize America's emancipatory achievements— as well as the recent end of the Franco-Prussian War and the onset of the Belle Époque in Europe, you might say that liberty was enjoying something of a golden age.

It is, therefore, somewhat surprising to find, less than a century and half later, that liberty has fallen out of fashion. Or at least the word has. Today it has been almost wholly supplanted by "freedom" in the lexicons of law, politics, philosophy, and social chatter.

As a matter of fact, both terms were used commonly, though sometimes with different connotations, by the greatest of our liberalist thinkers from the ancient Greeks to the mainstays of the European Enlightenment. Plato treated them synonymously. Thus, in *The Republic*, he warns against the "excess of freedom" and counsels that "all human freedom is limited by the laws of nature and of mind."[1] Loving freedom too much, he argued, blinds us to the ulterior motives of tyrants who promise to protect it. Thomas Hobbes, in *Leviathan*, focused on freedom *from* hindrance or opposition by defining freedom as a state of being without "external impediments."[2] John Locke also built his notion of freedom on the foundation of one's unrestricted capacity to exercise free will but added that an individual has freedom to take certain actions or have certain expectations—"to follow his own will," as he put it in his *Second Treatise on Government*.[3] Liberty, on the other hand, was envisioned by both Locke and Hobbes as the circumstance whereby some of our natural freedoms are relinquished to governmental authority (albeit that was an absolute monarchy in Hobbes's view) for the sole purpose that the state will enact and enforce laws that better protect the freedoms of all citizens. "Liberty," according to Locke, "is freedom from restraint and violence by others; and this can't be had where there is no law." Hobbes also subscribed to the importance of law and a "common power" or lawmaking authority (even if a king or queen), arguing that as law defines justice, its absence permits all manner of degradations of freedom to escape being labeled unjust.

Picking up the theme of "natural" freedoms, German rationalist philosopher Immanuel Kant held that freedom is the *only* innate right of humankind, calling this a "universal law." He defined freedom in terms of moral philosophy as constituting one's freedom of choice and action insofar as it can coexist with the same freedom of everyone else. Crucially, the political means by which such freedom is managed in practice—what Kant referred to as "freedom as a condition of rational actions"—was "to make public use of one's reason in all matters."[4] Liberty, in other words, is secured by people abiding by what he called "categorical" moral imperatives,[5] such as "Do not murder, even if it will help you achieve your goals," rather than following hypothetical imperatives, such as "If you don't want to go to prison, don't commit murder." Kant's idealism maintained that the rationality of people's mutual respect will act as a guarantor of social order and personal freedom, more than the protection offered by the force of state authorities.

The heydays for the waltz between liberty and freedom were undoubtedly during the cauldron of political revolution at the end of the eighteenth century. Two of the most passionate intellectual firebrands who ever waved the banner of liberty were at the heart of the politics of the time. Thomas Paine wrote *The Rights of Man* (1791) in celebration of the French Revolution in 1789 and drew inspiration from the American War of Independence before it and the US Constitutional Convention that had followed. Paine even dedicated his "small treatise" to President George Washington. Mary Wollstonecraft wrote *A Vindication of the Rights of Women* (1792) in direct response to the stark omission of the other half of humanity from the deliberations (including Paine's contribution) over people's rights and freedoms. Both publications were short but extraordinarily powerful defenses of individual liberty. Both were also iconoclastic.

Paine's *Rights of Man* caused him to be exiled from England, imprisoned, and sentenced to death in France (he despised the tyranny that followed the Revolution), and while narrowly escaping execution there, he was shunned by former American friends, including Washington, for his uncompromising promotion of individual freedoms, bordering (they thought) on subversion.[6] Wollstonecraft was no less forthright and shocking. Arguing that reason dictates that women are equal to men, no matter social conventions to the contrary, did not endear her to the establishment at the time. Yet her place as a groundbreaking feminist thinker was secured not only by the bravery and potency of her arguments but also by the elegance with which she delivered them. "Liberty is the mother of virtue," she wrote, "and if women are slaves by their very constitution, and not allowed to breathe the sharp invigorating air of freedom, they must always languish like exotics, and be regarded as beautiful flaws in nature."[7]

Unsurprisingly, liberty and freedom are both championed in many key constitutional instruments of modern history, including those of England (as it then was), France, and the United States. The 1689 English Bill of Rights refers to freedom three times and liberty once. The Déclaration des Droits de l'Homme et du Citoyen de 1789 contains five references to *liberté* (there being only one word in French for the term), while intriguingly the official English translation of the French assigns the word "freedom" to three of those and "liberty" to the other two. Surprisingly, both the US Declaration of Independence (1776) and the US Constitution as ratified in 1788 refer only once to liberty and not at all to freedom. The Bill of Rights, ratified three years later, comprising the first ten amendments to the US Constitution, does include one mention of freedom (of speech) and added another mention of liberty.

Liberty and freedom continued to share history throughout the nineteenth and early twentieth centuries, and not just in the words of foundational legal texts and on the plaques of inspiring monuments but in the clarion calls of leaders and writers alike. In noting that "we all declare for liberty," Abraham Lincoln was publicly debating what we all mean by the term.[8] At the same time across the Atlantic, John Stuart Mill was offering his definition based on equality of freedom and the "harm principle" in his landmark treatise *On Liberty.* Jeremy Bentham had earlier and passionately defended liberties of "the press" and of "public association" as essential to calling the power of government to account in what he considered to be its "sole object," namely "the greatest happiness of the greatest possible number of the community."[9] Seventy years later, in the lull between two world wars, Virginia Woolf's acerbic depictions of the injustice of denying women the same liberties as men made uncomfortable reading for society's elite just as Mary Wollstonecraft's words had done a century and a half before.[10]

Liberty's Conditional License

For me the appeal of liberty, then and now, lies in its inherent association of freedom *with* responsibility. It is true, as we shall see repeatedly, that many authors, including the most prominent and celebrated, use the words interchangeably. While understandable and to some extent unavoidable—there are, for example, many different interpretations of "freedom" which are perfectly acceptable[11]—I want to build my argument for the rehabilitation of liberty today on the basis that it is distinguishable from freedom simpliciter. That it is distinguishable from absolute or unconditional freedom, which is the freedom to do what you want without interference. Liberty, rather, is equivalent to freedom *within limits*, and those limits are born of responsibility. Liberty, in this sense, can be considered a license to be free, but one that is inescapably conditional.

To this end I draw support from the greats. I'm with Mill, who argued that responsibility is hardwired into liberty, sitting both on the shoulders of the freedom claimant to use freedom in ways that do not encroach unduly on the freedoms of others (the "harm principle") and on society and the representative state to police those boundaries accordingly.[12] Isaiah Berlin's notion of "positive liberty" in his "Two Concepts of Liberty" also makes sense to me insofar as it promotes the idea that liberty connotes more than freedom from interference (his other, "negative," liberty). The positive sense of liberty, according to Berlin, acknowledges that freedom can be controlled or interfered with but only after establishing the source of the legitimacy of those seeking to do so.[13] In more recent times, Philip Pettit elegantly portrays this perspective of freedom as being one of "nondomination," as opposed to noninterference.[14] The critical difference is that the former recognizes the need for limits on freedom as negotiated between free and equal individuals; the latter, ultimately, accepts no such interference with personal freedom.

It is true that there exist many differing views on what precisely constitutes liberty, not just within the canon of liberalism itself but among nonliberals too. "Just about every modern rival to liberalism has claimed to stand somewhere on the side of liberty," notes Edmund Fawcett in his work on the subject, from communism to fascism and everything in between. Yet the unifying principle that binds them all is that with freedom comes responsibility, even if interpretations of what such responsibility entails differ markedly. Liberty is "ordered," as Fawcett adds, driving home the point that whatever else liberty is, it is assuredly not unbounded freedom.[15] Others make the same point: "Although liberty implies the absence of (some particular) constraint, at the same time it implies a continuation of a surrounding network of restraint and order," as Hanna Fenichel Pitkin neatly argues.[16]

This two-part formula provides liberty with its greatest strength—namely, the prospect, when the mix is right, of a balanced allocation and use of freedom between us all. My freedoms are equal to yours in the sense intended by history's long line of liberty theorists from Plato to Mill. But the formula also contains the seeds of its greatest weakness. For if you get the mix wrong, the result can be catastrophic, either tending toward the anarchy of too much freedom and not enough responsibility, or the tyranny of too much responsibility and no or little freedom. So, just as when we misjudge the balance between adhesive and fixer when mixing two-pack epoxy glues, so it is with liberty. In both cases the result can become seriously unstuck.

If there was a competition for the moment in human history when liberty was most seriously unstuck, the first half of the twentieth century would be a top contender for the gold medal. The virulent ascent of both fascism and communism in that time was marked by a shared ingenuity for interpreting liberty to suit their own ends. Liberty's irresistible appeal is such that, as economist and libertarian Friedrich Hayek notes, there is "no end to the tricks by which people can be exhorted in the name of liberty to give up their liberty."[17] Thus, while both Adolf Hitler and Joseph Stalin were consummate exponents of the art of using systematic violence to pursue their goals, they were also drawn to the rhetorical power of invoking and twisting liberty to their respective causes. Hitler, for example, in a speech on May 1, 1939, intoned that "above the liberty of the individual . . . there stands the liberty of our Volk [people]. The liberty of the Reich [state] takes precedence over both."[18] Stalin, with no hint of irony, proclaimed three years earlier in an interview with an American journalist, "We did not build this society in order to restrict personal liberty but in order that the human individual may feel really free," and that is why, he added, "we want to give Soviet people complete freedom to vote for those they want to elect, for those whom they trust to safeguard their interests."[19] Whether through Stalin's artifice or the direct route chosen by Hitler, both pervert the meaning of liberty by subordinating individual freedom to individual responsibility to the state.[20]

It was, however, their actions rather than words before, during, and (in Stalin's case) also after the Second World War that created the impetus for reassessing the relationship between liberty and freedom. As a new international legal order began to emerge from the geopolitical ashes of the Second World War, a preference for the term "freedom" streaked ahead of liberty. "Freedom" went viral, as it were, propelled by an ardent appreciation of the virtues of freedom in the minds of everyone who had survived that war, coming so soon after "the war to end all wars," as the First World War had been so inaptly labeled.[21]

"Liking" Freedom

What made the period immediately following the Second World War so accommodating to the notion of freedom was the sense of optimism and even good will among nations that together they might build a better world. A world that respected the dignity of all human beings and not just that of the privileged and powerful. It was a short window of opportunity before the Cold War took hold of global politics, when suspicion and distrust replaced cooperation and camaraderie as the default mindset. But it was during that time that the most significant international agreement in human history was drafted in New York and Geneva and officially proclaimed in Paris in 1948.

Pronouncing itself to be "a common standard of achievement for all peoples and all nations" and referring to "free" or "freedom" no fewer than thirty times throughout its thirty articles, the Universal Declaration on Human Rights (UDHR) was nothing if not a tribute to freedom. A product of the recently created United Nations (and specifically of its Commission on Human Rights, chaired by Eleanor Roosevelt), the UDHR represented progress toward one of the UN's principal objectives—to reaffirm faith in human rights and in the dignity and worth of the individual. The 1945 charter establishing the UN was itself steeped in the fortifying merits of freedom, pronouncing that "social progress" and "better standards of life" were achievable only within "a larger freedom."[22]

The waves of human rights instruments that have since washed through international law have been no less devoted to the promotion of freedom. Freedom *for* women, children, Indigenous peoples, racial minorities, persons with a disability, and migrant workers. Freedom *of* expression, thought, religious belief, movement, association, and family, and freedom *from* hunger, neglect, discrimination, arbitrary detention, genocide, slavery, torture, and abduction ("forced disappearance"). Liberty barely gets a mention. True, it did make sporadic appearances throughout some of the lengthy drafting discussions,[23] and the term was retained in the text for rights against arbitrary arrest and detention, as well as, rather oddly, for the "liberty" of parents to choose to send their children to private schools should they wish to (and can afford to). But these instances aside, the tide of preferred terminology flowed overwhelmingly toward freedom.

In respect of so-called civil and political rights, this was to be expected given their focus on rendering space and opportunity for people to say and believe what they wanted, to move wherever and associate with whomever they wished, to be free from discrimination, and to have private lives.[24] What was more surprising, however, was the equally prevalent use of "freedom" in regard to economic, social, and cultural rights. These (then) newly minted human rights—a direct consequence of the international community's concern to ameliorate the deprivations of the poor and marginalized between and within all countries—focused on ensuring people were adequately fed, clothed, housed, and educated, had access to basic health care, and were protected against dangerous and exploitive working conditions.

The integral role of freedom in the fulfillment of all of these rights was captured most compellingly not by any of the international law texts but in President Franklin D. Roosevelt's "Four Freedoms" speech. Delivered in 1941, in part to galvanize support for America's entry into the war, FDR's impassioned plea for all people everywhere to be free from want and fear, while being free to speak and worship, expanded the bounds of states' responsibilities to include securing new levels of economic and social welfare alongside protecting more traditional civil and political freedoms. Indeed, throughout deliberations on the UDHR itself some six years later, Eleanor Roosevelt, as well as other members of the drafting committee, often harked back to the message and sentiments in FDR's words.

Freedom had, in effect, become the favored path toward achieving the twin goals of political emancipation and economic justice and, thereby, more fully respecting the dignity of all human beings. It certainly struck a chord with the various emancipatory movements that persisted or were initiated throughout the second half of the twentieth century. From decolonization and the immense challenges of newly independent governance for many states, to growing demands for racial, gender, and economic equality within states, landmark political protests and a new generation of constitutional proclamations extolled the virtues of freedom.

Commemorating one hundred years since Abraham Lincoln signed the Emancipation Proclamation, Martin Luther King Jr.'s "I have a dream" speech in front of the Lincoln Memorial in Washington, DC, on August 28, 1963, marked the highpoint in what King himself declared would be "the greatest demonstration for freedom in the history of our nation." He invoked freedom (or free) twenty-five times during the sixteen-minute speech, and liberty only twice—once quoting the Declaration of Independence, and again quoting the lyrics of "My country, 'tis of thee."

Betty Friedan's writings and speeches, including her mold-breaking *The Feminine Mystic*, also published in 1963, demanded that women *and* men be freed from gendered stereotypes that effectively imprisoned women in roles over which they had little or no choice. Emancipation was also at the heart of the revolutionary movements behind Charter 77 in then-Czechoslovakia and its progeny Charter 08 in China a decade later. In seeking release from the throttling grip of communism, both charters expatiated on freedom as a "universal value," without the flourishing of which "there can be no modern civilization of which to speak." This last quote comes from Charter 08, which, despite conceding that in China "individual economic freedom" has been "partially restored," laments the lack of political freedom. It then proceeds to call for or refer to freedom (or free) no fewer than thirty-five more times (and liberty not at all) throughout its nineteen articles, thereby guaranteeing its official proscription by Chinese authorities.[25]

Finally, in this catalogue of homages to freedom in revolutionary texts, there is no more striking example than South Africa's thoroughly modern and comprehensive 1996 constitution, which refers to freedom or free some forty-eight times, and not once to liberty. In so doing it reflects a nation's determination both to erase the obscenity of apartheid and to honor the struggle against it as epitomized by Nelson Mandela's "long walk" to freedom, a march no less noble and heartfelt than that trod by Reverend King.[26]

Freedom's elevation during this time was also evident in the language that dominated the political economy. For example, though focused initially on providing macro and micro financial assistance for the reconstruction of shattered economies after the Second World War, both the International Monetary Fund and the World Bank grew to become arch proponents of free market economics, especially in the 1980s and 1990s. Similarly, and despite the failure to establish an international trade organization to oversee its implementation, the 1947 General Agreement on Tariffs and Trade's explicit promotion of free trade provided sufficient legal framework for globalization of the world's economies. The eventual formation of such a global body in 1994—the World Trade Organization—added further impetus to free trade ideology, but not before history's most successful experiment in international economic cooperation had nailed its freedom colors to the mast.

In 1952, the founding instrument of what was to become the European Union (EU) announced that the European Economic Community (as it was then called) would be based on four guiding freedoms—the free movement of goods, services, people, and capital.[27] What is more, the EU has since expanded its commitment to freedom beyond economic matters with the proclamation in 2000 of the Charter of Fundamental Rights of the European Union, which, true to form as one of the world's most recent international human rights texts, is awash with references to freedom and free—forty-four in all, and just a single mention of liberty.

This litany of the propagandization of freedom at liberty's expense would not be complete without reference to "freedom fries." This briefly infamous renaming of French fries on US congressional cafeteria menus in 2003 was orchestrated by Ohio Republican representative and chair of the Committee on House Administration Bob Ney in retaliation against France's opposition to the US-led proposal (dubbed Operation Iraq Freedom) to invade Iraq that same year. "Freedom" was of course a convenient alliteration, but it was also a sign of the times.[28] During the First World War, in contrast, Americans had renamed sauerkraut "liberty cabbage" and dachshunds "liberty dogs," and—as linguist Geoffrey Nunberg notes—were buying "liberty bonds," building "liberty trucks," and planting "liberty gardens."[29] Not anymore; a century later the word is "freedom."

The Implications of Freedom

So what are the implications of this lexical tsunami of freedom?

Most of all it has instilled a sense of confidence, of hope even, by establishing what appear to be achievable aspirations. By way of a fulsome rejection of tyranny and discord, alongside a sincere commitment to economic and social justice, the preponderance of freedom language reflects both negative and positive dimensions. The overwhelming conception of freedom displayed in the preceding pages is one that promises *individual* freedom: freedom, that is, from interference by others or by the state. Yet in all the above examples, such individual freedom is assumed both to exist within a social setting and to be safeguarded by society (that is, through the state) itself. Social order, in other words, is required if personal freedom is to mean anything at all. It's a sort of "have your cake and eat it" approach.

The danger here is that freedom may be promising more than it can deliver. Or, rather, people's *perceptions* of what freedom promises are at odds with what it actually provides. The wholesale embrace of freedom by the language of human rights, in particular, has created problems of raised expectations whereby freedoms are interpreted more or less literally so that any restrictions on them are considered illegitimate. Such claims to uninhibited freedom necessarily ignore or dismiss any competing claims or interests.

Thus, for example, when free speech absolutists maintain that the right to free speech is the right to say anything you want, to whomever and whenever you want. When monotheistic fundamentalists assert their right to practice their religion, including freedom to punish heretics or apostates as they see fit. Or when the Second Amendment to the US Constitution protecting the right to bear arms is interpreted to mean freedom from any requirement to obtain a license to hold a firearm, as Dick Heller argued in his lawsuit against the District of Columbia's gun-licensing laws, a case that reached the US Supreme Court.[30]

The fact is, however, that in each of these cases, the asserted freedoms are not absolute and were never intended to be. Yelling "Fire!" in a crowded theater, broadcasting opinions that incite terrorism or violence based on racial or religious grounds, and uttering many other forms of offensive or defamatory speech or expression (though *not* lies or simply making stuff up in the world of politics) are commonly prohibited by legislation.[31]

In many countries, speech deemed to threaten national security is also prohibited, even if the grounds of what constitutes sufficient threat vary enormously between despots and democracies. In nearly all countries, religious zealots are no longer free to interrogate, torture, maim, or kill nonbelievers and other blasphemers, except, that is, in such theocracies as Afghanistan, Brunei, Iran, Saudi Arabia, and Sudan, where the death penalty still exists for apostasy and homosexuality (deemed blasphemous).[32] And, today, licensing laws for gun ownership and use are commonplace throughout most of the world not just because it stands to reason that if you need a license to own a dog or drive a car, you should surely need one to possess a gun, but also because gun laws demonstrably reduce gun-related deaths. The stark fact that the US states with the weakest guns laws have the highest firearms-related mortality rates demonstrably proves the point.[33]

The foremost implication of the enthusiastic rise in the rhetoric of freedom, therefore, is the imperative that we must manage the expectations that come with it. In its ordinary meaning the word evokes a sense of boundless opportunity,[34] of wide-open spaces (as seems to come to many people's minds when asked to picture freedom)[35] across which one can roam unencumbered. Yet borderlines there must and will always be. Certainly, their prescriptions will differ, often greatly, and their contours will be debated and sometimes hotly contested, as many of the examples explored in this book illustrate. But, in just about all cases, limitations of *some* form will be imposed. They are there, as we have just seen, even with the most ardently claimed freedoms, and so too they are present with the many more mundane but no less important freedoms we assume as we go about our day-to-day lives.

At base, the task of managing expectations comes down to an awareness of our social circumstances and a preparedness to see that the value of compromise lies not in what we might give up but in what we stand to gain. As individuals living together, we have multiple ends and aspirations. In consequence, as Isaiah Berlin observes, "the possibility of conflict—and of tragedy—can never wholly be eliminated from human life, either personal or social."[36] It is this possibility of conflict (or tragedy) that frames our negotiations on freedom and its limits. Freedom simpliciter makes no sense, argued Berlin's contemporary Karl Popper, since the absence of any constraint on freedom leads inevitably to *un*freedom. It "makes the bully free to enslave the meek,"[37] he explained, before concluding that freedom therefore must necessarily have restrictions. Your freedom to swing your fists must be restricted according to the position of your neighbor's nose, as Popper memorably put it.

Synonymity and Difference

It is here, at the point of navigating the frontiers of freedom, that the notion of liberty can help provide perspective. For no matter how often they are treated as such, I want to be clear that I do not consider the two words to be synonymous. Certainly, they share many important characteristics—foremost of which is the inherent dignity of individual choice—but it is what distinguishes them that is critical. While freedom focuses on the individual and shouts loud its promise to them, liberty remembers the collective and delivers a more nuanced message. It's like the single-minded enthusiasm of youth versus the prudence of age and experience—as indeed befits their respective etymologies. Freedom, after all, is the brash Anglo-Saxon newcomer, as compared to liberty's patrician Latin roots.

What liberty has to offer is more in tone and accent rather than in pure semantics. Liberty's commitment to freedom is no less, just differently composed. It sees the responsibilities that accompany your freedom and mine as necessary to ensuring the freedom of others, such that the sum of all freedom is shared as widely and deeply as possible and thereby its total is maximized.

As a matter of fact, at a broad level we already subscribe to liberty's vision of freedom. Personally, we may not always like the fact that our freedoms are limited, or approve of where precisely those limits are set. And yet, more often than not, we seem to abide by them. Why? Well, because most of us, most of the time, concede that for communities to work at all, costs must be borne and benefits enjoyed by everyone. Whether intellectually or intuitively, we understand the ethics of reciprocity. We acknowledge that in claiming our own rights to be free, the same claims can and will be made by others. Further, to settle any resulting disputes and to protect our common interests, we see the need for some formal, societal means to evaluate and arbitrate competing claims. To some degree, therefore, we seem perfectly capable of comprehending that freedom must always be qualified, never absolute.

That's the theory at any rate. Our record in practice, however, is less reassuring. The cases, examples, and circumstances discussed in this book represent a history of negotiating freedom, its borders and its responsibilities, that contains the bad and the ugly as well as the good. Where freedom's boundaries are settled between competing interests in ways that range from fair (or at least as fair as can reasonably be) to most foul. The state—that is, the organs of government—is always a player in these deliberations in the sense that it sets the rules and enforces them. But, in so doing, the state is also inescapably representing some private interests above others.

The levels of freedom we enjoy, therefore, are as much a matter of which private interests hold most sway over public power as they are about the negotiating of the rules themselves. What is more, such negotiations are likely to get harder in days to come as, individually and collectively, we face new challenges posed by declining levels of trust in public authorities and in one another,[38] and the ever-increasing ramifications of technology's impact on the scope and exercise of our personal freedoms.

Liberty's Added Value

So, what might the renovation of the notion of liberty do to help here? What will we gain from its reinstatement as the guiding principle in our relentless quest to define the liminal bounds of our freedoms? What, simply, is the added value of liberty? To begin to answer these questions, let me turn to the People's Republic of China.

A few years ago, I was speaking at an event in Tianjin, an hour's train ride southeast of Beijing. The occasion was noteworthy not only because it was a human rights workshop bringing together almost one hundred university professors from all over China who taught in the field, but also because of the range and frankness of the participants' opinions. Perhaps because the workshop was organized and sponsored by a coalition of determinedly open-minded Nordic aid agencies, I had conversations with several delegates (admittedly over tea or meal breaks rather than in open session) who were happy to debate the differences between, and reasons for, human rights freedoms in theory and in practice.

It was during one of these conversations that I was struck by a comment made by a Chinese colleague which, coincidentally, planted an idea in my head that lead eventually to my writing this book. We were talking about constitutionally protected freedoms, including the right to free speech in China and elsewhere when my colleague paused and, with a wry smile, said, "Of course our right to free speech is clearly stated in our Constitution [and so it is, in Article 35],[39] but it's a liberty with a price tag!"

Now, what he meant by this was that attached to the right are certain responsibilities. Namely, the constitutionally mandated duties of all Chinese citizens in exercising their rights and freedoms (including free speech) not to "infringe upon the interests of the State, of society or of the collective, or upon the lawful freedoms and rights of other citizens" (Article 51). In that way the Chinese state is empowered to restrict free speech insofar as it is deemed to threaten or endanger state interests. Then and (even more so) now, talk of democracy and, ironically, of the right to free speech itself on political matters is precisely the sort of speech that the state believes to threaten the stability and unity of the country and, above all, the power of China's ruling Communist Party.

You and I may scoff at this seemingly blatant expression of self-interest on the part of the Chinese government, and justifiably so. Examples of uncompromising suppression of free speech, especially in recent years under the tightening fist of President Xi Jinping's rule, are not hard to find. Journalists, writers, and poets have been jailed for criticizing the Party, social media sites have been shut down, civil society organizations have been fined into silence, up to 1 million Uyghur Muslims have been interned in "reeducation camps" for practicing their faith, and internet service providers, websites, and users have been "harmonized" (that is, silenced) or jailed for expressing what in most other countries would be considered unremarkable political points of view.[40]

But in terms of *form* these restrictions are little different from the ways Western states typically curtail the freedoms of their citizens. For they too use national security and the public interest as grounds for curbing rights and freedoms, albeit, usually, with different results. Such rights restrictions not only are commonly provided in many states' constitutions but are also expressly articulated in the world's principal international human rights instruments.[41] How and when these conditional clauses are used by states to regulate freedoms is discussed in depth in the following chapter and revisited time and again throughout the book.

Returning now to tea with my Chinese colleague: what had especially caught my attention was his choice of words. Liberty, he implied, is distinguished from freedom by the fact that liberty incurs a cost. Aside from reflecting his command of idiomatic English, his intention was to convey liberty's intrinsic accommodation of responsibility, of the need for reciprocity, and thereby of the acceptance that freedom operates within precincts. Deeper still, his remarks portrayed an engagement with the most fundamental of all questions regarding freedom: where does one draw lines between that which is properly the concern of the individual and that which is properly the concern of others, including and especially the state? Or "how much of human life should be assigned to individuality, and how much to society?" as John Stuart Mill quaintly puts it.[42]

In providing his own somewhat unhelpful answer to this question—"to individuality should belong the part of life in which it is chiefly the individual that is interested; to society, the part which chiefly interests society"—Mill is essentially admitting that there is no definitive demarcation line. Rather, the boundary is often fuzzy and always a matter of some negotiation. This is the work of liberty—recognizing, first, that individual freedoms have borders and, second, that they are flexible. Liberty therefore provides an essential optic through which to approach the task of defining freedom.

Every day and in a myriad of circumstances, we negotiate the terms of our freedom. Sometimes openly and formally, such as in policy debates about whether childhood vaccinations, community-wide quarantines or self-isolation, or voting, or wearing clothes should be compulsory; whether walls should be built to keep people out; whether we should tax inheritances and, if so, how much; or what levels of protection of our privacy we should expect when we are at home or online. More often our deliberations are discrete and informal, such as the implications of the promises we make and break, or our behavior toward others, whether they are friends, family, enemies, or strangers.

However we deliberate (and personal inclination plays a significant role in that regard), we do so within parameters established by legal rules or social norms. Some may be subliminal and assumed, such as the compromises we make in marriage, when walking in a busy street, queuing, or handing over personal details online; while others might be pressing and explicit, such as prohibitions on violence and theft, passport and immigration controls, stay-at-home orders in pandemics, age restrictions on drinking alcohol or criminal responsibility, or laws regarding adultery, bigamy, or incest. But in all these ways freedom and its limits are subject to a social contract in precisely the manner intended by Jean-Jacques Rousseau's *Social Contract*, whereby the protection of freedom by "the collective force of all" is achieved by way of each individual "uniting himself with others."[43] From liberty's perspective, one cedes some degree of individual freedom on condition of its preservation overall.

But is the condition honored? What are the consequences of our negotiations for us as individuals and for the societies in which we live? Is the freedom cost-benefit ratio a good one? Is it a fair one? Should we—*can* we—do better? These are the questions I explore throughout the book. I try to answer them by explaining how freedom is won, lost, and limited in the domains that are central to the ways we live our lives—how we attain and maintain our health; what makes us happy; how we accumulate wealth; how and why we work; what makes us feel safe and secure; what beliefs we hold and how we practice and voice them; who, what, and how we love; how we die; and who or what we respect and whether we can or should trust them. Drawing on liberty's insistence on the responsibilities that come with freedom is essential in these tasks because it places freedom in its proper context and provides the framework to manage its expectations.

So how do we make freedom responsible?

2

There Are No Robinson Crusoes

With freedom comes responsibility.
—Eleanor Roosevelt

Imagine you live just south of the equator on a small tropical island in the Indian Ocean forming part of the Seychelles archipelago. You live alone. Your closest companions are 120 giant tortoises (you keep the hatchlings in your bedroom), an abundance of bird life, and the fish in the warm, aquamarine expanse that surrounds you. A coral reef fringes the island's western shore and a teak forest occupies its center. Home is a weathered, two-story wood cabin, shabby-chic by necessity more than design, but with water, electricity, and a phone line. You have a boat. You thrive on the island's resources (fish, nuts, berries, and eggs) and the supplies you collect weekly from the markets in Victoria, the Seychelles capital, an hour away by boat. Visitors come and go fairly regularly, but only for the day; none stay the night. You've lived here for fifty years. You own the island. You bought it on a whim in 1962 for £8,000. It's now worth $50 million (as offered to you by one wealthy visitor some ten years ago). Money now occupies little place in your life—you draw on your modest savings to buy a few supplies and pay for basic utilities—but you have had fun looking for the pirated treasure reputedly buried somewhere on the island, though you're too canny to reveal whether you've found any.

This is not a fantasy. It is a description of Brendon Grimshaw's life on Moyenne Island.[1] In terms of a life of freedom, Mr. Grimshaw's sounds about as close as you can get. He was free to buy the island (granted he had the cash, being at the time an accomplished newspaper editor in his mid-thirties) and had a keen eye for adventure. He lived as he pleased, was answerable to no one, and could choose whether to receive visitors or make visits elsewhere himself. Ultimately, he was free to sell and give it all up. He never did succumb to the millions on offer—"they just want to build a big hotel"—succeeding instead in having the island designated a national park shortly before he died in 2012. He demanded little of the wider world save being left to live as he wished, and the wider world demanded little of him.

"I did what I wanted to do," he was fond of saying. And he wanted to do a lot. During his time on the island he reintroduced more than 2,000 birds (there were none when he arrived), bred and cared for the giant tortoises, and together with a Seychellois friend, cleared and constructed more than three miles of pathways across the island and planted 16,000 trees, including the teak forest. He also built his home.

Totally Free?

So is "doing what you want" an adequate definition of freedom? Well, yes, in theory it might be. But not in a practical sense, not in any kind of social setting where freedom is always limited. John Locke argued this very point three hundred years ago by strenuously denying that anyone can "do what he likes, to live as he pleases." Freedom, he insisted, "is constrained by laws both in the state of nature and political society." It is, in practice, never absolute. Individuals, as Locke held, don't exercise freedom in "a state of license," but rather (if they are fortunate) in "a state of liberty."[2] Certainly Grimshaw recognized his freedom's limits. Although his island home was his castle, as it were, he was still subject to Seychelles law. Relevant criminal laws, for example, reached into his home, as they do into all of ours. Unlike the rest of us, however, local tax laws were never going to trouble him given the Seychelles' somewhat notorious tax haven status.

But it's not just unavoidable legal limitations that impinged on Grimshaw's freedom. Certain things he wanted to do required the engagement or even permission of others. His title of ownership of the island had to be properly registered. To make his home "habitable," as was his declared intention, he had to apply and pay for the extension of electricity, water, and phone connections to the island. He used basic financial services to transfer money from his bank account in the United Kingdom to pay for utilities and other supplies, as well as for his boat and its upkeep. He also had to engage in protracted and at times painful negotiations with Seychelles authorities to win the island's national park status.

Freedom, in other words, *necessarily* comes with responsibilities. Even for those in such circumstances of relative isolation and minimal encumbrance as Grimshaw enjoyed, life inescapably involves engagement, negotiation, compromise, and compliance. For all the rest of us, of course, the breadth and depth of these interactions are of a different magnitude altogether. Daily, hourly, even by the minute, our freedom of choice is curtailed by, or conditional on, the varying demands of others. Sacrifices made in the protection of the freedom of others are the price each of us must pay for the preservation of our own. "Those who expect to reap the blessings of freedom . . . must undergo the fatigues of supporting it," as philosopher Thomas Paine put it, drawing on his intimate observations of the American and French Revolutions.

His words still ring true. It may seem counterintuitive, therefore, but freedom is the product of the limitations that we impose on ourselves.

Tyranny and Doing What You Want

But what of tyrants? you might ask.[3] Are they not free to do as they please, cost free? If there is a common thread running through the history of tyrants, it is that they acquire and use power for the sole purpose of satisfying their own desires and wishes, whatever the cost to others. Caligula plumbed the depths of depravity and self-indulgence so completely during his four-year rule of the Roman Empire that he declared himself a living God and laid plans to have his horse Incitatus appointed consul, which position presided over the Senate and was invested with certain judicial powers. Wont to proclaim, "Remember that I have the right to do anything to anybody," he often and extravagantly exercised the right, summarily executing anyone he pleased and frequently mixing gluttony and orgies with torture and rape.[4] Eventually, however, Rome lost patience with him, and he was assassinated in 41 AD at the age of twenty-eight (before Incitatus could take office).

The twentieth century spawned a horrifying array of tyrants whose narcissistic and freedom-exploiting traits devastated whole countries, peoples, races, and religions. From Leopold II of Belgium, Hitler, Mussolini, and Stalin, to Mao Tse-tung, Idi Amin, Nicolae Ceaușescu, Pol Pot, Augusto Pinochet, Suharto, Ferdinand Marcos, Kim Il-sung, and Francisco Macías Nguema of Equatorial Guinea (who, not to be outdone by Caligula, declared himself the *only* God), their trail of malevolent indulgence was long and terrible. The autocrats of our present century—Saddam Hussein, Muammar Gaddafi, Robert Mugabe, Bashar al-Assad, Omar al-Bashir, Alexander Lukashenko, Kim Jong-un, Vladimir

Putin, and Xi Jinping—have been no less intemperate. And if, as history so clearly indicates, pathological selfishness is indeed an essential characteristic of despots, then its lavish flourishing in such seats of democracy as 1600 Pennsylvania Avenue between 2016 and 2020 is cause for alarm.[5]

During their dictatorial reigns none of the above individuals showed (or show) much restraint in pursuing their every whim or deeply held conviction, no matter what the consequences. Their freedom to do whatever they wanted seemed to have few bounds. It might seem reasonable to expect, therefore, that their chosen actions would have brought some joy to them, some increase in happiness, or at least contentment.

Yet unbounded freedom appears to have yielded precious little happiness or contentment to any of them. Caligula was sick, insane, perpetually fearful, and so insecure about his abundant body hair that he prohibited the use of the word "goat" in his presence. Hitler was sexually impotent, liable to fits of uncontrollable rage and increasing paranoia, and so contemptuous and impossibly demanding that he was seldom satisfied. Even at the moment of his greatest victory, when he orchestrated France's surrender in June 1940 to take place in the very same railway carriage as Germany had been forced to sign the Armistice ending the First World War in November 1918, his face was described by CBS reporter William Shirer, who witnessed the event, as "afire with scorn, anger, hate, revenge, triumph."[6] Stalin also suffered from paranoia, as well as depression and loneliness. Mao, according to his personal physician, was often ill with worry, bedridden for months at a time, plagued by insomnia and a theatrically erratic libido, and constantly dosed with barbiturates.[7] And so the list goes on. Even Kim Jong-un, apparently one of our happier despots (his former Swiss boarding school classmates recall him having a good sense of humor as well as an impressive collection of Nike trainers) conceals a darkness beneath his sunny, choreographed public image. An indulgent lifestyle of deific gluttony has reportedly left the still young Kim with a litany of physical ailments, including gout, diabetes, heart disease, kidney disease, and hypertension, as well as stratospheric levels of paranoia. "The tyrant never tastes of true freedom or friendship," as Plato tartly put it.[8]

Evidently, then, while unbridled power may bequeath great freedom, neither guarantees happiness, health, or personal fulfillment. But what does that mean for the status of freedom for all the rest of us with more modest reserves of power and more limited capacity to act on our desires? Brendon Grimshaw's chosen path to do what he wanted may be both cheerier and closer to what you and I might consider achievable and desirable when compared to the lives of history's autocrats, but it still begs the question whether freedom boils down to simply doing what we want.

Free Will

One way to approach this question is to look to Socrates for assistance, for he was much concerned by the derivative problem of intention. That is, do any of us—even near-omnipotent tyrants—really *do* what we *want*? To this question Socrates provided an intriguing answer.[9] He argued not only that our daily lives are littered with examples of us *not* doing what we want, but that we may well be incapable of doing otherwise. What he meant is that we are forever taking actions intended to help achieve some further outcome, rather than merely to achieve the outcome of the action itself. He cited examples of imbibing unpleasant medicines in order to improve our health and undertaking perilous sea journeys (he was a Greek after all) in order to gain wealth. He called these "in between actions"—doing something we don't necessarily want to do for the sake of something we do want. To Socrates's examples of actions committed, we might add actions omitted—like resisting the temptation to retaliate so as to preserve a friendship and refraining from speeding so as to maintain road safety and avoid penalties. You get the point, I'm sure.

But what of his additional claim that we might be incapable of doing what we want? Here Socrates expands "in-between actions" to cover just about all actions. In other words, he's saying that we seldom act in a way that seeks only the outcome of that particular action, but rather we nearly always employ that action (and its outcome) in pursuit, in part, of some other outcome. That other outcome is what he called "our real good," or what we believe to be in our own best interests. Thus we eat and drink to stay alive, we exercise to stay healthy, we socially distance to avoid disease; we read, watch, and listen to entertain and educate ourselves; we communicate in order to convey meaning; we pray to appease and honor our gods; we dance, draw, design, and write to promote and create; and we argue and fight to resist and destroy. We even kill to avenge, defend, or (chillingly) gratify.

Consistently, therefore, we employ tangible means to achieve intangible ends. While this is not how Socrates puts it, it remains true to his message. Namely, that in all that we do, we possess an ulterior motive, such that no matter how enjoyable or unpleasant the actions we presently take are, they themselves are not what we truly want. What we want is what we hope those actions will lead to.

The link between what we desire and our freedom to get it is the perplexing notion of "free will." Characteristics of both freedom and our wants and desires are to be found in our exercise of free will, but free will is not the same as either. Thus, while it is true that when pursuing our goals we must be, to some extent, engaging our free will to do so, we can also freely decide to take actions we'd rather not take (such as medicines and dangerous journeys, as Socrates suggested). Freedom, on the other hand, while necessarily constituting a part of free will in the sense that some level of choice is available in both, is nonetheless a much broader concept that encompasses social as well as personal dimensions.

To put it another way, *free will* focuses on the impact of your individual personality on the choices you make—from what to eat or wear and when to lie or tell the truth, to whether you believe in God or capital punishment. *Freedom* focuses on the wider social and political forces that impact those same choices (and many others)—for example, what rules or restrictions limit our choices of food or clothing, if and when it is OK to lie, and what philosophical, cultural, or religious beliefs we might hold.

As a matter of fact, the degree to which any of us really exercises free will is the subject of intense dispute. Psychologists question whether we have much room left for truly free will after all our predispositions are taken into account. Some argue that whether as a consequence of nature (our genes) or nurture (our circumstances), our predispositions to everything from chocolate to murder effectively determine our every choice of action. On this reading we have no free will at all. Others reject such extreme determinism, holding that in fact we do have significant capacity to exercise free will and to choose whether to indulge in chocolate or murder.

Obviously, whichever perspective is preferred has profound implications for whether we take responsibility for our expanding waistlines or the blood on our hands. Which is one reason why criminal lawyers and health professionals, as well as psychologists, are especially interested in these debates.[10] Many others also ponder the conundrum of free will—philosophers, economists, political scientists, theologians, linguists, ethicists, and marketing managers. We shall encounter all of these in one way or another throughout this book as we explore the intersections between freedom and free will in the chapters focusing on happiness (can we choose to be happy?), voice (do we practice what we preach?), security (is a deluded killer any less culpable?), and love (do we have any control over who or what we love?).

The Politics of Making Freedom Equal

That said, while our investigations of freedom will inevitably take us inside our own heads to examine what preconditions we impose on its exercise, much of the book is concerned with the limitations that *others* put on our individual spheres of freedom, while conceding that the two are not mutually exclusive.

The reason is that it is essentially meaningless for us to talk of freedom outside some form of social setting—does anyone live entirely alone, utterly isolated from any human interaction whatsoever? Freedom is in practice an intensely social and therefore political concept, intelligible only when the individual is in community with others. Indeed, so essential is this connection, argues nineteenth-century German philosopher G. W. F. Hegel, that one's very individual identity is only realizable as such within a social order where interpersonal relations (including freedoms and responsibilities) are possible. Absent such political community we have no individual identity to speak of and nothing (or no one) to be free from or responsible to.[11] Hannah Arendt also stresses the ineluctable nature of political relations to individual freedoms, in her classic essay *Freedom and Politics*, holding not only that "the *raison d'être* of politics is freedom" but that the concept of freedom is never free from politics.[12] It follows, therefore, that defining freedom as a circumstance whereby one's choice of action is unhindered to the extent it can coexist with the freedom of others to do the very same necessarily involves a process of unending social and political negotiation. It is here that we begin to see what is meant by making freedom responsible—that is framing it as liberty—as well as why and how to make it so.

Freedom must be fair and respectful of others if it is to exist at all. "Freedom is indivisible," declared John F. Kennedy in his iconic June 1963 speech before more than 400,000 West Berliners, "and when one man is enslaved, all are not free." Although leaning heavily on uncompromising rhetoric, Kennedy's point is essentially sound. In its dispersal and exercise, freedom must apply universally, it must be open to all, and be regulated accordingly. In short, access to freedom must be based on the principles of equality and fairness. Where dictators or the privileged few have abundant freedom and all the rest have little or none, undeniably humanity as a whole suffers. As communities of human beings we fare much better the wider and more equally freedom is spread, when we strive for "equality in liberty," as Alexis de Tocqueville urged us to do. If we all wish to draw on the benefits of civilized society, we each have an obligation to negotiate our freedoms within it. The challenge is, and always has been, to define what that means in practice. By what rules do we or should we negotiate?

Teaching a law class on development and human rights in Nepal most years over the past decade has meant that I spend long hours sitting in Kathmandu's traffic. I don't choose to do so— the course has many site visits—but it does have some upsides. First, it teaches you to be patient. Second, you learn that out of free-for-all chaos can come responsible order. The city's roads are perpetually clogged, broken, dirty, dangerous, and, seemingly, anarchic. Cars, trucks, taxis, buses, motorbikes, horse-drawn carts, bicycles, dogs and (sacred) cows, and above all people are everywhere on the roads, moving in all directions and all at once.[13] There are almost no road signs, no lane markings, no sidewalks, no pedestrian crossings, effectively no speed limits, and sometimes no road at all. There are few traffic lights (and even fewer of those work), frequent roadblocks, impromptu protests, and permanent and peripatetic maintenance work. And then there are the silent assassins—motor bikers who cut their engines and freewheel downhill to save fuel.

Yet, beneath the frenzied surface, there is a semblance of order. Most of the time speed is limited naturally by the sheer volume of traffic, and there are traffic lights or traffic police operating during peak hours (if such are discernible) at some of the city's busiest intersections—all of which helps. But what is truly impressive are the unwritten rules of road etiquette that otherwise apply. Merging and giving way are matters of negotiation, with size and maneuverability being the main determining factors rather than purely driver aggression. Horns are used primarily to alert others rather to admonish them, and overtaking is typically a collaboration between the drivers, using horns, headlights, and speed adjustments to communicate intentions, warnings, and opportunities. Provided that pedestrians are bold and predictable, vehicles will yield to them and even stop to let the especially young or infirm cross the road. At times the pantomime is terrifying, but after a while one begins to appreciate the etiquette involved. A perpetual process of freedoms claimed and responsibilities counterclaimed results in a much better road safety record than in most similarly poor countries.[14]

This tale of Nepali road etiquette helps us understand the possibility of unregulated social interaction on matters of personal freedom (your unhindered passage from A to B), even in the most unlikely of circumstances. But we don't have to venture onto the streets of Kathmandu to witness continuous, negotiated settlements between the users of public places and inhabitants of shared spaces. We experience it every day—queuing, sidewalk manners, working or playing in teams, interacting with officialdom, dealing with abusive family members, handling humor, arguing with neighbors, working with colleagues, befriending and loving, the whole alternative universe of social media etiquette, and much more.

Such socialized civility stems from a sense of shared equality, a concoction of selfishness, mutual respect, and altruism, which satisfies nearly everyone nearly all the time. By an appeal to enlightened self-interest, small compromises to everyone's individual freedom help both to distribute freedom fairly and to preserve its enjoyment overall. This is the essence of just about all our political negotiations over personal freedoms, be it on the road, in halls of government, in the boardrooms of businesses, or in the family home. Sometimes, when the balance is right between motives, objectives, processes, and above all vested interests, the impact on freedom is tolerated and supported. But when the equation is skewed unjustifiably toward satisfying the vested interests of a few to the detriment of many, the impact will be scorned and resisted.

This is the very art of politics. It is the difficult practice of government as prosecuted under the demands of the rule of law, as illustrated in the many examples of negotiated freedom explored in this book. For in making freedom responsible—that is, by reinstating the bounded notion of liberty at the heart of our social relations—we necessarily engage low politics with high principles whereby we may yield to pragmatism or compromise but do so within limits perceived to be fair and just.

Negotiating Liberty

Our stewardship of liberty is guided and sometimes directed by a broad combination of formal (written) and informal (unwritten) laws. We use these both to define and thereby limit our freedoms and to continually refine them. They act like traffic lights, telling us when we are free to go, when to stop, and when to exercise caution.

Formal laws are usually quite explicit in the way they intrude on our freedoms. "Every law is an infraction of liberty," as Jeremy Bentham put it, but it is an infraction that may nevertheless be justifiable. "The law, which restrains a man from doing mischief to his fellow citizens, though it diminishes the natural, increases the civil liberty of mankind," argued the great English jurist, and contemporary of Bentham, William Blackstone.[15] Thus, criminal laws limit how far we can encroach on the interests of the community as a whole, and tort (or duty of care) laws delineate how far we are responsible for the consequences of our actions that affect others. Employment and consumer protection laws limit the freedom of some to exploit others, and contract laws enshrine the notion of trust by making your word your bond. There are also human rights laws which, as discussed below, operate as a sort of normative umbrella protecting both freedom and equality but doing so by limiting both where they overlap or contradict each other.

In our behavior toward one another we are also guided and corralled, often without realizing it, by informal laws. Social and cultural mores set standards of whether, when, and how we impinge on the freedoms of others. These unwritten rules are everywhere, acting sometimes in concert with the formal, written rules, at other times as qualifiers to them. Most often they operate in circumstances where little or no formal law exists. Some are relatively trivial, like the censure of displays of selfishness at work or play, or with friends or family, or the highly nuanced boundaries of acceptable humor and satire. There are also the many protocols surrounding social interaction, from dating, conversation, and personal hygiene to sharing public spaces and audience and crowd behavior. Other such rules are more serious, such as intolerance of zealotry, bigotry, and bullying; entitlements to privacy; caring for the young, elderly, and sick; and a general expectation of mutual respect, equal treatment, and fair play.

Our individual spheres of freedom, therefore, are determined as much by community standards as by statutes and rule books. The burden of making freedom responsible in this way is no trifling matter. It can be onerous and never-ending and, for many of us, unappealing. "Liberty means responsibility. That is why most men dread it," as George Bernard Shaw saw it.[16] Sigmund Freud went even further, holding that what psychoanalysis had taught him was that most people are "uncomfortable" with the freedom civilization affords them, precisely because they are frightened of the additional responsibilities that come with it.[17] It is, in other words, liberty, not pure freedom, that worries us.

Yet, when it comes to responsibilities, what choice do we really have? Quite obviously you cannot avoid them if you live in servitude or under tyranny. But nor will you escape responsibilities in any other form of society that lies on the spectrum between enslavement and the freest of lives, like Brendon Grimshaw's. Obedience, respect, and recognition are all required of us to varying degrees in all aspects of social order. The greatest promise offered by those societies at the freer end of the spectrum is that you get more for your responsibility buck, as it were. The reasoning being that if one's responsibilities to state, community, church or temple, employer, family, and fellow citizens are unavoidable, it is better that you gain some appreciable level of personal freedom in compensation.

To flip it around, we are back to where we started—the price of freedom is responsibility. It is a price that demands effort, empathy, and compromise, and it is inescapable. No one can legitimately claim their rights to freedom without paying the responsibility price tag. Popular proclamations that individual *liberty* (rather than pure or hypothetical freedom) equates to "doing whatever you want" are misguidedly incoherent at best and quite simply tyrannical at worst.[18] Even the doyens of modern libertarian thought accept that much.

David Boaz, head of the Cato Institute and author of *The Libertarian Mind*, believes that "we should all be free to live our lives as we choose, so long as we respect the equal rights of others," which distinguishes him not at all from just about anyone else who believes in individual freedom. It is in how the qualifier "respecting the equal rights of others" is intended that he and libertarians like him purport to differ. The cardinal principle for Boaz is that "the burden of proof ought to be on those who want to limit *our* freedom [my emphasis]."[19] The clear implication here is that there is an "us and them" divide. But this doesn't make sense. "Our freedom" is in fact everyone's freedom. Each one of us is, at one and the same time, both a freedom holder or exerciser *and* one of those securing or seeking limitations on the freedoms of others. Why? Well, for the ironclad reason that as none of us chooses to live life in exactly the same way as does another, so there are always clashes between chosen life paths. Clashes that can be resolved only through compromises of the freedoms of some or all concerned.[20]

In this way right-wing libertarians are no different from left-wing proponents of freedom. Their true point of distinction—no matter how they protest otherwise—is in the manner or form of determining the scope of the "equal right of others" to freedom. And that issue so often boils down to a debate about the size and role of the state, which, while important, is not the same as a debate about the nature of freedom itself.[21]

To hint at or even perpetuate the notion that one's freedom in society means independence from others, still less complete sovereignty over oneself and one's affairs, is fundamentally to misinterpret the concept. Hannah Arendt is quite right to assert that in practical reality freedom is neither independence nor sovereignty. On the contrary, freedom in social settings requires dependency on others, albeit to varying degrees, and it does so in ways that necessarily intrude upon one's personal sovereignty or control. This is the process of liberty. We all live in the company of others, whether close or distant, and it is both our individual freedoms and their limitations that underpin the social orders we inhabit (of whatever kind) and help frame the lives we each lead.

This assertion is never truer than in times of crisis. When in March 2020 governments across the globe began in earnest to clamp down on citizens' freedoms in response to the exponential spread of COVID-19, most people understood the reasons and accepted the restrictions despite the hardships. But not all. Some, like Katie Williams, a Las Vegan running for election to a local school board, vehemently asserted their rights to freedom above all (and anybody) else. "This is America," Williams tweeted, in response to widespread calls to stop going to restaurants, "and I'll do what I want."[22] Predictably, her tweet went viral with no shortage of supporters alongside her many detractors. Such farcical myopia has, of course, become a hallmark of responses to the pandemic even in the highest echelons of government, no more so than in Florida where in August 2021 Governor Ron DeSantis, in defiance of the delta variant of the coronavirus then ravaging the state, threatened to defund any school that mandated the wearing of masks by staff and pupils.[23]

Respecting people's equal rights to freedom is undeniably difficult as it requires striking a delicate balance between the demands of individuals separately and their demands together as a community. That task in turn requires an unavoidably imperfect reconciliation of people's many and varied perspectives on what it is to be human or, more especially, to be a human living in a society of humans. To this grand project much of the edifice of human rights has been dedicated.

The Bendability of Human Rights

For all its earnest and loudly trumpeted commitment to freedom, the international human rights movement is nonetheless an important repository of freedom's limitations. Alongside the promulgation of specific rights and freedoms, duties, responsibilities, and straight-out qualifications to freedoms are all hardwired into human rights' legal texts. Human rights, in other words, are necessarily bendable, not rigid and straightjacketed.[24]

This is seen most clearly in international human rights law (which is commonly incorporated or otherwise reflected in domestic laws). The Universal Declaration on Human Rights (UDHR; 1948), for example, declares (in Article 29) that "everyone has duties to the community in which alone the free and full development of his personality is possible" and that in their exercise of their rights and freedoms, "everyone shall be subject only to such limitations as are determined by law solely for the purpose of securing due recognition and respect for the rights and freedoms of others and of meeting the just requirements of morality, public order and the general welfare." Such conditions placed on human rights are no mere consequences of political expediency, bowing to the demands of states. Rather they reflect a philosophical commitment to bounded freedom—a commitment, that is, to liberty. "Freedom makes a huge requirement of every human being," as Eleanor Roosevelt counseled during the drafting process of the UDHR.

The steady stream of international human rights instruments coming thereafter have followed broadly the same script. As chapter 1 shows, civil and political freedoms to speech, belief, religion, movement, association, assembly, and privacy are typically first proclaimed and then qualified to the effect that such freedoms carry duties and responsibilities and that they may be subject to restrictions necessary for the protection of national security, public order, or public health or public morals.[25] We are all familiar with these "permissible" limitations to our freedoms: Defamation laws and prohibitions on hate speech. The removal of privacy protections in criminal matters. Age restrictions on employment, voting, drinking alcohol, watching movies, driving, sex, and marriage. The imposition of travel restrictions or quarantines to control the spread of disease. The proscription of criminal, terrorist, or other associations deemed to be security threats.

All these restrictions of freedoms are, or can be, justified by the wording of the relevant human rights laws themselves. And the extent to which any such restrictions are deemed justified in practice is always a matter of debate. The widespread and extraordinary restrictions on people's movement throughout the COVID-19 crisis, for example, have been broadly accepted as appropriate and necessary in the face of the grave danger the pandemic poses for public health. Indeed, if anything, many (and especially health specialists) have argued that the constraints are not enough or, at least, were not imposed quickly enough, given the speed, severity, and mutability of the disease. The boundaries of our individual rights, therefore, are flexible, and necessarily so to fit the demands of the societies we live in. The question, from a human rights point of view, is always whether and how well those demands are explained and justified by governments and accepted by society as a whole.

Economic, social, and cultural "freedoms" are expressed somewhat differently in international law than are civil and political rights, but the effect is much the same. Freedom from destitution, hunger, ignorance, homelessness, and ill health are implied in the rights to food, housing, education, adequate health care, and fair labor practices.[26] But typically these rights are subject to potentially extensive qualifications regarding their "full realization." The UN's International Covenant on Economic, Social, and Cultural Rights, for example, stipulates that states must "take steps" toward the "progressive" implementation of the covenant's rights by utilizing the "maximum of [their] available resources." Thus, while the intent to promote people's freedom is clear, so is the elbow room allowed states to fulfill their responsibilities according to their political, social, and, especially, economic circumstances.

What lies at the heart of these responsibilities and restrictions of freedom are the twin issues of, first, securing everyone's equal access to, or exercise of, freedoms and, second, reconciling conflicts between individual freedoms and competing community interests. Human rights' built-in limitations are not optional extras; they are integral to the freedom they promise to everyone. The rights and freedoms themselves are important, but so are their limitations. That the positions of freedom's boundaries are contestable in human rights discussions is neither regrettable nor a failing. Such contestation is precisely what legitimates the content and extent of our freedoms.

It is each one of us, as freedom holders or claimants, who must do the contesting. We must engage in freedom debates, whether directly or indirectly through those who represent us. Here again we find freedom inexorably associated with responsibility, and therefore properly labeled "liberty" to my way of thinking. Here the responsibility is an obligation of "participation," albeit an obligation with benefits. As Charles Malik, one of the drafters of the UDHR, insisted during debates on the declaration, there are "no Robinson Crusoes."[27] We all live in societies, not alone in the sense Daniel Defoe bestowed on Crusoe. This, for Malik, was the foundation for him arguing, successfully as it turned out, for "person" to be used throughout the UDHR's text in preference to "individual." His intention, and as it is translated into the dec-laration, was to stress the social dimension of personhood.

Freedoms as expressed in human rights terms are, therefore, un-avoidably political. How we negotiate freedoms and responsibili-ties in our various domains of life, what reasoning or principles we bring to the table when doing so, and what compels us to come to the table in the first place (if we come at all) are all political questions. Questions, that is, of fairness and equity that endure in any human society, no matter what its level of sophistication or technological advancement. In fact, the advance of technology is itself providing us with some new ideas and challenges as to how we go about addressing these age-old problems.

The Responsibilities of Technology

Technology—and especially our responses to it—is provoking debates beyond science and its applications to include growing concerns about freedom, responsibility, and ethics, as exemplified by the following tale of AI overreach.

Amid a host of impressive innovations unveiled by Google CEO Sundar Pichai, at the company's "I/O [input/output] Con-ference" in Mountain View, California, in May 2018, one stood out. To the collective wows of an adoring audience, Pichai put "Duplex"—a voice system and the latest addition to Google As-sistant's gadget armory—through its paces. He showed it calling a hair salon and then a restaurant to book an appointment and a reservation. It was very convincing. The thoroughly human-sounding voice included typical conversational ticks—*ums*, *ahs*, and *mm-hmms*—and could respond to and navigate diverse complexities, such as unavailable dates or times, booking condi-tions (minimum of five people for the restaurant), and waiting times. The robot certainly convinced the humans on the other end of the phone. Pichai was puffed up and proud, telling the assembled that Duplex was indicative of a future where bots and AI will deliver more freedom by saving people time and businesses money. Techies lapped it up. Leading technology media network *The Verge* was typical of the sector's fulsome praise in calling the demonstration "stunning," "incredible," "jaw-dropping," and "next level AI stuff."[28]

But there was a problem, and in the following days the reaction was swift and brutal. Many people, including some technology specialists, were horrified at the intentional deception at the core of Duplex's design. Had anyone at Google thought past the intriguing technical challenge of a lifelike voice system to the human consequences of its use? some asked. Others cut to the chase and called it a sign of Silicon Valley's continuing ethical deficit: "Here we are again being shown the same tired tech industry playbook applauding engineering capabilities in a shiny bubble, stripped of human context and societal consideration, and dangled in front of an uncritical audience to see how loud they'll cheer," as *TechCrunch*, another industry media outlet, weighed in. "Deception is not cool," the article's author, Natasha Lomas, continued. "Not in humans. And absolutely not in AIs that are supposed to be helping us."[29] Purported freedoms, it seems, were being offered at the expense of commensurate responsibilities.

Not knowing whether we are conversing with a bot or a pulse bearer influences how we interact with others and whether we trust them. Indeed, we may tend toward not conversing at all if we suspect there's a machine at the other end. How many of us immediately punch the "off" button when we receive calls from a recorded voice service? Quite a few, I suspect. And, if we do decide to talk, who among us remonstrate (even rudely) with automated menu filters? Ditto. Our parents used to argue with the TV, but at least they knew they were being ridiculous (I think!). We now swear at chatbots, but soon we might not be so sure what or who we're insulting. Meanwhile, propensities to troll, bully, lie, and vituperate online already show how comfortable some of us are with insulting and abusing others, as does the sobering fact that the more outrageous, the content the more clicks it attracts.[30]

Google's fix for Duplex was to have it declare, up front, that it is automated and that the call is being recorded. Honestly, though, in the time it takes you to instruct Google Assistant, consider the alternative options it anticipates might arise, and receive confirmation (or otherwise) of the booking, you could have placed the call yourself and maybe even drawn comfort from interacting with another human being. In any case, solutions for other ethically questionable AI initiatives may not be quite so easy, as illustrated by the hyperventilated debates over whether and how to respond to the indefinite implications of ChatGPT for the provenance and veracity of the written word.[31] As fast as new technologies are expanding their footprint on our daily lives, so are the questions they raise about the appropriateness of the foot and the consequences of the imprint.

A new class of geek has emerged in response. "Tech ethicists," says David Polgar, a pioneer in the field, view technology very differently. Engineers, he says, "typically see a societal problem that they try to craft a solution to, whereas a tech ethicist sees the solution that was created and finds the problems with that." Robert Oppenheimer's profound realization of the sheer scale of destructive power that his pioneering work on atom splitting could lead to is perhaps history's most famous example of a scientific second thought. What people like Polgar and Tristan Harris—former design ethicist at Google (they have them) and cofounder of the Center for Humane Technology—want to see are not ex post facto ethical revelations, but ethical perspectives being built in up front at the conception and design stages of technological innovation.[32] They are not alone.

In 2016 the British Standards Institution issued BS 8611, "Ethics Design and Application Robots," which aims to help identify potential ethical harm and provides guidelines for safe design of robots. In 2018 the European Union's European Commission flagged the urgency of the moral questions raised by the speed and opacity of AI innovations and proposed a set of fundamental ethical principles on which to base AI design, development, and applications. And in 2019 the Institute of Electrical and Electronics Engineers (IEEE) published the first edition of *Ethically Aligned Design* as part of its global initiative to ensure that technology is advanced for the benefit of humanity by prioritizing ethical considerations in its design and development. To this end both the EU and the IEEE stress the importance of widening stakeholder involvement, something also championed by David Polgar, who talks of the pressing need for societal engagement with the creation and deployment of new technologies. Such engagement will not only help shine light on technology's blind spots but also help find them in the first place.[33]

Two decades into the digital age there are now real signs of pushback. The honeymoon of convenience, interconnectedness, automation, information, and entertainment-oriented besottedness has ripened into heightened expectations not only of technological capacity but also of its conscience. Alongside the burgeoning public debate on the ethics of data and AI use,[34] we now see outrage over the online harvesting, use, misuse, and abuse of personal information; inquiries into the role of media platforms in spreading hate speech, violence, and misinformation; reports on the implications of an increasingly automated workplace; and forehead-smacking revelations of algorithmic and machine-learned failures and biases, and how to combat them.[35] The trustworthiness of technology is also central to ongoing debates over whether and how surveillance technologies are used in tracking people's movements to prevent or control disease outbreaks, and even more relevant to the question of whether today we can really believe what we see with our own eyes. On that last score, Nina Schick's revelatory investigation of the frankly mind-blowing online world of "deep fake" videos (such as the now infamous clips of Barack Obama and Tom Cruise[36]) leads her to conclude that we live on the edge of an "infocalypse" where already "up to 90 per cent of all online video could be synthetically generated."[37] Or, in a word, faked.

All this is new terrain for debates about freedom and its responsibilities. It is not the only terrain, but it is a crucial and, as revealed throughout the book, an increasingly pervasive one. Whether or not new technologies will deliver to us a life that is freer has as much to do with the debates we must have about what freedom means, for whom, and under what conditions. That is why these signs of wider public engagement on the social and political implications of technology are to be welcomed and fostered. Discussions about privacy, trust, truth, dignity, fairness, the financialization and weaponization of data, and the automation of human actions or thoughts are, at base, discussions of freedom—yours, mine, and everyone else's—and of what responsibilities come with it.

We have reached a critical juncture in the march of technology into our spheres of freedom. One that demands our rapt attention by the very fact of our technological dependency. We are aware, at some deep level, of the dangers of such dependency, which we deal with, as Shoshana Zuboff observes, by way of a "psychic numbing that inures us to the realities of being tracked, parsed, mined, and modified."[38] Zuboff's engrossing work on what she calls "surveillance capitalism" and how to resist its insidious malignancies is directed toward awakening our critical faculties, of pulling our heads out of the sand and engaging with matters vital to the preservation of our own individual freedoms and to the freedom of the societies in which we live.[39] What might prompt such reawakening, she argues, is indignation. Indignation born of a widening and deepening realization of the freedoms we stand to lose as well as those we might gain in the name of technological progress. For too long we have bought into the tunnel vision of a digital future that will, inevitably, enhance our lot. It appears now that we are seriously contemplating the other side of the ledger.

Our preparedness to do so will have ramifications beyond the technological realm, precisely because of its significance, and will encompass negotiations of freedom across the full spectrum of our quotidian existence. What use we make of social interactions, of the apparatus of government, and of the opportunities and limitations afforded by laws and by human rights standards to define and delimit freedom—that is, to make it responsible—are concerns common to all of life's staple domains. It is to an examination of how well we tackle these concerns that we now turn.

PART II
Negotiating Liberty

In which I examine how well we negotiate the myriad encounters with freedom and its limits in eight staple domains of life—namely, health, happiness, wealth, work, security, voice, love, and death.

3

Health

Knowing What's Good for You

In health there is freedom. Health is the first of all liberties.
—Henri Frederic Amiel

The vote to catapult Clement Attlee's Labour Party into government on July 26, 1945, had been a long time in the making. Coming less than two months after the end of the war in Europe, Attlee's landslide victory was especially remarkable for the fact that voters had chosen him over Winston Churchill, then at the zenith of his reputation as the United Kingdom's wartime savior. But grateful though they were to Churchill, the overwhelming majority of Britons did not want to return to business as usual in peacetime. For the ordinary man and woman, the bitter memories of the decade-long Great Depression that preceded the Second World War were still raw, compounding the sacrifices that so many of their parents had made during the First World War twenty years before that. They were not just keen but desperate to conquer what William Beveridge, in his iconic report on the national welfare published in 1942, labeled society's five "giant evils" of want, disease, ignorance, squalor, and idleness.[1]

With the Blitz in full swing and the very existence of the country in peril, Beveridge, a bookish civil servant with degrees in mathematics, classics, and law, presided over a committee that compiled and produced what was both an excoriating critique of the abject state of British society and a viable blueprint for its redemption. Health—or more particularly health *care*—was at the heart of it.

By incorporating the Beveridge Report into his political mandate, Attlee had captured the electorate's imagination of what a new United Kingdom could look like—that is, free, caring, healthy, prosperous, and above all "inspired by something greater than materialism." The appalling levels of people's health in the country had been recognized for some time. Medical checks conducted during the recruitment (and later conscription) of British troops for the First World War had revealed truly shocking levels of poor health throughout the general community. Nearly 40 percent of all volunteers were rejected on medical grounds, and malnutrition was found to be widespread, resulting in stunted growth, among other problems. The mean height for working-class fifteen-year-old boys at that time was 160 centimeters, while for upper-class boys the same age it was 171 centimeters (which is the average today across all fifteen-year-old boys in the UK).[2] A popular story from the period—that when first encountering regular Australian soldiers drafted into the war, British regulars saluted them assuming from their height and build that they were well-fed officers—underlined the point. A number of social surveys undertaken between the two wars, and upon which Beveridge drew heavily, confirmed the toll that poverty, bad diet, and meager to nonexistent health care was taking on the welfare of the country's population.[3]

The recommendations of the Beveridge Report were the harbingers of the United Kingdom's welfare state that followed, with the National Health Service at its core and a promise to citizens to provide them with care "from the cradle to the grave." It also reflected and inspired similar welfare reforms across Western Europe at the time that have since developed into full-blown welfare states in all countries wealthy and motivated enough to maintain them.

Health Care Opportunities

The central objective of any publicly funded health care program is to enhance people's welfare and thereby provide them with security and opportunities that they might not otherwise be able to access. By and large the services such programs offer are voluntary: within limits, you have the freedom to choose whether to opt in. Most of us do, precisely because of the benefits on offer, but also because it is our taxes that helped pay for it. And yet, in the process of achieving their objectives, health care programs have become victims of their own success. In many countries, especially the richer ones with aging populations, demand is enormous and so, correspondingly, is the health care bill, commanding a significant and growing proportion of public and private expenditures, at an average of 9.9 percent of gross domestic product (GDP) in countries belonging to the Organisation for Economic Co-operation and Development, or OECD.[4] The pressure on health care programs today comes from the inevitable clash between people's heightened expectations and mounting demands on one hand and the limits of medical science and public coffers on the other.

The freedoms bestowed on individuals to whom health care is available are, therefore, not unlimited. The intense and continuous scrutiny and debate over the prescribed lists of which services and medicines a state funds is but one example of both why and how lines are drawn. The right to adequate health care (notably not the right to *be* healthy) is now a well-established human right, with a growing body of case law illustrating just how hard such line drawing can be.[5]

For example, is it fair for a provincial health authority in South Africa to deny a man's access to a renal dialysis machine on the basis that demand far outstrips supply and not everyone can be accommodated? Well, yes, as it turned out. The local authority had implemented a policy of giving priority to younger patients with acute renal problems, which effectively excluded the man in question (Mr. Soobramoney), who was older (forty-one) and suffering from chronic renal failure. Despite the South African Constitution's guarantee of the right of access to health care services, including that "no one may be refused emergency medical treatment," the Constitutional Court of South Africa sided with the provincial government. Where medical resources are scarce, the Court held, preferential access to them is inevitable and, provided such access is based on sound medical reasoning and does not otherwise arbitrarily discriminate (on grounds, for example, of race or gender), then it is also justified.[6] The decision was not good news for Mr. Soobramoney, but you can see where the Court is coming from. The reality of limited budgets in rich countries as well as relatively poor ones like South Africa cannot be ignored, even if it can be contested and debated.

That said, sometimes the right (or freedom) to individual health care is elevated above budgetary concerns and above the competing rights of others. Thus the right of children to access adequate health care under the Colombian Constitution has been enforced by the country's Constitutional Court against both public and private health providers to cover the costs of specialized medical treatment overseas when (a) the treatment is not available in Colombia, (b) there is a strong likelihood of its success, and (c) the individuals are unable to cover the costs themselves.[7] That even though the Constitution also obliges the state to ensure delivery of health services that are "efficient, universal and co-operative." Here again, the Court's choice is an invidious one, and once more, you can see the reasonableness of the decision whether you agree with it or not.

Deciding how much, on whom, and on what to spend health care dollars is an especially critical matter in times of crisis, such as the HIV/AIDS and COVID-19 pandemics, when health care systems are overwhelmed. In such situations tough, often unconscionable decisions have to be made. Medical professionals, health care bureaucrats, and, above all, governments are put to the test on two counts. First, their leadership, as noted by *New Yorker* journalist Amy Davidson-Sorkin in writing about failed government responses to COVID-19 in the United States; and, second, the "test of values" it puts them to, she asserts, "because it [the pandemic] preys most fiercely on the vulnerable."[8] Her point is that while organization, planning, and efficiency are essential in dire circumstances, they are not alone sufficient. When the crunch comes, compassion, selflessness, and a keen sense of fairness are agonizingly vital when deciding who gets treatment and how much and, ultimately, who lives and who dies.

In such dire circumstances the responsibilities of governments and health care providers become paramount. Their singular duty is to protect people's health and welfare as best they can and be judged accordingly. In the case of COVID-19, we must ask whether governments were adequately prepared, or initiated testing for infections quickly and widely enough, or imposed appropriate and effective restrictions on people's movements and socializing, or administered vaccination programs efficiently and fairly. Are they putting people before profit when deciding whether and how to secure more medical supplies, build extra hospitals, or develop vaccines? Are they drawing on the advice of health experts or on their own hunches or the opinions of political spin-doctors? Are they telling the truth, distorting it, or hiding it? And, above all, how much do we trust them? Given the breadth and depth of the continuing impact of COVID-19, the answers to these questions will be long and complicated.[9] But the questions themselves—focusing on cost and benefits, transparency and fairness, rationality and veracity—are essentially the same as those asked about the freedom-responsibility trade-offs in any health matter.

Healthy Liberty

This is the negotiation of liberty in action. For many of us our freedoms in the domain of health are considerable—certainly, that is, compared to our ancestors. In particular, we have more freedom than ever to choose whether and how we approach our own health. In this we are left pretty much alone. Some of us obsess about our health to an extent that is, well, unhealthy, but all of us pay some regard to our well-being. What we eat and drink, how much, and when. Whether we exercise, and, if so, how many miles, steps or reps per day, and which activities are best for which bits of us we want to tame, inflame, or eliminate. Whether and how to think yourself bigger or thinner or healthier or happier or wiser. What supplements or stimulants to use, which medications to take, how much sun, how much sleep, if and when to use opioids or pray, and the existential question of whether dark chocolate and red wine are good or bad for you.

On the matter of what is indeed bad for our health, we are also especially animated. The question of how much is too much food, drink, exercise, screen time, work, medication, psychiatry, homeopathy, religion, or even wealth may (or may not) be in our thoughts even as we overindulge.[10] Too little of any of these might also affect our well-being. Embracing what we know or suspect is bad for us is evidently part of human nature, whether it is drugs, alcohol, smoking, gambling, dangerous jobs, extreme sports, criminal behavior, willful ignorance, or trusting politicians.

Alongside all of these concerns, there is seemingly no end to our appetite for hearing what others have to say about how we ought to manage our own health and well-being. Book shelves, magazine racks, the internet, and social media groan under the weight of this industry's output, such that there are now self-help books that suggest self-help books are bad for you![11] That said, we are largely free to choose how we approach the promotion (or abuse) of our health. Largely, but not entirely. Some acts or indulgences may be outlawed, such as proscribed drugs, underage drinking or gambling, and suicide (which topic I discuss in more detail in chapter 10, on death). Some vices are taxed to dissuade certain health-harming behavior (tobacco, alcohol, and, increasingly, sugar),[12] and if that doesn't work, our health insurance, whether public or private, may be restricted or unavailable for the treatment of medical complaints associated with smoking, alcoholism, or obesity. Likewise, the sporty types who break bones or tear ligaments may find their access to remedial elective surgery circumscribed or prohibitively expensive.

More controversially, while there have nearly always been limits imposed on a woman's freedom to choose to terminate a pregnancy (most notably during the third trimester, based on concerns for the health of both mother and fetus), the idea that the state should be able to prohibit abortion more broadly, at any stage and for any reason,[13] is now widely considered not only an unjustified restriction on a woman's freedom to choose but also an unconscionable invasion of her privacy in matters of her own bodily autonomy.[14] On which point and in light of the recent (and distinctly unpopular) dismantling of abortion rights in United States,[15] it is grimly ironic to note the striking correlation presented by many anti-vaxxers who also deny women the right to choose to terminate a pregnancy. For these folk, it seems, "my body, my choice" applies only when it suits them.[16]

All these limits on our freedom to do as we wish with our own health are effective only so far as we might seek to rely on public health services to treat our ailments and promote our well-being. For those who choose to eschew health services or, alternatively, to seek only private health care where available, they are more or less free to act as they wish. For many of us, however, it is via the public health system that the state intrudes most obviously on our health choices.[17] It does so by way of a curious and delicately poised balance between essentially demanding that each of us has consideration for others and, at the same time, providing health care that enables us to pursue our health-related choices with relative freedom. Community considerations, in other words, are the price we pay for whatever level of health care services we enjoy. And those levels have been rising for nearly everyone. Indeed, global health has improved dramatically, especially over the past fifty years or so, in terms of increasing life expectancy and decreasing child and maternal mortality.[18]

Wonder Drugs

There have been many reasons for the incredible changes in the state of global health, including aggregate increases in global wealth, education, and sanitation standards, more enlightened and better-implemented public health policies, and huge advances in medical science. But the two most important health care initiatives over the past half century—which are in truth combinations of all these factors—have been the development and widespread use of antibiotics and vaccines. Together, these two innovations have revolutionized the worlds of medicine and health care. They have been instrumental in controlling and even eliminating some of humankind's most virulent infectious and parasitic diseases, in drastically reducing infant mortality, and in vastly increasing life expectancy.[19] Until the mid-twentieth century, for example, two of the world's greatest killers were pneumonia and diarrhea. Both are treatable with antibiotics and also, in the case of pneumonia, vaccines. Today people still succumb to one or the other, but in far fewer numbers.[20] Diarrhea is now hardly ever the cause of death in developed countries and retains its lethality only with young children and where sanitation is poor and antibiotics are unavailable. Pneumonia, once dubbed "the captain of death," is now typically seldom deadly in the West, with only the very young, very old, or already chronically ill remaining especially vulnerable. In some developing countries it is still a significant scourge due largely to the lack or absence of adequate health care.[21]

While, evidently, the very young still face considerable health risks, antibiotics and vaccines have nevertheless saved hundreds of millions from premature death. Infant mortality rates have plummeted from a global average of 16 percent in 1950 for children under five years old to 2.9 percent today. In rich countries, the average rate is now 0.39 percent (with the United States being the worst performer among Western countries).[22] Average life expectancy across the globe has also improved, rocketing from 48 years in 1955 to 72 years today; again, in the West, the average is better still, presently standing at 83 for women and 78 for men.[23] According to France's National Institute of Demographic Studies, while there were only 200 centenarians in France in 1950, current trends indicate that by 2050, there will be around 140,000—a 700-fold increase in 100 years.[24] No doubt the Gallic diet has something to do with that, but much more is due to vast improvements in sanitation and medical and health care services in France, as elsewhere.

The freedoms bequeathed to us by the fact that today we not only live longer but also live healthier lives is hard to overestimate. Yet these extraordinary advances in health care are not without problems and setbacks. Novel and virulent diseases like COVID-19, SARS before it, and whatever scourges lie ahead remain grave threats to all humankind regardless of borders or wealth. New health challenges and complications have replaced many of the old ones and so-called First World diseases are now spreading throughout the developing world. Obesity is now a greater global health problem than hunger;[25] noncommunicable diseases (heart attacks, strokes, renal failure, cancers, diabetes, and respiratory afflictions) have overtaken communicable diseases (such as HIV/AIDS, tuberculosis, pneumonia, infectious diarrhea, and malaria) as the primary causes of death worldwide.[26] And our overuse of antibiotics has prompted nature to do what it does best—namely, to adapt and create antibiotic-resistant strains of diseases previously readily susceptible to antibiotic treatment, including pneumonia, tuberculosis, gonorrhea, and salmonellosis, *Escherichia coli* (*E. coli*), staphylococcus, and streptococcus infections.[27]

Anti-vaxxer Exceptionalism

In the realm of health and freedom, we have also encountered the pernicious impact of an anti-vaccination movement. For despite the incontrovertible proof of their efficacy in combatting some of the greatest blights on human civilization, vaccination programs have also attracted hostility because of their intrusive, demanding, and sometimes compulsory nature. The insistence on near-universal, mandatory application of such programs is precisely what makes them so effective. That was the principal reason why smallpox and rinderpest were successfully eradicated. It is also the reason why such diseases as polio, tuberculosis, diphtheria, and tetanus are now almost nonexistent in most developed countries where once they were rife: today there are so few people who have *not* been inoculated. In such cases we have developed what immunologists call "herd immunity," where communities maintain high levels of immunity (acquired either through previous exposure to the disease or by vaccination) of around 90 percent or more of the total population, thereby essentially protecting everyone.[28]

There also used to be herd immunity control of measles, mumps, and rubella (MMR). But today this triumvirate of diseases is making a comeback in Western countries due to growing distrust in the MMR vaccine (or the three vaccines given separately) that for nearly fifty years has been winning the battle against these previously pervasive and highly contagious diseases.[29] Vaccine skepticism or hesitancy is now considered to be one of the top ten health treats worldwide, according to the World Health Organization (WHO).[30] Yet, remarkably, the threat is emanating almost exclusively from the very places where vaccinations have had their greatest health-liberating impact. In an extensive pre-COVID-19 global survey published in 2018 involving 140,000 people in 144 countries conducted jointly by the Wellcome Foundation and Gallup, it was the citizens of the rich countries that displayed the greatest cynicism.[31] Fully 22 percent of people from across high-income Western European countries said they considered vaccines to be "unsafe," with France returning the highest percentage (33 percent) of distrust in vaccine safety of any single country. Twelve percent of North Americans and 11 percent of Northern Europeans believed vaccines were unsafe. In contrast, populations in low-income countries were much more trusting. Ninety-five percent of South Asians and 92 percent East Africans believed that vaccines were safe, with both Bangladesh and Rwanda recording near 100 percent confidence in their safety.

Interestingly, uptake levels of COVID-19 vaccinations among populations worldwide have largely followed this pattern, with studies showing higher approval rates in low- and middle-income

countries (LMICs) than richer states. The results of one extensive survey of 44,260 individuals published in *Nature Medicine*
in July 2021 showed that in ten LMICs spread across Asia, Africa, and South America the mean of those willing to get a vaccine stood at 80.3 percent (in Nepal, where the disease has been
especially rampant, the figure was 98 percent).[32] By contrast, in
the United States the study found that just 64.6 percent of people
were willing to get vaccinated against COVID-19.[33] That more
than one-third of Americans were skeptical about vaccines for this
particular disease, when barely a handful of years earlier only
12 percent declared themselves to be skeptical of vaccines generally, shows just how scurrilous the concerted campaign to politicize
COVID-19 has been in the United States (and elsewhere), without regard to the dire consequences to people's health, welfare,
and freedoms.[34]

Overall, these differences in perspective do not reflect greater
awareness among populations in Western states of any problems
with vaccines. Quite the contrary: they may have little awareness
or understanding of the protection that vaccines provide them.
It's a "complacency effect," as Imran Khan, head of public engagement at the Wellcome Foundation, puts it. People in low-income
countries, on the other hand, are very pro-vaccine precisely because
they "can see what happens if you don't vaccinate," Khan adds
poignantly.[35] Bangladesh, for example, carries one of the heaviest
tuberculosis (TB) disease burdens in the world, with more than
360,000 new and existing incidences of the disease recorded in
2020. Bangladesh's annual mortality rate for TB stands at 27
deaths per 100,000 population, or roughly 44,000 people per year,
out of a population of 165 million.[36] This is not good, but rates
of vaccination against TB and rates of successful treatment once
contracted have been steadily climbing (and mortality rates duly
declining) over the past ten years. Why? Well, fundamentally,

because the government and people of Bangladesh are all too familiar with the ravages of TB and so take little convincing of the merits of prevention through widespread vaccination. They see clearly, in other words, that their individual freedom to choose not to take a vaccine is outweighed by their individual responsibility to society to choose to take it.

My Body, My Choice

Vaccination skeptics and anti-vaxxers are in fact exercising the fundamental freedom of choice regarding one's bodily integrity— whether that choice is based on philosophical, religious, medical, conspiratorial, or bogus beliefs. There is something different about being urged or required to ingest or be injected with a foreign substance from, say, being urged or required to wear a seat belt or bike helmet, to refrain from smoking or drinking alcohol, to respect speed limits, or to be subject to security checks at airports. While each of these demands is also aimed at safeguarding our individual and collective health and well-being, the *bodily* intrusion is minimal. Anti-vax advocates talk of people being "allowed to have measles if they want to have measles," and they object to the "coercion" behind making admission to school conditional on children being vaccinated.[37] Some also make outrageous and, frankly, offensive claims such as dubbing vaccines "a holocaust of poison on our children's minds."[38] But, in any event, what is also different about vaccinations is the preponderance of their service to the common good.

This much has been recognized from the earliest days of public vaccination programs: In 1905, in the landmark case of *Jacobson v. Massachusetts*, the US Supreme Court ruled that the Commonwealth of Massachusetts's program of compulsory vaccination of all adults against smallpox was constitutionally valid no matter the claims made by Mr. Jacobson that the Equal Protection Clause in the Constitution's Fourteenth Amendment guaranteed his absolute right to refuse the smallpox vaccine and further that he could prove the "injurious or dangerous effects of vaccination." So compelling is the Court's reasoning in this case on the general necessity of balancing individual freedoms against public interests that it is worth quoting in full:

> The liberty secured by the Constitution of the United States to every person within its jurisdiction does not import an absolute right in each person to be, at all times and in all circumstances, wholly freed from restraint. There are manifold restraints to which every person is necessarily subject for the common good. On any other basis, organized society could not exist with safety to its members. Society based on the rule that each one is a law unto himself would soon be confronted with disorder and anarchy. Real liberty for all could not exist under the operation of a principle which recognizes the right of each individual person to use his own, whether in respect of his person or his property, regardless of the injury that may be done to others.[39]

Indeed, in this short passage the justices of the Supreme Court show how ruminations on the legitimacy of compulsory vaccination are in fact talismanic investigations of the question of freedom and its limits. They capture all the essential antagonisms associated with the idea of liberty as are aired throughout this book. Individual interests *versus* the community's common good; one person's right to freedom *versus* another's equal right to health and safety; the societal order of the rule of law *versus* the disorder of anarchy. There is even the juxtaposition—if not exactly antagonism—of absolute freedom and liberty's limitations, as reflected in the Court's careful use of the term "*real* liberty" to distinguish the notion of liberty (and its inherent responsibilities) from the idea of freedom without constraint. This is precisely the distinction with which I am concerned in this book, and for very much the same reasons.

The Importance of Information and Argument

Negotiating these overlapping parameters of the vaccination question is an essential and important task within the wider arena of health and freedom. In this fundamentally democratic task, we must embrace all sides of the debate—whether emotionally charged balderdash or ascetic science, or anything in between—and then decide on the most appropriate action. The Supreme Court was explicit on this point in the *Jacobson* case, noting that its decision was not a determination of whether or not any particular vaccination program is a good thing, but rather merely a pronouncement on the constitutional validity of such programs: "It is for the legislature, and not for the courts, to determine . . . whether vaccination is or is not the best mode for the prevention of smallpox and the protection of the public health."[40] The European Court of Human Rights argued along similar lines in a 2021 judgment upholding the legal authority of the Czech Republic to fine parents who refuse to have their children vaccinated and to exclude unvaccinated children from preschool. While the court recognized the importance of the individual right to privacy, it concluded that "the pressing social need to protect individual and public health" was sufficient to justify the restrictions on the free exercise of that right as imposed by the relevant Czech laws.[41]

In terms of negotiating such freedoms and boundaries, one might start with the proposition that people are free to believe what they want about vaccinations and free to argue as they wish. Their body; their choice. But when the consequences of what they believe in and argue for directly affect the very same health and well-being of others as they are claiming for themselves, then re-ciprocal responsibilities come into play. Certain rules, or at least expectations, are rightly imposed on the debate. Suspicions, concerns, and beliefs can (and should) be sincerely held, but they must also be based on some level of rationality, on some body of evidence to back them up. Given the gravity of the implications for others of the decisions that you or I make based on our personal views, surely nothing less suffices. Yet many vaccination debates today are dominated by cant, mis- and disinformation, accusation and counteraccusation. Most serious of all, the debates have been thoroughly infected by bogus science, in which world Andrew Wakefield is a messianic figure.

A nondescript and, as it turned out, corrupt British gastroenterologist, Wakefield was the lead author of a paper published in 1998 linking MMR (measles, mumps, and rubella) vaccines to instances of autism in children. The facts that the study was based on a sample of only twelve children, artfully rather than randomly selected, that the data were falsified, and that Wakefield was being funded by lawyers acting for parents involved in lawsuits against vaccine manufacturers should have been enough to consign the paper to the reject pile of any serious science journal. Yet, not only was it published, but it was published in *The Lancet*, one of the world's most prestigious medical journals. *The Lancet*'s editors failed in their duty to review the paper properly and in fact fully retracted it only some twelve years later, after a *Sunday Times* journalist revealed the extent of Wakefield's malpractice and fraud.[42] Shortly thereafter Wakefield was also struck off the British Medical Registry, but by then the damage had been done.

No matter that in the meantime dozens of researchers had categorically disproven Wakefield's incendiary claims, the fire had already caught in circles far outside medical research. Parents of children with autism, some understandably troubled and desperate for answers, were susceptible to apparently scientifically based evidence that pointed a finger of causation at MMR vaccines. Traumatic tales, anecdotes, conspiracy theories, and further fabrications flourished, feeding an anti-vax fervor that soon moved from the fringe to the mainstream of vaccination debates. Today books promoting the mantra that vaccines cause autism or Crohn's disease, or that they contain unsafe toxins and additives, or that they are unnecessary because naturally acquired immunity suffices, pepper the Amazon best-seller list, including two by Wakefield, who now occupies folk-hero status within the anti-vaxxer movement.

The pro-vaccination establishment has, naturally, countered. Mainly by appealing to the enormous body of medical evidence that supports the benefits of vaccinations. Public health authorities worldwide try to debunk vaccine myths by highlighting the before-and-after statistics of instances of vaccine-treatable diseases. According to the US Centers for Disease Control and Prevention (CDC), for example, an epidemic of rubella in 1964–65 infected 12.5 million Americans, killed 2,000 babies, and caused 11,000 miscarriages.[43] The near-universal administration of the rubella vaccine has since reduced reported infections in the United States to single-digit figures each year. Measles used to be endemic, like a cold. Everyone got it. But since the rollout of measles vaccine programs throughout the developed world in the 1960s and '70s, doctors there now hardly ever see a case (though millions are still infected with measles each year in developing countries).[44] While certainly there are acknowledged cases of undesirable side-effects or inappropriate administration of vaccines, these are typically so few—including the COVID-19 vaccinations—as to be statistically inconsequential when set against the overwhelming numbers of infections avoided or quelled and lives saved.[45]

Other than school immunizations, few vaccination programs are universally compulsory (though COVID-19 vaccine mandates for certain community sectors and activities are now common-place).[46] Rather, as is typically the case in the West, they are largely or fully funded and strongly recommended by public health authorities, as well as being widely supported by the community. There are legitimate reasons for some people to refuse or be exempted from vaccines, such as religious conviction, age or infirmity, or medical condition, but these numbers alone should not threaten a community's critical herd immunity. Hitherto, exceptions such as the measles outbreaks in California in the mid-2010s after the vaccine rate dropped to 90 percent (which figure was quickly corrected after removal of the religious and "personal belief" exemptions by the state's legislature), tended to prove this rule.[47] But with sizable cohorts of COVID-19 vaccine skeptics in some countries (especially Western) we may yet see a serious and preventable global disease become endemic in certain communities based on ill-informed truculence or conspiratorial prejudice.[48]

Free to Believe

Despite all the noise and heat generated by the anti-vax movement, overall vaccination rates in developed economies remain relatively high, even in those countries referred to earlier as containing significant populations of vaccination skeptics. To be sure, anti-vaxxers have had some negative impact, but across the developed world vaccination rates for many major diseases (polio, meningitis, tuberculosis, hepatitis, diphtheria, tetanus, and pertussis) hover between 90 percent and the herd immunity target of 95 percent. Even for the falsely maligned MMR vaccinations, the uptake rates across the thirty-five member countries of the OECD are all around or above 90 percent (with the sole exception of Poland, at 80 percent), at an average of 95 percent for the bloc as a whole.[49] Localized low rates of vaccination in rich countries tend to be concentrated in certain areas, often bearing clear socially definable characteristics. In the United States, for example, such sectors includes ultraorthodox Jewish communities in New York, Amish in Ohio, and immigrant Somalis in Minnesota, as well as "affluent boho-yoga moms, evangelical Christians, [and] Area 51 insurgents,"[50] as Nick Paumgarten acidly quips in the *New Yorker*.

The above-mentioned resistance to COVID-19 vaccines in certain communities would appear to spoil this general tendency toward conformity, but even there it is evident that as the pandemic has begun to slide from front-page news, so vaccine skepticism has waned as people begin to heed mainstream scientists more than fringe-dwelling politicians and shock-jocks, such that vaccination rates are rising to levels that provide extensive community protection.[51]

Indeed, what is most striking about attitudes toward vaccines generally is that despite evident skepticism as to their safety, there remains widespread confidence in their effectiveness. People's belief in the inoculative capacity of vaccines is high, sitting at 84 percent worldwide. Pre-COVID-19, 83 percent of Americans said they believed in the effectiveness of vaccines, as did 84 percent of Northern Europeans. Even in France, where only 47 percent of people said they believed vaccines were safe, 68 percent nevertheless thought they were effective, and 76 percent agreed that vaccines were important for children to have.[52] People's perceptions of COVID-19 vaccines have in fact followed much the same pattern, with 85 percent of Americans now believing them to be effective (even though only 73 percent consider them to be safe). Perhaps most striking of all, in Russia (traditionally a highly vaccine-skeptical state), while only 48 percent of people thought COVID-19 vaccines were safe, 67 percent believed them to be effective and 80 percent thought they were important for children.[53] Folk seem continually to be wrestling with the conflict between taking vaccines and facing the diseases against which the vaccines provide protection. Most people are pretty sure about the gravity of the latter, but that doesn't stop them from also being wary of the possibility, however remote, of the vaccines themselves causing health problems.

This cognitive dissonance is in fact a basis for hope rather than despondency in respect to vaccines specifically and in the realm of freedom and health more generally. For the important point to grasp here is that people feel free to exercise their choice, or at least to express it in the form of protest or revolt, and yet, in the end, most comply. Of the full complement of vaccine skeptics, most are the silent or private doubters, and most of them end up eventually joining vaccine programs, albeit reluctantly or late, or both. The need for public health authorities to resort to compulsion, as in the *Jacobson* smallpox case or the response to the 2019 measles outbreaks in California and New York, as well as in France, Greece and Italy, is still relatively rare. Even COVID-19 vaccine programs are largely voluntary, being typically mandated only for health care workers or, more exceptionally, for certain activities like travel and teaching in primary and secondary schools.[54]

This doesn't mean that disease outbreaks among unvaccinated and nonimmune communities are harmless or peripheral. The mutating ravages of a new disease like COVID-19 have certainly made that clear. The latent potential for harm that lies behind outbreaks of old diseases is equally devastating; such outbreaks are the "the eyes of the hippopotamus" as immunologist Mark Mulligan puts it.[55] But what our apparently abiding belief in the importance of vaccine programs does indicate is how vital the free, frank, and full exchange of information is to any negotiations over the extent to which personal freedoms may be limited by the demands of public health. Above all we must take care to value the lessons of experience. As a *Los Angeles Times* editorial on anti-vaxxers counseled during the early days of COVID-19, "Come the time when vaccines have rendered COVID-19 just a memory, it's frightening to think that future generations who did not live through it may think of the vaccine as more problematic than the disease."[56]

Intimate Relations with Strangers

Decisions taken about our bodies, our minds, and our health are intensely personal. That is why choice, or at the very least perceptions of choice, is so vital when together we navigate the boundary between individual and community well-being. The vaccination debate happens to be an especially graphic illustration of the political as well as personal dimensions of that task. It reminds us, as Meghan O'Rourke writes, that "our bodies, like the body politic, are fatefully interconnected."[57] But there are many instances of such a connection regarding our health. To the lists of what we are and are not free to do with our own health, bearing in mind the indirect consequences for the health and welfare of others, we must add the freedom to do that which directly affects the health and welfare of others. That is, more especially, the freedom to act with the *express intention* to impact directly the health and welfare of others. As a general rule, of course, we are not free to act in ways that harm others. But what of our freedom to act intentionally to protect or promote the health of others—our family, friends, colleagues, communities, or even strangers?

Here the health-related intimacy is not personal, not inwardly focused on oneself, but empathetic and outwardly focused, based on one's love, respect, or concern for the welfare of another. This is in fact a key feature of our social relations. An essential, caring glue that binds us in large groups and small. Parents worry about the health of their children (including whether or not to vaccinate them); partners look out and care for each other; friends help friends in need; public servants such as police, doctors, welfare officers, and even politicians are mandated to care for the public's well-being; and businesses are required to safeguard the health and welfare of customers, clients, and employees.

The parable of the Good Samaritan represents an expectation shared across all cultures that people help those in need.[58] That we should "not pass by on the other side" of the sick or stricken, whether fellow citizens or foreigners. In this regard refugees and many migrants today occupy a special place. By definition, each of the world's 30 million or so refugees is fleeing "a well-founded fear of persecution."[59] Global migrants, on the other hand, are much more numerous and can be on the move for a host of reasons that have nothing to do with persecution and trauma, though some are nevertheless desperate and helpless. Whatever the reason, moving between countries can be a perilous experience. Refugees and migrants alike can find their health and welfare endangered. In such circumstances, you might feel certain that your freedom to render assistance to those in need would be unhindered. And mostly you'd be right to think so. But not entirely. Laws that prevent you from doing so, laws that, in effect, criminalize your Good Samaritan instincts, can stand in your way.

The US Harboring Aliens Statute, for example, which was originally enacted in 1907, prohibits the smuggling or transportation of unauthorized aliens, concealing or harboring them, encouraging or inducing their entry into the United States, or conspiring to undertake, aiding, or abetting any such acts.[60] In itself, this statute is not unusual and nearly all countries have similar laws. Certainly, and in line with an abiding theme of this book, our personal freedoms are limited by what is legally prohibited. Aside from breaking the law, the business of people smuggling is often cruel and exploitative. That said, to use the statute to target genuine Good Samaritans would be cruel and perverse. Yet this is precisely what happened following an instruction to federal prosecutors issued by former US attorney general Jeff Sessions in 2017 that they prioritize such harboring cases.[61]

Texas county attorney Teresa Todd, for example, was arrested for stopping one night in February 2019 to help three sick and distressed individuals marooned on the roadside and pleading for assistance. That they turned out to be migrants was irrelevant to Todd: "I can't just leave [them] on the side of the road. I have to see if I can help."[62] In another case, Scott Warren, a teacher and volunteer with a humanitarian aid organization called No More Deaths, was arrested and charged with conspiracy to smuggle aliens for having left water and aid supplies in places in the Arizona desert where it is known that hundreds of migrants die each year due to dehydration and exposure. On one occasion, Warren also provided a place to sleep for two young male migrants for three days in a place known as the Barn in Aja, a small town forty miles from the Mexican border.

The combination of these actions by Warren led federal prosecutors to proclaim: "This is not a case about humanitarian aid" but a case involving conspiracy to break the law by shielding the two men for Border Patrol officers. On this basis they sought Warren's conviction and a possible jail sentence of twenty years.[63] As Warren's defense counsel made abundantly clear (by displaying the word "INTENT" in large red letters on the Tucson courtroom's PowerPoint projector in his opening statement), his client's sole intent was to render aid to those in need. The case eventually ended in a mistrial in June 2019 after the jury deadlocked, but the message federal prosecutors and their superiors wanted to convey was resoundingly clear: American citizens are not free to care for the health of another human being, no matter how dire their circumstances, if they happen to be an unauthorized migrant. Furthermore, federal authorities will interpret legislation in the widest possible manner to punish citizens who do so.[64]

In the unavoidably contested realm of negotiating personal freedoms regarding our own or another's health, there are many examples of intrusions by governmental authorities, some more justified than others. The nature and extent of publicly funded health care, for example; activities restricted or prohibited on grounds of health (such as drug use, pedophilia, or traveling during pandemic lockdowns); actions recommended or required on grounds of health (such as vaccinations, seat belts, and condoms); and education on alcohol and drugs, sex, sanitation, nutrition, and fitness. The draconian deployment of criminal laws that endanger health and life by proscribing one's freedom (some might say "obligation") to act as a humanitarian surely marks a regrettable low point of such contestation. Yet, as in all the examples explored in this chapter, debate and contestation there must always be.

Viewing freedom through the lens of health is a visceral experience for most if not all of us. It is (literally) a sore point. For while each of us jealously guards the freedom to make our own health choices, we must also accept limits on doing so born of the equal right of others to claim the same freedom *and* the impact our choices might have on their health. Defining these limits itself requires the freedom to exchange information and opinions, as well as recognition of the limits of resources, science, and medicine. But above all what the debate requires is a sense of empathy: not only recognition of others' circumstances but also respect for them as fellow human beings whose health is in some way connected to our own. "Humanitarian Aid Is Never a Crime," as some Tucson residents chose to express their outrage on signs in their windows during Scott Warren's trial,[65] which in the context of all our ongoing debates on health and freedom, captures both the spirit of such empathy and the obstacles it faces.[66]

4

Happiness
Of Miserable Grumps and Graceful Oysters

Stupidity, selfishness and good health are the three
prerequisites of happiness, though if stupidity is lacking
the others are useless.

—Gustave Flaubert

International Day of Happiness (yes, there is one) in 2018 was a special day for Anne Brokenbrow. Aged 104 and then living in a nursing home in Bristol in the west of England, Brokenbrow had led an exemplary life, apparently full and satisfying. But privately something was missing; something gnawed at her soul. This was the day the matter would be settled. She was duly arrested and handcuffed by three police officers, trundled out to the squad car in her wheelchair, and taken for a spin downtown with lights flashing and sirens wailing.

Some weeks earlier, in a response to a call from a local charity collecting the wishes of people living in care homes, Anne had submitted her greatest wish: "To be arrested. I am 104 and I have never been on the wrong side of the law." She was charged with "being a good citizen" and after a quick visit to the police station and photo op of her wearing a police hat and waving cheerily to the small band of media waiting outside, she was carefully deposited back in the care home. "I wouldn't have missed it for the world," she said.[1]

It takes all sorts.

Our freedom to pursue happiness is seldom unconditional. It nearly always involves the presence or actions of some, or the absence or inaction of others, even if indirectly and facilitative. Indeed, often, it is the very togetherness of the pursuit that creates the joy (as video footage makes evident in the case of Anne with the men and women of the Avon and Somerset police force). We are social animals. Many of us find the greatest pleasures when we are together, whether it is sharing a drink or a meal, attending a show or concert, playing a sport or watching it (though depending on which sport and what team, this can bring more pain that joy), sex, dancing, exchanging deep and meaningful opinions or talking drivel, or just being out and about in the company of others.[2] Happiness derived from virtual socializing—through social media and online gaming—might be included here too, even if it distresses parents of teens or preteens to concede as much. In any event, insofar as we are doing such things collectively, we have, individually, freely chosen to do so.

Equally, of course, many of us also enjoy solitary pursuits, whether reading a book, going for a walk or run, listening to music, meditating, staring at the stars, or the solo versions of the pursuits I list in the previous paragraph. Here again, we normally choose these activities. A big part of the happiness we draw from them is the very fact that we are free to pursue them. Unsurprisingly, when we are not free in our choice of activity (or perceive ourselves not to be so), the lack of freedom is often associated with unhappiness or, at best, not an increase in happiness. On this score research shows that what does not give us pleasure is being ill, caring for infirm adults, working or studying (even if we often say otherwise), queuing or waiting, and doing administrative tasks or tax returns, and commuting.[3]

These perspectives on happiness or unhappiness are all taken from the personal standpoint—they begin and end with the question, What makes *me* happy? But there is another perspective on the matter, which in the context of this book is in fact more important. It is the collective perspective—a concern for the social consequences of our individual happiness choices. How, in other words, do those choices affect others? And how free ought we to be in making them?

Everyone's Happiness

The balancing of collective and individual happiness was at the heart of Jeremy Bentham's utilitarian philosophy, which was founded on the beguilingly simple goal of securing the greatest happiness of the greatest number. As a measure of what is "right" and what is "wrong," both morals and laws ought to subscribe to this end, argued Bentham, and insofar as they do so, society will be fair and just.[4] He even devised a basic formula to measure the happiness quotient of any proposed act, since labeled (by others) the "felicific calculus" or "utility calculus." Bentham laid out a set of seven vectors that he suggested allows us to calculate the pain or pleasure to be derived from a contemplated action.[5] They are worth describing in full, not because they constitute a workable algorithm for leading a happy life (Bentham himself accepted that they were idealistic rather than practicable), but because, unlike much of what occupies today's gargantuan self-help literature, they are concerned with the pursuit of collective, not just individual, happiness.

Considerations of the *intensity* and *duration* of pleasurable or painful sensations were the starting points for Bentham. To these he added the need to reflect on the sensation's *fecundity* (the likelihood that it will be followed by more sensations of the same kind) and *purity* (the likelihood that it will be followed by sensations of the opposite kind). How certain can we be that the pleasure or pain will occur (what he called its *certainty*), and when that is likely to occur (its *propinquity*), were his fifth and sixth enumerated factors. His seventh and final factor is the most important for Bentham's utilitarian sensibilities, for it speaks in aggregate terms rather than in terms of the individual. What is the *extent* of the sensation? he asks. Who and how many are affected by it? In this he is seeking out the aggregate quantum of pleasure or pain—taking note, that is, of not only how many are likely to experience pleasure from one act or pain from another, but also how the one act (uninhibited free speech, for example) may elicit pleasure in some people and pain in others.

Splendid as this calculus may be in theory, it is as difficult, if not impossible, to put into practice today as it was in Bentham's day. What any one of us—let alone all of us collectively—considers to be a state of happiness is hard enough to say. Pinpointing what really makes us happy is still more complicated, often beyond rational explanation. Indeed, the very fact of the inscrutability of happiness is a large part of its endearment. We are all aware, for example, of times when pleasure and pain seem to be operating in tandem—the "bright side of pain" when pushing ourselves physically or speaking in public, or the "dark side of pleasure" when flirting turns into an affair or we overindulge in drugs or alcohol. Even frustration can be an important part of enjoyment, as psychoanalyst Adam Phillips points out in his fascinating book *Missing Out*, being the prelude to so many pleasures that ultimately heightens their effect.[6] In the end, however, we may have to accept that we are psychologically ill-equipped to solve the happiness question. What makes the task so tricky, as Clive James sardonically pondered, "is that we are given both the capacity for personal happiness and the sense of proportion to realize that it is an offence against common reason."[7]

Trying to Smile

Inscrutable it may be, but that hasn't stopped us trying to find the answer to the happiness puzzle. We are all forever seeking happiness at some level or another. Pleasure, gratification, contentment, comfort, security, or simply the avoidance or minimization of pain are variously hardwired into our motivations, our goals, how we behave, and what we say and do. Battalions of psychologists, psychiatrists, philosophers, poets, politicians, and preachers purport to help, guide, advise, or tell us how to increase our happiness quotient throughout life and by the minute. We are urged (and we urge ourselves) to "smile," "be happy," "laugh more," and "don't worry." Yet we often worry—openly or more likely furtively—that we are not happy enough, or not as happy as we ought to be or as others seem to be. How we deal with disappointment, including disappointment in ourselves for not being sufficiently happy, is itself a crucial indicator of our capacity for happiness. And so it goes on.

Amid all the "how to be happy" cacophony, Emiliana Simon-Thomas is one of those voices worth listening to. A neuroscientist and a director of the Greater Good Science Center at the University of California, Berkeley, Simon-Thomas teaches a hugely popular course, The Science of Happiness. Her insights into what makes us happy are drawn from what she sees our brains and bodies react to as we go about our daily lives. Fundamentally, she argues, happiness stems from "having satisfaction and meaning in your life . . . a propensity to feel positive emotions, the capacity to recover from negative emotions quickly, and holding a sense of purpose."[8] The recipe for happiness, she ventures "is not having a lot of privilege or money. It's not constant pleasure. It's a

broader thing: our ability to connect with others, to have meaningful relationships, to have a community. Time and again—
across decades of research and across all studies—people who say
they're happy have strong connections with community and with
other people."

Happiness around the World

Certainly, even a quick glance at Gallup's annual world happiness polls bears out this point. Fiji was the happiest country in
2017, and Finland the happiest in the five years thereafter.[9] A striking characteristic that both these countries shared is their peoples'
strong senses of community—communities to which they actively
contribute and from which they readily draw comfort. Fijians, for
example, like many Pacific Islanders, invest enormously in their
cultural traditions of close family and tribal ties, which seemingly
repay them with security, contentment, and above all a sense of
belonging.

Finns also apparently really care about one another. Economist
and coeditor of the UN's *World Happiness Report*, John Helliwell
believes that among the reasons why Finns are such a happy bunch
is that they are "generous with each other."[10] They also have a
charmingly understated, self-deprecating sense of humor (one of
my favorite jokes from anywhere was told to me by a Finn [in a
sauna!] in Helsinki: "Q: What's the definition of an extrovert
Finn? A: They look at *your* shoes when they're talking to you").
These characteristics, together with the fact that Finns "pay high
taxes for a social safety net, they trust their government, and they
live in freedom," means that Finland is the kind of place where
people want to live.[11] Even Finland's immigrant population is happier than the immigrant communities in any other country: "It's
not about Finnish DNA," notes Helliwell, underling the point:
"it's the way life is lived."

A combination of personal freedom and security, it seems, is necessary both to be happy and to strive for it. Freedom, that is, to pursue goals and activities that make us happy, that satisfy or provide contentment, that elate or bring joy. And while, in the spirit of liberty, we recognize that our freedom to do so is conditional, we rightly expect that any hindrance, whether from public authorities or private entities and other individuals, will be fair and reasonable. Security—in the sense of personal safety, adequate health and welfare, and an overall confidence in the apparatus of government—is also needed. As is a basic level of financial security, though interestingly, beyond providing bare minimum levels of comfort, the importance of wealth in achieving happiness diminishes as wealth increases.[12] In fact, one of the many curious features of the discipline of happiness studies is that, time and again, surveys show the spread of happy and unhappy people to be very similar across all wealth categories.[13] There are, in other words, proportionally as many happy poor as there are happy rich.

The Tyranny of Happiness

Some of what makes us happy has got to do with personality traits. Individually we are all to some extent predisposed to being happy or unhappy, no matter what our circumstances and to some extent age.[14] But much is also due to that most fundamental of psychosocial characteristics—our seemingly insatiable need to compare ourselves to others. "Keeping up with the Joneses" is an especially powerful determinant of our perceived levels of happiness when the Joneses in question are our neighbors and peers. How we fare compared to those more or less immediately around us is apparently a critical yardstick of our personal sense of accomplishment and satisfaction, or lack thereof.

Aside from the fact that it might simply be easier to be a miserable grump,[15] the practical applications of this particular theory of relativity are profound and perplexing. Perhaps the most remarkable example of both is the tenacity of our so-called set point for happiness. This is the point psychologists refer to as one's natural or normal level of happiness (where you sit on a scale of one to ten) and around which we fluctuate daily and for as long as we live. It is also the point to which we nearly always eventually return, regardless of what befalls us in the meantime. Thus, it has been shown that even after events of enormous good fortune (winning the lottery, for example) or catastrophe (an accident that leaves you paralyzed) people's happiness register will eventually return to its baseline—that is, its long-term average. True, there is a spike upward or downward immediately after either event, but consistently in both cases, happiness levels start to head back toward individuals' respective set points after the shock wears off.[16]

We adapt to the circumstances we find ourselves in. Many of us do this very well,[17] others less so, but whichever the case, our capacity for happiness is directly affected by our surroundings. Those of us who best deal with the slings and arrows of fortune, however outrageous, prove to be the most resiliently cheery. Much of our capacity for adaptation boils down to how we handle expectations. It is not hard to imagine how someone staring at their lottery winner's check might be seduced by all those zeros into believing that life henceforth will be a bed of roses, while another staring at limbs rendered suddenly immobile might be tempted to despair of their future. Yet for the lucky rich the trials and tribulations of life continue (even if differently composed than those endured by the rest of us), and for the disabled, new challenges can bring forth new triumphs. The world is not short of the wealthy whingers, nor of paralyzed optimists. As George Vaillant, who oversaw one of the most extensive longitudinal studies of happiness ever undertaken, put it so elegantly, "Analogous to the involuntary grace by which an oyster, coping with an irritating grain of sand, creates a pearl," so humans, "when confronted with irritants, engage in unconscious but often creative behavior."[18]

The state of happiness across the globe is in fact full of paradoxes, as happiness researcher Carol Graham shows in her work on the topic, including "the paradox of happy peasants and miserable millionaires."[19] "Frustrated achievers," as she calls rich-world discontents, are that way precisely because of unmet expectations, while "happy peasants" are contented souls because they have satisfied their expectations. Happiness, of course, is also to be found in the rich world, just as misery exists in poor states, but the point is that neither can money secure happiness nor its scarcity guarantee gloom. Rather, it is our skill in managing expectations, our upward and downward adaptations of them on a daily or longer-term basis, that really sets the tone of our levels of individual contentment.[20]

What individual freedom has to do with our quest for individual happiness is equally intriguing, as it too has much to do with how we handle our expectations. For the freedom associated with happiness is not, and cannot be, that which *begets* happiness; our freedom is not to *be* happy. As we see with freedom's relationship to other notable circumstances of the human condition explored in this book—one's health, wealth, and stocks in love, for example—there can be no cast-iron outcome, no assured happy ending. Instead, the freedom in question is, and must be, in the *pursuit* of happiness, whatever the actual result.

In Pursuit of Happiness

Of course, the very freedom to pursue is itself a critical ingredient in the happiness recipe. Where folk are largely free to go about their business in ways that they believe please them as much as possible, they are more likely to be content with the actual outcome no matter what. Where they are not so free, where their actions are crimped and circumscribed, even apparently success-ful outcomes may be tainted.

On one hand, consider the relative freedom Americans enjoy to possess firearms. This, apparently, brings great comfort and pleasure to many citizens. As the chapter on security shows, thirty-six of the fifty US states have little or no licensing requirements, and an esti-mated 393 million firearms are now in the hands of American ci-vilians (more than one gun each).[21] At the same time, the United States boasts by far the highest firearm mortality rate in the West-ern world.[22] Depending on your perspective (and I make mine clear in chapter 7, on security), either this extraordinary propensity toward gun violence is propelled by the easy access to firearms, or it justifies the reason for having a gun cited by more than two-thirds of gun owners—namely, "protection."[23] Either way, and despite the horrifying results of so much firepower in their homes and on their streets, a substantial minority, 42 percent, of *all* Americans say they are happy with gun laws as they currently stand.[24] Evidently, the freedom from infringement on the right to bear arms in the Second Amendment is as cherished as it is costly.

On the other hand, curtailing one's freedom to act as one pleases in ways that seem unfair or heavy-handed can skewer any resulting pleasure. One of the many run-ins between France's national policy of secularism, *laïcité*, and its resident Muslim population—over what Muslim women choose to wear— illustrates the point. On this occasion the dress in question was the burkini. On a hot day in June 2019, a group of seven women entered a public baths in Grenoble wearing the head-to-toe gear in defiance of local municipal regulations which required women to wear either a one piece swimsuit or a bikini. Pictures of the seven women laughing and splashing about in the pool among other bathers who either applauded them or were simply nonplussed didn't sway the authorities, who called the police, whereupon the seven were duly ejected from the pool, fined €35 each, and banned from all pools in the area for a month.[25]

Opinion in France was divided on the matter, but with no national policy or regulation specifically governing burkinis in public pools, local municipalities are free to choose whether or not to ban them.[26] Alongside Grenoble several have done so, but many others have not. No one denies that in the name of *liberté*, French law can impose dress restrictions on bathers in public pools (for example, prohibiting shoes, motor bike helmets, or wearing too little or nothing at all), it is just whether by so doing it gets the mix right between secularism, the rights of women, and religious culture when banning burkinis. For while Muslim women in France are still free to swim legally in some public pools wearing a burkini, they can hardly do so discreetly and comfortably given the profile such an apparently simple act now attracts.

The freedom coefficient of happiness seems to matter more to those who are accustomed to having freedom.[27] In this respect, one's familiarity with freedom is like one's familiarity with wealth—the more you have, the more you expect of it. The conditions imposed on freedom in the name of liberty, therefore, can have markedly different effects. Even relatively minor infringements on one's erstwhile freedom to pursue a chosen path can, for some, become major irritations—the introduction of licensing requirements to fish or own a dog, for example. Conversely, the existence of seriously restricted opportunities to choose one's path—say, in circumstances of poverty, discrimination, rampant crime, or corruption—may be tolerated. In this latter respect there is evidence that such tolerance is for some worn as a badge of pride, their resilience giving them a sense of satisfaction that they can make do come what may.[28]

Evidently, precisely what makes us happy is ineffably difficult to define. That is certainly the case for society as a whole, but it is also true for each of us individually. What we get in life is not always what we want, but even when we do get what we want, it may disappoint, either because our expectations of it were unrealistic or because we don't understand ourselves well enough. Most likely it is a combination of the two. The elephant of our unconscious mind, as Jonathan Haidt puts it in his 2006 book, *The Happiness Hypothesis*, is forever upsetting the best intentions of the driver that is our conscious mind.

So asking anyone what they really want or need to make them happy is fraught with problems. In terms of deciding how we might best organize ourselves to pursue happiness individually and collectively, however, it is the obvious place to start. It also has the inestimable merit of investing in each of us the agency of self-awareness to choose as we wish rather than have someone else choose for us. For, as Immanuel Kant argued, despite the universal importance of happiness to all of us, the concept is not specific enough to denote any particular set of universal human desires such as might warrant claims to know what must be done to achieve it.[29]

This is not to say that each of us must be given entirely free rein in our search for happiness. Instead, we—like Kant—must focus on what such freedom means in practice. In keeping with this book's argument that liberty means negotiating freedom in the company of others, our desired pathways to contentment must be scrutinized for crossovers and clashes with those of our neighbors, and consideration must be given to how happiness if faring throughout the community as a whole. In these balancing tasks we are helped by some generalized perceptions of what happiness entails.

While many thinkers, including Kant, are undoubtedly correct to say that happiness evades *precise* definition, certain broad features are discernible. Surveying the views of philosophers ancient and modern, father and son duo Anthony and Charles Kenny conclude that happiness comprises three essential components: welfare, dignity, and contentment.[30] That said, they accept that the composition and respective proportions of each can vary greatly from person to person. The Kennys' essential point is that together the three are necessary, if indistinct, features of personal happiness.

Can the State Help You Find Happiness?

Defining happiness by way of this triumvirate puts it at the heart of the meaning of life. It secures happiness as a matter of enormous personal and social importance, maybe even the ultimate good—the summum bonum. Philosophers from Cicero and Aristotle to Kant and Bentham have entertained that very question in their various attempts to understand whether and how we ought to pursue the goal. It is an appealing concept. Like kindness and doing good, not evil, it is hard not to agree with it as fundamentally desirable. More recently, some states have toyed with the prospect of enshrining the happiness goal in public policy deliberations. Bhutan's King Jigme Singye Wangchuck declared in 1972 that "gross national happiness [GNH] is more important than gross domestic product" and set about establishing an index by which it could be measured. His monarchical successors have maintained the country's fealty to GNH, which over the years has boiled down to a conscientiously welfarist economy with free education and health care for all and heavily subsidized electricity for many.[31] Bhutan also sponsored a UN General Assembly resolution in 2011 that urged all states to "give more importance to happiness and well-being in determining how to achieve and measure social and economic development."[32] The resolution prompted the first *World Happiness Report* in 2012, though Bhutan itself has always languished well down (or not featured at all) in the world happiness rankings published in the report each year.[33]

In response to the rising popularity of happiness studies in the early 2000s, both the French (under Nicolas Sarkozy) and the British (under David Cameron) introduced "well-being frameworks" into their policy agendas. These too focused on welfare concerns, albeit by way of actively tracking such indicators as poverty, income inequality, and health standards, as well as life satisfaction (United Kingdom)[34] and carbon footprint (France), rather than necessarily directing more resources toward them. In 2019, Jacinda Ardern's Labour government in New Zealand announced its intention to champion well-being over the traditional economic markers of growth and monetary policy in its latest budget. Here again the approach is welfare oriented, focusing on addressing problems in mental health, poverty, and child suicide, rather than the decidedly more elusive "contentment" and "dignity."[35]

The roles that governments and lawmakers can and do play in curating our freedom to pursue personal paths toward happiness do seem to be somewhat limited. And so it has been for millennia. The globe-trotting bon vivant Irishman Oliver Goldsmith's 1764 poem *The Traveller (or a Prospect of Society)* offers his reflections on the state of happiness across many nations and what, if anything, different forms of government have to do with it. His conclusion that, frankly, governments don't have much to offer us is best summed up in this stanza near the end of the piece:

How small of all that human hearts endure,
That part which laws or kings can cause or cure.
Still to ourselves in every place consign'd,
Our own felicity we make or find.

That said, as Goldsmith lived much of his guilelessly colorful life free of officialdom—either because he flouted it (being perpetually pursued by creditors) or was oblivious to it (twice failing to emigrate to America, the second time because he missed the boat)[36]—we might beg to differ, as today governments and lawmakers have important roles to play in the happiness space. The pursuit of happiness is often a matter of negotiated liberty, whether tacit or overt, not of unbridled freedom to do whatever one pleases, and it therefore demands some level of regulation and standard setting. First of all, our rulers need to ensure that basic welfare needs are met, especially for those not otherwise able to do so unaided. They must set boundaries—proscribing pursuits that are cruel, destructive, or dangerous to others, for example. They can stipulate conditions and responsibilities for how people act or behave when engaged in happiness pursuits (whether gambling, trainspotting, extreme sports, or religious practices), and they typically act as arbiters when conflicts arise (think of hunting, music festivals, culture mores, and risqué comedy). So, while the state may not mandate what it is that you must or must not do in order to *be* happy, it can stipulate certain conditions under which we negotiate among ourselves our respective quests toward happiness.

The state can and should do more with respect to happiness. It is not all about setting limits. There are also legitimate expectations that our rulers facilitate our chosen paths, that they accommodate, encourage, and promote individual and collective happiness. This was the very thinking behind Bentham's felicific calculus, discussed earlier. It is also a derivation of what American psychology professor Abraham Maslow argued in his monumentally influential paper "A Theory of Human Motivation," published in *Psychological Review* in 1943. His pyramidal "Hierarchy of Needs" starts at its base with the essential physiological requirements of food, water, health, and safety before heading upward through the needs of love and belonging, self-esteem, and finally, at the pyramid's peak, to a state of self-actualization where you fulfill your entire potential. "What a man can be, he must be," as Maslow put it.

Setting aside the fact that, initially at least, Maslow believed these layers of needs were cumulative, in that the higher-level needs cannot be fully realized without first the lower-level needs being met (evidence points to their being more fluid and interchangeable than that), in fact his hierarchy popularized an articulation of what people expect from life: that matters of love and belonging are vital to building happiness (as Fiji shows us) and that self-esteem or dignity (as it is expressed in human rights terms) is not an optional extra but something critical to our well-being and contentment. Each of us, from personal experience, appreciates the importance of these higher needs, and many of us spend a good deal of our lives striving for them. In this we expect, or ought to expect, that our leaders, in representing us and in respecting our needs, act in ways that promote our sense of community and of individual dignity, as well as health and safety. This is, after all, the very stuff of government, the essence of the social contract.

Self-actualization in the absolute terms conveyed by Maslow is best seen as an ideal, something aspirational rather than truly attainable (are you, or have you ever met, someone who has fulfilled their entire potential?). It is a process, an accumulation of the lower level needs, that, while never ending, is nonetheless eminently worthwhile pursuing. It is no accident that Thomas Jefferson insisted on "the *pursuit* of happiness" as one of the truths held to be self-evident in the US Declaration of Independence, not happiness itself. Our own responsibility for negotiating that pursuit or process, along with that of our governments to facilitate it, is no different from the way I describe above.

What this means in practice is that a government's policies and their implementation must reflect a society's values; they must represent what it is that people stand for if they are to succeed in providing an environment in which happiness can flourish. If the aim is (as it ought to be) to provide people with freedoms that achieve the greatest happiness for the greatest number, this twining of societal values with government policies begs a number of important questions about responsibility. What are a society's values, and who decides what they are? Whose happiness stands to gain most from these values or policies, and how are either modified or changed? The ways one might address these questions are legion, but for our purposes two stand out as concerning fundamental inequalities that reflect just how difficult the negotiation of happiness can be. The first concerns inequalities in wealth and safety, and the second focuses on gender inequality.

Wealth, Women, and Well-Being

The happiness consequences of wealth and safety inequalities boil down to the obscenities of poverty. Two of the happiness paradoxes discussed earlier bear out the problem. One—the paradox of social resilience—encapsulates Carol Graham's "happy peasant" epithet, where the poor or disadvantaged seem content with their lot, a contentment born of a dogged sense of pride in being able to cope with inadequate or even appalling circumstances. Lack of basic amenities, high levels of crime or corruption, and endemic discrimination are factored into the life expectations of many living in poverty, lowering them to a point where they are in fact satisfactorily met.

I've seen this coping mechanism in action in many countries (both rich and poor), including Nepal, where decades-long delays in a project aiming to divert water from the Melamchi River to the water-starved Kathmandu Valley has caused enormous hardship. Neither the farming and fishing communities living along the Melamchi River whose livelihoods are seriously affected by the diversion, nor the 5 million inhabitants of Kathmandu Valley who face chronic water shortages and sanitation problems have fared well during this saga, which has been plagued by incompetence, mismanagement, and corruption. Yet, over the many years I, my colleagues, and our students have been observing the project, nearly all the ordinary families we talk to demonstrate the same levels of extraordinary resilience and fortitude. Many have complaints—including lack of information, promises not kept, missing or inadequate compensation, or worsening sanitation situations—but when you ask them about what they have done or might do to seek redress, many shrug and smile, and say they are just getting on with life, seemingly resigned to their plight.[37]

The other paradox—like the reverse side of the coin—encapsulates Graham's "frustrated achiever" model, touched on earlier. Here the apparent unhappiness absurdities of affluence are highlighted. For, while it is clear that an absence or stark scarcity of wealth can stunt happiness, beyond a certain minimum level of comfort and security-buying wealth, it is the *relative* lack of riches and good fortune that so often irritates and perturbs. Is not such discomfort mere pettiness, you might ask? Thoroughly deserving of its "First World problem" tag? Yet the competitive unease experienced by the comfortable in not keeping pace with one's apparently more fortunate neighbors or fellow citizens is real and is felt by many.

At its extremes, however, the happiness-wealth question of "How much is enough?" takes on more profound and troubling dimensions. That is when the breadth of wealth disparity is so searing as to affront people's dignity and sense of fairness to the point, as underlined in the following chapter, that people respond in political, economic, or civic rebellion.[38] The freedoms and opportunities afforded to the world's richest 0.1 percent or even 1 percent (approximately 8 million and 80 million people, respectively) in their pursuit of happiness are ridiculously many and varied compared to the rest of humanity (and certainly to the 700 million or so who still live in abject poverty),[39] no matter whether the financially fortunate are in fact happy or not.

The happiness consequences of persistent gender inequalities have been lamented by feminist writers and others at least since Mary Wollstonecraft's *A Vindication of the Rights of Women*, published in 1792, and Olympe de Gouges's Déclaration des droits de la Femme et de la Citoyenne, released one year earlier (and for which, in part, she was guillotined shortly thereafter).[40] If we are to take seriously talk of striving for the greatest happiness of the greatest number, then we must pay more attention to prevalent or systemic barriers that stand in the way of that goal for many or even most of us in society. The happiness of women in this respect is of paramount importance. Or at least it should be. Jill Filipovic, for example, protests that for too long our societies have side-stepped, belittled, or simply ignored what she calls women's "H-Spot."[41]

In her study of women's happiness in America today, Filipovic concludes that "the ideal of women as self-sacrificing buoys for important male work survives to the present," such that for women to actively seek pleasure and fulfillment beyond such boundaries "remains an act of rebellion." The chimera that today women can "have it all" is not so much liberation or equality but a piling up of burden and expectation.[42] "What seems to be making women miserable is being pulled in too many directions and dedicating too many hours of the day . . . to unpleasant activities rather than pleasant ones." It doesn't have to be this way, she argues, not least because, for all the embedded biases in our views regarding the happiness of women, the matter is fundamentally a political one and therefore, like gross wealth disparities, not beyond reform or even revolution.

The currently fraught debates over when and how to regulate transgender rights and freedoms show just how difficult such reform can sometimes be.[43] As one's free expression of gender identity is central to one's being and therefore foundational to quests for personal fulfillment and happiness, so any exercise of authority that affects such free expression is rightly a matter of concern. Recognizing and respecting transgender people, as well as facilitating their inclusion and guarding against discrimination, are hallmarks of a society based on empathy and equality. But as is so often with the miscellany of the human condition, such noble ideals can be fearsomely complicated to implement in practice, when, for example, they bump into other people's legitimate freedom claims. On which point the imbroglio concerning what regulations should govern participation of transgender women in women's sports and how they should balance the respective rights of trans and cis women is but one vivid and highly charged illustration.[44]

The discriminatory effects of both prosperity and gender are matters that governments as well as individuals and communities at large negotiate every day and can change if they are so minded. Negotiations within and between all levels of society about what makes people happy or unhappy effectively determine the quantum, quality, and dispersal of personal and societal contentment. Whether it be bucket list wishes like Anne Brokenbrow's faux arrest, or obsessions, hobbies, pastimes, sexual expressions, religious experiences, or any of the opportunities enabled by wealth, health, genes, gender, education, or just pure chance, our freedom to pursue our chosen pleasures is in fact a liberty. It is always, to some extent, limited. Most often we do not test these boundaries, but we are nevertheless aware of them. They are, or should be, set and reset by our social and political institutions of governance, not so much to dictate what will make us happy as to articulate the boundaries that exist to protect reasonable expectations for the welfare and happiness of others as well as ourselves.

Brokering Boundaries

Bright lines of proscription exist, of course, regarding crimes such as pedophilia, rape, gratuitous violence, enslavement, racial vilification, theft, and fraud, no matter the "pleasure" that protagonists might claim to derive from such abhorrent or aberrant behavior. At the same time, the curtailment of other pleasure-seeking activities is genuinely ambiguous and debatable—like smoking, drug use, certain sexual proclivities, cultural practices, ribald comedy, sedition, or voicing extreme opinions. Certainly, such matters as the social consequences of excessive wealth disparities and entrenched gender bias should be on the table for the very reason that they can and do inhibit the happiness opportunities of so many.

The extent to which each one of us feels a sense of freedom is itself a barometer of our own levels of happiness. Alongside the unloved and the lonely, the unfree, as we have learnt, tend to be unhappy. The act of balancing potentially conflicting claims in the pursuit of happiness is, ultimately, the task of our institutions of governance, no matter that they focus on broad social policy or guidance rather than on micromanaged personal interventions. So smoking is discouraged by high taxes, nonsmoking zones, and public information campaigns, but it is not banned altogether for those who enjoy it. And while nudism is prohibited in public, you can let it all hang out in private if that makes you happy. Government's happiness interventions also tend to take a long- rather than short-term perspective. They look to the social and economic costs of the health consequences of smoking and take seriously the long-standing and cross-cultural mores regarding the wearing of clothes, regardless of passing fads. Within these boundaries, your freedoms and mine to choose whether to smoke or wear clothes become matters of negotiation over the responsibilities we owe one another.[45]

5

Wealth

Is Freedom for Sale?

If we command our wealth, we shall be rich and free.
If our wealth commands us, we are poor indeed.
—Edmund Burke

In 1928, just as autumn was turning into winter and the Fens began their annual ritual of greeting and ending the days shrouded in mist, a middle-aged woman of somewhat austere appearance and manner arrived in Cambridge to deliver a pair of lectures at the university's two women's colleges, Girton and Newnham. Grimly determined more than enthusiastic at the prospect, Virginia Woolf was nonetheless about to lay the groundwork for what was to become her most celebrated work and foremost feminist critique. *A Room of One's Own*, published a year later, is more than a caustic lament of the continuing suppression of women in Georgian England; it is also a homily on the benefits of wealth, the opportunities it provides, and the freedom it bestows. "That is why I have laid so much stress on money and on a room of one's own," writes Woolf.[1] In fact, she spends much of the book investigating what might be done if she had the same independence and freedom to pursue her craft as wealth typically affords to men, and while she unapologetically focuses on her own, comparatively privileged circumstances, Woolf does so in a way that speaks to the poverty of all women in terms of freedom.

Virginia Woolf is here referring to the first of two aspects of freedom regularly associated with wealth—that is, what wealth buys you, what you can do with it or make with it. It is concerned with the *freedom derived from* wealth. The second aspect of freedom's association with wealth refers to how wealth is made; the freedom that permits the generation of wealth in the first place. It is, in other words, concerned with the *freedom to create* wealth. Combined, the two aspects form a sort of sandwich, with wealth as the filling between two slices of freedom.

The two freedoms are intimately linked. The supposed necessity of the freedom to make wealth is strongly predicated on the belief that the resulting wealth will provide the means to garner greater personal freedom by offering us more opportunity and more choice. The two freedoms are neither entirely separable nor entirely equal. The freedom wealth buys (or we hope it buys) is, it seems, elevated above the freedom to make wealth precisely because of its perceived utility. What you can do with wealth rather than its mere accumulation is, therefore, the most important axis between freedom and wealth, the driver behind their association. I must say, though, that in the many years I have been working in the field of finance and human rights, what truly stands out among financiers is their devotion to the making of money. The intrinsic thrill of it, that is, rather than merely its utility, especially if they make more than their competitors or colleagues. And the higher up you go in the financial sector pecking order, the more pronounced the devotion. "It comes with the territory," I was frequently told, which may be true but is no less alarming because of all that is trampled along the way.[2]

Most of the rest of us, I'd say, see more value in the utility of wealth. We're more excited about the freedoms we hope to gain from having some wealth and spending it than we are about the manner of its creation. We're focused on having the freedom to choose more education or more shoes, less or different work, or more or better food, as well as eager for the freedoms acquired by wealth—greater voice and influence, more travel or security, or whatever. Flippant (and hardly short of a dollar) though Gianni Versace might have been when he said, "I have a fantastic relationship with money; I use it to buy my freedom," I suspect there is more than a little truth in that for all of us. Indeed, we see ample evidence of it throughout this chapter, but before getting there, we must be careful not to overlook the rhetorical power of the prefatory side of the sandwich—namely, the arguments for the freedom to make money. For such arguments have deeply influenced the ways our economies, societies, and personal lives are organized today.

The Sandwich Filling

Should you care to dip into the enormous and ever-growing mountain of literature devoted to the coalition of wealth and freedom, you will find a great deal of attention paid to the creative side of the sandwich by philosophers and economists, politicians and potentates. And among the many keen advocates of financial wealth expounding on the importance of both creative and derivative freedoms to their cause, you will also find no shortage of grand claims made about the relationship between the two.

Perhaps the grandest of all claims are those which bind the wealth-freedom sandwich to the fortunes (literally) of capitalism. Namely, that both the freedom we enjoy to accumulate wealth and the freedom born of wealth itself are possible only through capitalist enterprise.[3] Capitalism, according to this line of thinking, is an integral part of the Enlightenment philosophy of liberalism. Indeed, it is true that the intellectual crucible of the

Enlightenment forged the notions of individuals striving for both societal and economic freedom. Working in tandem—so the liberalist ideal dictates—one's social and political freedoms extend into the economic sphere, where choices of action are theoretically available to all.

The Enlightenment's greatest and most influential exponent of this interpretation of the freedom-wealth relationship was Adam Smith, who extolled the virtues of freedom across two monumental treatises. *The Wealth of Nations*, which appeared in 1776, focused on the economic potential of market freedom to *create* wealth, and *The Theory of Moral Sentiments*, published some seventeen years earlier, deliberated on the necessity for a wider, deeper, and fairer *distribution* of the freedom-enhancing benefits of greater societal wealth.[4]

What Smith essentially did in *Moral Sentiments* was to map out the principles by which we should live our lives in the company of others—shared and interlocking degrees of mutual respect, fairness, freedom, and equity. In *The Wealth of Nations*, he set about articulating the most efficient and effective means by which to deliver the economic wherewithal to satisfy those principles. It is, therefore, a cardinal mistake to read Smith simply and only as a zealous advocate of the free market. That is only half the story. His commitment to market freedom was premised, crucially, on what it could deliver for society as a whole—for the poor and weak as well as the rich and powerful.[5]

The driving force of market freedom at the center of Smith's endeavor is a means to an end, not an end in itself. "The obvious and simple system of natural liberty," coupled with "the industry of private people," as he put it, leads "towards employments most suitable to the interest of society."[6] It is certainly true that Smith distrusted the capacity of the directorial hand of government to cultivate such conditions and achieve such an outcome (preferring, as he put it, the market's "invisible hand" to do the job), but he was nonetheless adamant that the outcome—the betterment of society—was the point of the whole enterprise. The free and open competition generated by people's industry was, he argued, the surest way not just to provide what the market wants but also, at least potentially, to provide what society needs through the generation of a greater quantity of aggregate wealth.

Given the resonance of these words and sentiments today, it is truly astounding to remind ourselves of the times in which they were written. The sort of political and social economy with which Smith was familiar some 250 years ago is almost unrecognizable to us today. Commercial trade, including across borders, was flourishing, but it was small scale and limited in scope. Industry was in its infancy, completely overshadowed by agriculture, with large-scale steam power and transport mechanization still decades away. The mills, mines, factories, and railways of the industrial revolution were yet to make their mark in Europe and North America. Most people lived in rural areas, and towns and cities were still relatively small. Few folk were employed. Most worked for themselves, were feudal serfs or in some other form of debt bondage, or were enslaved. Beyond a handful of megacolonial enterprises such as the British and Dutch East India companies and the British North America Company, companies were rare, and corporations and employment laws nonexistent.

Wealth was highly concentrated and entrenched, taxation was irregular and regressive, education was the privilege of a very few, and there was no such thing as health care. Social stratification was rigid, the power and authority of the Church still considerable, and the rights of ordinary people few and far between. Democracy in any form like how we now view it was more of an idea than reality nearly everywhere. At the time Smith published his *Wealth of Nations*, the Parliament of Great Britain (as it was then) lacked universal suffrage, with only the rich, landed, and male able to vote. The American Revolution was ongoing and the French Revolution still a decade away, while most of the rest of Europe was still under monarchical rule.

Compared to today, then, the overwhelming majority of people during Smith's time were poor, illiterate, short-lived, and unfree. It took a considerable leap of imagination and of faith for Enlightenment thinkers such as Smith not only to envisage a world where ordinary "private people" could be liberated but to believe that they possessed within themselves the capacity to be so despite all that constrained them. But, of course, that is why this extraordinary epoch in the evolution of philosophy is called the Enlightenment. Still, in terms of the relationship between wealth and freedom, the movement's leading lights didn't get everything right.

The presumption that an expanded freedom *to make* wealth will result in expanded freedoms *created by* wealth relies heavily on the assumption that increases in prosperity will be distributed widely and fairly. Free market capitalism by no means guarantees such an outcome. We know this to be true, but we have the benefit of 250 years of hindsight. For Smith, this second part of the equation was built on what he believed the free market *could* provide, rather than on any clear and available evidence of what it *does* provide. Thus, in one of his pivotal statements regarding the work of the invisible hand, Smith declares:

> The rich . . . consume little more than the poor, and in spite of their natural selfishness and rapacity though they mean only their own conveniency, though the sole end which they propose from the labours of all the thousands whom they employ, be the gratification of their own vain and insatiable desires, they divide with the poor the produce of all their improvements. They are led by

an invisible hand to make nearly the same distribution of the necessaries of life, which would have been made, had the earth been divided into equal portions among all its inhabitants, and thus without intending it, without knowing it, advance the interest of the society, and afford means to the multiplication of the species.[7]

On the face of it, this is a remarkable claim. For, while today we see clearly how imperfectly the rich have distributed life's essentials (and certainly in nothing like "equal portions"), surely during his own time Smith was witness to the divisive rather than unifying consequences of the "selfishness and rapacity" of the rich. Assuredly, it seems, he witnessed such inequity, if we are to take at face value the disparaging terms he uses to describe the rich and the fact that throughout his work Smith devotes so much attention to investigating the nature and role of greed in human relations. So, then, what does he mean by the above statement? The answer is locked within the virtues he attributes to the market's invisible hand. Despite themselves, Smith seemed to believe, and without them so intending—"invisibly," in other words—the rich redistribute the life-enhancing benefits of commerce by their very participation in free market enterprise. He hammers home the point by saying that even (indeed *especially*) when a merchant single-mindedly pursues his own interest, intending only to promote his own security and his own gain, "he frequently promotes that of society more effectually than when he really intends to promote it."[8]

The free market's invisible hand, therefore, was expected to do some seriously heavy lifting. Such an ambitious theory demanded substantial proof in practice, which, alas, is not something Smith himself saw in his lifetime. He died in 1790, just as the industrial revolution began and long before industrialized capitalism appropriated his theory as its raison d'être. As a matter of fact, many of the claims made today of the relationship between freedom and wealth are similar to those made more than two hundred years ago, though they are now expressed somewhat differently, and both the nature of commerce and the way it is regulated have changed beyond all recognition.

The Visible Hand of Liberty

Industrialization, globalization, and technologization have increased the size and reach of trade and commerce exponentially. And, while free market incantations are still voiced loudly and often, they are pitted against strong countervailing forces. First, the inexorable tendency of free market players is not toward efficient competition of the sort envisaged by Adam Smith but rather toward monopolistic concentration, as the corporate behemoths of banking, mining, industry, and technology today and across the past century bear ample testimony.[9] Second, governmental intervention in the market is unavoidable and often substantial. Whether it is to combat corporate concentration and promote (free) competition, or to regulate the operation or impact of the market by way, for example, of taxation, quality control, environmental regulations, workplace health and safety standards, or minimum wage policies.[10]

In other words, the "free market" is in reality anything but totally free. A market without rules and limitations may indeed permit the fittest to survive and the most efficient to thrive, but it also allows the opportunity for the fittest, most efficient, or simply the keenest and meanest to dominate and destroy. "Destruction" is not itself necessarily bad, at least not in market terms. Joseph Schumpeter, one of the twentieth century's most revered economists—coined the phrase "creative destruction" to encapsulate the dynamic rise and fall of products and services, producers and service providers as the whims of the market dictate. The free market, so this argument goes, rewards innovation, responsiveness, and efficiency and discards that which fails in these respects.

But where, for example, a market for a particular product or service is dominated by one or a handful of producers or service providers, the rewards are skewed and the freedom of the market necessarily compromised. Efficiency may also suffer—at least in terms of price and quality—in the absence of viable competitors because monopoly (or oligopoly) holders may have little reason to drop prices or improve quality. Think of oligopolistic oil companies and gas/petrol prices, or banks and interest rates, or (until recently) cell phone and internet service provider charges.

Alongside the key concerns of market freedom and market efficiency, therefore, there is a third matter of critical importance—fairness. Fairness regarding who or what can access a market, under what conditions, at what cost, with what rewards. It is based on the matter of fairness—or at least purported fairness—that governments most often justify their market interventions. To ensure freer access by countering anti-competitive behavior, such as with laws restricting cross-media ownership. Or to ensure wider access by countering market tendencies to underserve unprofitable sectors of society, such as laws compelling or compensating essential service providers (of power, water, health care, and sanitation, for example) to serve poorer or rural and remote communities, not just richer areas and urban dwellers. In some cases, as with the establishment of universal health care programs, the concern is not merely to ensure fairness but also to alleviate unnecessary suffering and save lives.

Together the intersections of freedom, efficiency, and fairness yield a wide variety of market formats: from the relatively free market economies of the United States, Singapore, Australia, and

Hong Kong to the more regulated market economies of the European Union and the mixed economies of Latin America, such as Argentina, Brazil, and Chile. The state-directed and still substantially state-owned (or -controlled) market economies of China and Vietnam, the neofeudalist, oil economies of the Persian Gulf states, and the crony-kleptocracies of Cambodia, Russia, and Zimbabwe (both past and present). Despite their manifest differences all of these essentially market economies share the characteristic of not being fully free; all are hedged, all bear the marks of the visible hand of the state. More accurately, then, they are "liberty" markets—based on the notion and practice of an individual's commercial freedom but all nonetheless limited by the interests of others and the community as a whole, no matter how perverted the definition of those common interests might be.

Wealth Benefits

Well, so much for the (limited) freedom of the market to *make* wealth. The freedom that market-gained wealth *buys* is just as controversial and just as variously curbed. As indicated earlier, this side of the freedom-wealth sandwich is dominated by the question of wealth distribution: to whom does wealth accrue, under what conditions, and who or what decides how it is disposed? Here again, interventions by governments are based on notions of fairness, both to those possessing wealth and those possessing little or none of it. What is "fair" is itself, unsurprisingly, a matter of contestation.

One way to approach the question of the fairness of wealth-allocated freedom is to look at the big picture. In broad terms, the capacity of the market's invisible hand to deliver on Adam Smith's expectations of enhanced and distributed benefits for everyone has changed dramatically over the past two centuries, and so has the market's capacity to confound them. Thus, the extraordinary wealth gains worldwide in that time have changed the lives of the vast majority of human beings in ways that would be barely credible to Smith and his contemporaries. Since the very earliest days of the industrial revolution, around the time Smith was writing, aggregate global wealth (as measured by combined national GDPs) has increased spectacularly from approximately $1 trillion in 1820 to $125 trillion in 2020.[11] This has coincided with a tenfold decline in the percentages of the world's population living in extreme poverty—from approximately 90 percent to around 9 percent.[12] The wealth-welfare correlation is even more dramatically apparent when we look at the global figures in more recent times—that is over the past forty years. Thus, the reduction in the global poverty rate of more than 40 percent in 1980 to 9 percent today tracked closely the quadruple increase in global wealth over the same period.[13] As a consequence, wealth inequality *between* countries has decreased substantially, albeit at the cost of increases in wealth inequality *within* countries, especially in Western economies but also in China and India.[14]

People's freedom worldwide has also followed a positive upward trend over the past half century. Although freedom is harder to measure than states' aggregate wealth, the US-based Freedom House has attempted to measure it across the globe annually since 1973. Classifying countries' levels of freedom according to their performance against an array of civil and political rights,[15] the organization estimates that today 42 percent of states are "free," 30 percent are "partially free," and 28 percent "not free." Across the same three categories, the figures in 1973 were near enough the reverse at 30 percent, 24 percent, and 46 percent, respectively.[16] There is, then, a clear correlation between rising levels of wealth and freedom, but it is by no means consistent or inevitable. For, while the number of democracies has risen impressively worldwide since 1945 (when only 11 percent of the world's population lived in countries so classified; today that figure is 56 percent),[17] there are indications that democracies might lose their global economic dominance with the expanding influence of authoritarian capitalism in states like China, Brazil, Russia, the oil-based potentates of the Middle East and in a growing coterie of smaller economies such as the Philippines, Hungary, Poland, and Turkey.[18] Indeed, based on recent International Monetary Fund (IMF) data and projections of shifts in global economic power, we have long passed the point when democracy was seen as the best or only path to prosperity.[19]

Spending Freely

Perceptions of the freedoms purchased by wealth are not, of course, always related to our civil and political rights. For most people most of the time, their concerns are more prosaic. They may be practical or spiritual, long- or short-term in perspective, selfish and indulgent or altruistic and thoughtful. But at base our basic concerns revolve around our health, safety, comfort, and happiness. In fact, our freedom to spend whatever wealth we might have on whatever we want is as enthusiastically asserted as it is infinite in variety.[20] To a surprisingly significant degree we accept this self-centeredness in others as much as we do in ourselves. I say "surprisingly" because of our remarkable toleration of even the most outrageous and egregiously unequal differences between the levels of freedom people enjoy due entirely to their respective levels of affluence. Warren Buffett agrees. As the CEO of Berkshire Hathaway and one of the world's richest human beings, he often expresses his amazement at how readily people seem to accept extremely regressive tax rates which enormously benefit the rich in ways that he describes as "very unfair."[21]

Indeed, the wealth of the world's richest 0.1 percent of adults (some 5.5 million people, each worth more than US$5 million)[22] provides them with the freedom to live in extraordinary opulence, enabling them not only to buy more and better of just about anything but also to essentially privatize their lives. They create what is in effect an alternative universe. Education, health, housing, and land are all obtained or owned privately, as well as travel (including by air), personal security, entertainment and fitness, personal and household staff, and even beaches (an especially shocking notion to any "public dominion"–minded community).[23] The rich are free to cocoon themselves within private walls—literally (as in gated communities from Los Angeles to Mumbai) as well as figuratively—separating themselves as much as possible from the public and public spaces.

Most of the rest of us forgive such behavior most of the time, in part because we do some of the same things ourselves, or we would if we could. But also, in part, because of our expectation or resignation that this is the way of things in a free market capitalist economy. Capital begets capital in a cycle that is designed to reward investors, including the foolish as well as the prudent, or the lucky as well as the smart. But either way, the inevitable result is some margin of wealth inequality. The inequalities of freedom that duly flow therefrom are likewise wide and often viewed as unavoidable.

We have a begrudging fascination, even a perverse admiration, for the seemingly free abandon with which the rich and celebrated conduct themselves: the reality soap opera excesses of movie stars' mansions, tycoons' yachts, sporting heroes' cars, and the wardrobes, exercise regimes, and private lives of just about anyone famous. We are even obliged to pay for such indulgence by our leaders or rulers. Thus the 298 days President Trump spent at golf resorts during the four years of his presidency cost the American taxpayer more than $148 million in security, travel, and accommodation expenses.[24] British taxpayers have become used to having to foot the bill for royal family whims, as well as for the official duties that members of the extended family undertake. "Economising isn't a royal thing," notes *Private Eye*. Where once upon a time, royal court officials would loftily proclaim that the luxury of keeping the royals (*minus* security expenses) cost no more than the price of a bag of crisps per UK resident per year, that equation has now doubled to a price tag of £1.24 per person per year. And if you add the approximately £110 million per annum in security costs, it rises to nearly £3.00 per person.[25]

The wealth of the well-healed buys influence and power over others, including the authorities that govern us. Money doesn't just talk; it persuades and even compels others to listen and act accordingly. That is certainly often the intention, even if it doesn't always work out that way. "We bought the son of a bitch," as archetypal finance tycoon J. P. Morgan said of his financial backing of President Theodore Roosevelt's earlier political campaigns; "but he wouldn't stay bought," he grumbled when in 1902 Roosevelt began breaking up the sorts of powerful corporate trusts presided over by Morgan and his like.[26]

More than anything, what money "says" is directed at making more money or keeping the money you already have, but in either event the overarching objective is to enhance the freedom and opportunities available to the wealthy. Buying political influence is itself an enormous industry but practiced by very few. In the United States, for example, although the 2020 presidential and congressional elections were highly contentious and far and away the most expensive in history,[27] just 1.44 percent of the population made political donations of over $200. Of these 4.7 million people, only 104,000 donated more than $10,000, but together this cohort contributed $8.1 billion to political campaign coffers, accounting for 43 percent of all such contributions in that year.

That's a lot of political influence for just 0.03 percent of the country's citizens.[28]

The freedoms being promoted by such individuals and the groups they fund or represent vary hugely, but all, obviously, seek to advance their own position. Measuring how successful they are in doing so is no easy task, but one can be certain that the wealthy have overall been extraordinarily effective in protecting and indeed extending their own wealth. One study comparing the increases in wealth of the top 10 percent and bottom 50 percent of American households showed that whereas the former had risen by nearly 200 percent between 1971 and 2016, the latter's roller-coaster ride showed an increase of 0 (zero!) percent across the same time frame.[29] It is no accident that during those same years lawmakers were persuaded to change the tax laws in ways that enormously benefit the rich not only by reductions in both income and capital gains tax rates, but also through rafts of generous deductions, exemptions, and credits.[30] The COVID-19 pandemic increased this disparity in the United States, spawning what was dubbed a "K-shaped" recovery.[31] That is, the fortunes of the mainly white-collar rich headed up the northeast arm of the *K*, bolstered by job security, historically low mortgage rates, and a booming stock market, while the wealth of the rest headed down the southeast arm in the face of job losses and little or no exposure to the benefits of mortgage refinancing and diversified stock portfolios.[32]

In the face of such manifest disparities in wealth and in the comforts and freedoms it affords, our levels of tolerance do indeed seem to be wide, but they are not infinitely elastic. Political rhetoric, social expectations, and legal standards mark out boundaries between what the rich are free to do with their money and how great a burden the rest must bear to enable them to do so.

Unfreedoms

Economist and philosopher Amartya Sen regards such bound-aries in terms of freedom or, more specifically, freedoms and *un-*freedoms. The freedoms of opportunity and choice that the well-off enjoy are not just different in terms of frequency and quan-tity. How many pairs of shoes? Which private school or health care provider? Am I free to say what I want? Should I buy or sell real estate (Greenland aside)?[33] They differ in form too. Such freedoms are positive freedoms, in that they are potential or actual enhancements of one's life. Unfreedoms are the opposite—negatives, not only in terms of lacking opportunity but also as hindrances, not just standing still but going backward. For those with little or no wealth, freedoms are often quashed or limited—additional shoes (if any at all) are not an option, school-ing and health care (if available at all) are each a Hobson's choice, speaking your mind may be dangerous. And buying or selling land is out of the question. Sen does not consider such privations to be the fault of the rich (though they could be at fault, depend-ing on the economic means and political system that enriched them in the first place); rather their freedoms demonstrate what others are missing out on. Freedom, according to Sen, is a critical component in what constitutes "development" *alongside* economic prosperity. Freedom thus requires "removal of major sources of un-freedom: poverty as well as tyranny, poor economic opportunities as well as systematic deprivation, neglect of public facilities as well as intolerance or over-activity of repressive states."[34]

In this sense, the world's poorest are not only economically de-prived but also deprived of basic civil and political freedoms. And they are not few in number. For, while the decline in global poverty over the past two centuries is impressive in terms of population percentages, in terms of the raw numbers of our fellow human beings living in extreme poverty the dial has barely shifted. Of today's 8 billion people on the planet, approximately 730 million (or roughly 9 percent) live unfree without sufficient food; without adequate sanitation, shelter, or security; and with little or no health care or formal education.[35] In 1820, the world's population was estimated at 1.1 billion, of which 96 percent were living in poverty, including some 870 million (that is, 79 percent of the total) barely subsisting in abject poverty.[36]

Great disparities in wealth and freedom exist in richer countries as well as poor. India, the world's sixth largest economy, possesses the largest cohort of extremely poor (109–151 million people according to World Bank estimates) of any country,[37] and it is home to 104 of the world's 3,311 or so billionaires.[38] Just under 11.6 percent of Americans live beneath the national poverty line, alongside the wealthiest 1 percent of any country's population in history (including 927 billionaires).[39] China's booming economy has spawned a huge and growing gap of wealth inequality,[40] and even the European Union, the world's largest and wealthiest bloc of welfare economies, struggles with 6.8 percent of its people facing "severe material and social deprivation" and a widening disparity between the richest haves and the poorest have-nots.[41]

The distinction of bearing the greatest levels of wealth inequality on Earth belongs to South Africa, which, twenty-five years after the end of Apartheid, is blighted by stark divisions of wealth.[42] The relative poverty in which more than half the country's population lives has a crippling effect on those people's aspirations and sense of freedom. In a telling story regarding the making of her photo-documentary of the children of the "rainbow nation," *Born Free—Mandela's Generation of Hope*, Dutch photographer Ilvy Njiokiktjien recalls the reaction of a bookmaker on hearing the title of the project. "Born free?" he said. "We should call it Break Free. Our generation, we're not born free, we're born into shit and we're breaking free."[43]

The point is that in all societies the distribution of wealth and freedom is unequal to some extent, even if less than in the case of South Africa. In any given community *relative* poverty can stunt people's freedoms, just as much as poverty can in absolute terms. It is the nature of your circumstances in relation to those of your neighbor or fellow citizen that often matters most, for that, typically, determines whether and how free a life you lead. Such relativity is especially keenly felt by those on the wrong side of the relationship. Their discontentment, over absent opportunities and curtailment of basic freedoms to choose viable life paths when compared to others whose paths are gilded in comparison, is packed into powder kegs of political volatility. France's *gilets jaunes* (yellow vest) protesters, the United Kingdom's (or rather, principally, England's) Brexiters, Brazil's 11 million Flat Earth believers (including the monumentally whacky Olavo de Carvalho, so admired by the country's former president Jair Bolsonaro),[44] and the election in 2016 of a renegade charlatan to the US presidency were all stark illustrations of the disappointment and frustration felt by many. French economist Thomas Piketty, along with others, has been right to warn of the social and political ramifications of economic policies that have encouraged wealth disparities in developed and developing nations to expand to levels not seen since before the First World War in Europe.[45]

Dramatic responses such as these are symptomatic of deeper and broader concerns over the fairness of wealth distributions, precisely because people's freedoms are so often closely associated with their financial sufficiency. Societies built on notions of promoting individual freedom are therefore under an obligation first to recognize the importance of wealth disparities and then to address those that are unfair, unjust, or outrageous. We all have responsibilities here, within our own communities and spheres of influence. Those in positions of leadership and government, of course, have special responsibilities in terms of responding to widespread and strongly held opinions about wealth and freedom, but also in terms of providing options, offering directions, and setting the tone of debates and policy making.

This is true of big-ticket items, such as taxation, minimum wage rates, levels of social welfare, law and order standards, and the quality and extent of publicly provided health care and education. But it also applies to the apparently small stuff too, matters that often act as lightning rods for bigger and broader issues.

The *gilets jaunes* protests in France, for example, were sparked by rises in the fuel tax in 2018, which impacted poorer households more that the better-off, yet they developed into a broad-based platform of complaint against a range of economic policies that ignored or disadvantaged ordinary working people. Their disaffection was neatly captured in a slogan I saw scrawled on walls and yellow vests in Paris during my time there writing this book— "C'est jaune, c'est moche, ça ne va avec rien, mais ça peut vous sauver la vie."[46] Or, to put it more bluntly, "Look at me, I exist!" The US college admissions scandal in 2019 was in fact merely a garden-variety form of bribery and fraud, but the blatancy with which the rich and famous perpetrated the deception betrayed what was seen by many as a perfect example of an attitude of arrogant entitlement rife among those with money and connections. The fact that, with or without fraud, as Daniel Markovits reports, "Harvard, Princeton, Stanford and Yale collectively enroll more students from households in the top 1 percent of the income distribution than from households in the bottom 60 percent"[47] underscores just how entrenched Ivy League prejudice is against the less well-off. Wealth, power, and entitlement are also what lies behind the #MeToo movement, which began when the lid was lifted on sexual abuse in Hollywood, but which quickly extended to all those who sexually harass or harm others simply because the positions they hold or prevailing social expectations at any particular time allow them to believe they may do so. Whether on the casting couch, in the office, at school, or in a garish Palm Beach, Florida, resort, some men (as it almost always is) consider themselves free to let their genitals do the thinking when they assault women (as their victims usually are).

All these instances, and the many others that can be added to the list, prompt discussion of the nature and extent of freedom's relationship with, or dependency on, wealth. All are worthy of debate by each of us and by those who govern us. The notion of liberty demands that lines be drawn and, as the above examples illustrate, continually be redrawn regarding what are fair and just levels of freedom for those with wealth and those without. "Fair" and "just," as we've established, are not fixed terms; they are relative and to a large degree subjective. But they are not meaningless. Extremes of wealth and freedom and the extreme reactions they evoke help to point the way as to our freedoms both to make wealth and to spend it.

The Fight over Fairness

Negotiating the fairness of freedoms and their limits in the domain of wealth, as in all the other domains covered in this book, is often fraught and never ending. But the distance between disputants may be less than many presume, which gives us all cause for some hope that common ground can be found. Indeed, it can be difficult at times to differentiate between the champions of the free market and its critics. So let me draw this chapter toward a conclusion by asking you this: With a choice between Nelson Mandela and Milton Friedman, who do you think said,

"Money won't create success, the freedom to make it will"? And furthermore, which of the two professed that "government is essential both as a forum for determining the 'rules of the game' and as an umpire to interpret and enforce the rules decided on"? Well, surprisingly perhaps, the first quote is from Mandela—he was referring to the dignity of working for oneself rather than someone else,[48] and the second was Friedman—his reasoning being that to ensure a market economy is kept free and open, certain government-enforced rules are essential.[49]

Both men were ardent advocates of freedom albeit, it would seem, for very different reasons. Thus, Mandela, the longtime Marxist, protested that capitalism in Apartheid South Africa meant "the ruling class paid African labour a subsistence wage and then added value to the cost of the goods, which they retained for themselves."[50] Friedman, on the other hand, the doyen of free market economics, famously held that "few trends could so thoroughly undermine the very foundations of our free society as the acceptance by corporate officials of a social responsibility other than to make as much money for their stockholders as possible."[51]

Context, as ever, is critical. For it is perfectly possible to interpret Mandela and Friedman in ways that narrow the apparent distance between them. Both make clear in the above quotes their conviction that people be allowed the freedom to make and spend money in a market economy, but both also believe that such freedom must necessarily be limited. For Mandela this requires laws against the exploitation of workers, while Freidman wants laws that keep the market free from criminal and anti-competitive behavior. Fairness, as this chapter repeatedly points out, is at the heart of the concerns of both viewpoints. There is no reason to believe that shareholders' interests must *necessarily* be opposed to the interests of other stakeholders in a free market economy, whether workers, customers and clients, or the community at large. Indeed, the prevalence of "corporate social responsibility" claims made in business today would seem to hammer home that very point, despite Friedman's scorn of it some fifty years ago.

So, for Friedman and Mandela, and many like them on both sides, the differences are in reality more matters of degree than of irreconcilable substance. The freedoms associated with wealth are indeed essential elements of our social, political, and economic lives, but they are bounded by notions of fairness and equity as well as efficacy and efficiency. This is what liberty demands. Our levels of personal wealth, like the freedoms that come with them, do not exist in isolation. Nor do we, the possessors of wealth and freedom in whatever proportions, live alone, but rather in community with others. And so, it is with, alongside, and through others that each of us must negotiate the eternal question, How much is enough? Of wealth and of freedom.

6

Work
Bullshit or Beatific?

For there are many great deeds done in the small
struggles of life.

—Victor Hugo

Suzanne has never really been employed except for a couple of years in her early twenties (a job she was legally obliged to relinquish when she got married), but she's worked nonstop for nearly all her adult life. Raising children, cooking, cleaning, washing, setting fires daily to heat the house and clearing them afterward, and then, for ten of her prime middle years, becoming the full-time caregiver for a succession of four elderly and infirm relatives (her own parents and then her husband's mother and aunt) who came one after the other to live, slowly wither, and die in her home. No sooner had that demanding chapter of her life closed than another opened when her husband fell ill, had to quit his job, became house-bound, and required her constant care for a further nine years until he too succumbed. By then she was nearly sixty years old and tired. I know because Suzanne is my mother, now in her late eighties, still fiercely independent, and disinclined to read anything I write because, as she so delicately puts it, "I've already worked hard enough, thank you."

What Is Work?

Like many millions of her contemporaries across the globe and many billions before her, this mother, wife, and daughter worked hard as a homemaker and caregiver. Unpaid, informal, and seldom fully appreciated, it is undeniably work, and work, what is more, indispensable to the sustainability of families and social orders. Yet traditionally the label has not been attached to it. It still isn't in some places. Private, uncontracted, and undertaken mainly by women, such toil wasn't considered work "masculine-style," as Gloria Steinem puts it, because it wasn't "labor[ing] outside the home for money."[1] But that, as we should know better now thanks not least to the efforts of feminists like Steinem, is a mistake, being both false and unjust.

Work is hugely varied in scope and purpose. It can be paid or unpaid, pursued in public or in private, volunteered or forced, physical or cerebral, undemanding or exhausting, satisfying or indescribably dull, useful or utterly pointless. It can also be sickeningly false. *Arbeit Macht Frei* (Work sets you free), inscribed above the entrance to Auschwitz-Birkenau, as well as many other Nazi concentration camps, is perhaps the most infamous deceit of all time.

For our ancestors the work of hunting and gathering food was so essential—literally a matter of survival—that it was not called work. The tasks associated with these acts—fashioning tools for hunting and food preparation—were the real chores.[2] As human societies evolved and grew, so did the variety and scope of the jobs that were considered "work," even if their essence—to satisfy needs and desires—remained the same. Self-subsistence enterprise was gradually replaced by divisions of labor and of ownership and working for others, under serfdom in agrarian economies and by employment in industrial economies, and in slavery in both. As science and technology inserted themselves ever further into our social relations and economic endeavors, so professional and services sectors expanded and grew. Today, more people than ever work as employees, and work itself has become less manual and more automated, less labor-intensive and more systems and process oriented.

Some jobs have stayed essentially the same over the millennia—from politics, prostitution and the law, to priests, painters, and entertainers. Others remain the same in name while their modi operandi have been revolutionized—farmers, fishers, teachers, builders, medics, money lenders, document handlers, people managers, and clothes makers. Others have disappeared entirely, like night soil men, stokers, scythers and threshers, knocker-uppers (not what you might think), typists, and switchboard operators. And some have been entirely reinvented—snake oil sellers have been replaced by online influencers, military spotters by drone operators, bankers by algorithmists, and factory workers by machines. There are also the jobs that we know little or nothing about, even though they will dominate the working lives of our children. While widely cited suggestions that 65 percent of near-future jobs have not yet been invented have since been debunked,[3] even the more robust projected estimates (based on recent past changes in job types) of at least one-third of all jobs being entirely new fifteen years from now are startling enough.[4]

Whatever the nature of work, a great many of us might consider questions of what freedoms and responsibilities are associated with it and whether and how we negotiate the balance between them beside the point. For most people, most of the time, work is a responsibility first and foremost. Freedom seems to have little to do with it. We see work as a necessary and unavoidable part of human existence, essential for our survival and the thing that gets us out of bed in the morning (or night). Global and national surveys consistently show that, when we do get up, we spend between one-fourth and one-third of our waking hours at work. And that's just paid employment—what we habitually call our "jobs." If you factor in all the rest of what we do that falls within the broader definition of work described above—housework, preparing meals, caring for others, and furthering one's education—then obviously that time commitment increases significantly.[5] The extent to which we are truly free to engage in our labors is therefore a moot point. We *need* to work for a host of reasons.

Why Do We Do It?

Typically, work gets a bad rap. Tolerated rather than embraced. Bemoaned more than loved. A duty more than a right. Voltaire saw it principally as a way to keep us occupied, preserving us from the "three great evils [of] weariness, vice, and want." Superficially there is indeed a strong tendency to view work as a means to other ends. Most notably, it provides the financial wherewithal by which we can get on with the rest of our lives. To a degree this is of course true. But in light of the fact that paid work occupies so much of our lives (leaving less life to be lived on its proceeds), there must be more to it than that. At least you'd hope so. As a matter of fact, we do seem to be motivated to work for compelling reasons other than pay. An exception helps to prove this rule. One survey of workers both inside and outside the United Kingdom's financial services sector found that while only 16 percent of non-finance workers nominated pay as their biggest driver at work, those in finance were twice as motivated by the size of their paycheck.[6] Upon reading this, I dare say, many of you are muttering "No surprise there," but the 16 percent figure for nonfinance workers does underline my general point.

In another study by a career consultancy firm of more than 7,300 workers worldwide and across nine industry sectors, results pointed toward personal and professional fulfillment as key driving factors.[7] These workplace rewards included career growth, incentives, and recognition, as well as pay. One part of the survey compared differences between generations of workers.[8] Older workers (classified as baby boomers and Generation Xers) were more concerned with material benefits—levels of pay, health insurance coverage, benefits, and job security, whereas Generation Y employees were more concerned with advancement opportunities, professional development, and working in a fun environment, though they too valued job security.

Perhaps the most surprising disparity between the two sets was in their attitudes toward meaningful work. This was significantly more important to older workers (especially baby boomers) than it was for Generation Y millennials. Contemplating one's legacy, it seems—what does your work contribute to society and how stands your personal balance sheet of positive and negative impacts?—grows more pronounced as you age.[9]

A job can and surely should fulfill a social function while also contributing to our individual well-being by helping provide us with position or status in society. A job can thereby enhance our sense of self-worth and personal fulfillment, by providing "the chance to find yourself," as Joseph Conrad saw it,[10] as well as supply us with the economic security of an income. Jobs can promote social interactions, collegiality, and friendship; they can advance our learning and life skills and afford us opportunities to escape, reinvent, travel, and test ourselves. A job can encompass some or all of these positive attributes, whether by design or accident.

Equally, however, a job can poorly provide for any one or more of these outcomes, or worse, it can undermine or negate them.

"Workism," for example, can make us miserable or at least narrow-minded. This term, coined by journalist Derek Thompson, denotes "the belief that work is not only necessary to economic production, but also the centerpiece of one's identity and life's purpose; and the belief that any policy to promote human welfare must *always* encourage more work."[11] An affliction borne especially by the college-educated elite, workism converts otherwise apparently fortunate and well-rounded individuals into monofocal maniacs whose definition of self is inextricably tied to their job, which often, Thompson argues, fails to deliver. This need not be all bad, as the work involved might still be fulfilling for the individual and useful to society. A worse fate assuredly awaits those engaged in work that delivers neither personal satisfaction nor social utility.

Anthropologist David Graeber's excoriating book *Bullshit Jobs* doesn't so much spotlight jobs that are completely pointless as it exposes the uselessness, inanity, or pernicious nonsense that constitutes so many jobs, though admittedly some more than others. It's an eye-popping read, but uncomfortable too, either because you are acquainted with such features in your own work (in which case it may be rather painful) or because you've suffered at the hands of others whose work fits the bill (which, on reflection, is equally painful). Among the caustically labeled categories of workers Graeber takes aims at are "goons," whose jobs require them to promote aggressively their employers or clients' interests (for example, lobbyists, advertising and sales personnel, telemarketers, and corporate lawyers); "box tickers," who employ paperwork and lip service to disguise the fact that organizations are not doing what they are supposed to do (public relations specialists, performance managers, customer/client/employee satisfaction analysts); and "task masters," who use their managerial position to manufacture extra work for those who don't need it (middle managers, management consultants, and executive coaches).[12] Many of you may all too readily recognize these traits in workplaces past and present. As do I, having borne close witness over some thirty years to the way universities all over the world are now managed by metastasizing bureaucracies. Wherever these beasts are to be found (and universities are of course not alone in this regard), they all boil down to cadres of administrators mastering the rather neat trick of expanding in size in direct proportion to their capacity to justify their own existence.[13]

Some of the hundreds of stories people told Graeber read like pages from Franz Kafka's *The Trial*—mind-numbing officialdom, procedural dead ends, red tape madness, form filling for the sake of it, and gargantuan wastages of money, time, and above all, human beings. "I contribute nothing to this world and am utterly miserable all of the time," wrote one correspondent (a corporate lawyer, no less), and another (a computer programmer), lamented that her "workplaces . . . [were] cults designed to eat your life."[14] Such occupations seem to imprison more than they liberate, downgrading any sense of freedom they might otherwise deliver.

Profligate and enervating though such jobs are, they are different from those that are positively horrific. Cruelly exploitative and health or life threatening, these jobs have no redeeming features. When you see working conditions in the ubiquitous brick kilns of South Asia or listen to the details of abuse and neglect of workers on Thai fishing trawlers (to which we will return later when discussing modern slavery), one recognizes labor that is more feudal servitude than employment, more abhorrent and destructive than meaningless and banal.

The brick kilns of India, Bangladesh, Pakistan, and Nepal have changed little in centuries.[15] I've visited many over the years, so I should be used to them, yet each time the sight takes my breath away. As big as football fields, six to eight meters deep, and topped by huge coal-fired smokestacks, the still-smoldering sarcophagal kilns are broken open by hand and shovel to reveal towering stacks of hundreds of thousands of red-fired bricks. Men, women, and children then scramble back and forth across the kiln walls balancing up to 15 bricks at a time on their heads as they carry them away through curtains of brick dust to waiting donkeys or trucks. Each brick weighs three to four kilograms. The workers are uniformly clothed in rags, the few not barefoot are wearing flip-flops, their faces and hair are caked in red dust; some sport bandanas across their nose and mouth, but most don't bother. They are paid per (unbroken) brick that reaches the depot; each worker needs to work at least twelve hours a day to carry around 3,000 bricks to make the equivalent of $10 to $12. Many are bonded laborers, so a portion, and at times all, of this sum is taken by the employer or broker who secured them the job in the first place until the debt (or bond) is paid off.

The kiln workers are nearly always migrants, trucked in from rural provinces during the dry season; whole families make the trip, meaning that in the absence of either schooling or day care (and both are a rarity for such migrant workers), the children roam free or more likely work alongside their parents, no matter what local laws say about prohibiting child labor.[16] They live in crude tin-roofed huts they build themselves using unfired "green bricks" (it is their first and most important duty to form from wet clay when they arrive at the kiln site), with little or (more likely) no power, scavenged wood for cooking, shared standpipe water, and only that which they were able to bring with them for bedding. The tiny market stalls that pop up in the kiln sites tend toward selling escapism more than staple goods, with candy, tobacco, and alcohol (in India and Nepal) on prominent display.[17]

The International Labour Organization estimates there are between 4.4 and 5.2 million brick kiln workers across South Asia,[18] so not, you might say, an insignificant number. Yet they are only a fraction of the tens of millions of people worldwide who work in appalling conditions—in garment-making sweatshops, on tech assembly lines in export-processing zones, in primitive slaughter-houses, as migrant domestic workers or laborers in and around the Arabian Peninsula, as sex workers in Europe and India, on palm oil plantations or illegal logging stations in Southeast Asia and South America, and on commercial fishing boats in the South China Sea. Many of these jobs and the people who do them are found in developing countries, but not all, by any means. So why do they do the work? Why take the job in the first place? Have they no choice? Do any of us?

Can We Choose?

In fact, improbable though it may seem, when it comes to our freedom to choose gainful employment, we share much in common with the benighted workers just described insofar as we are all prisoners of circumstance. It is precisely their poverty, power-lessness, geographical remoteness, and lack of education, their eth-nicity or caste, the inadequacy of public services, and the failures of governments that consign the brick kiln workers to their fate. They have few, if any, other options if they want to survive. The circumstances of anyone reading these words are, I dare say, very different. Whatever your levels of education, wealth, and social status, wherever you come from and whatever public services and quality of governance you've enjoyed, all are equal determinants of the employment options open to you, albeit with conse-quences far less grave. I'm not saying that we can never tran-scend these circumstantial boundaries; rather I'm underlining the fact that they are undeniably central to what each of us can and cannot do in terms of work. There are, in other words, parameters to our freedom of choice of jobs, parameters that, for the fortunate, are very widely cast but that, for others, are narrow to nonexistent.

This is the reality of our liberty when it comes to work. It is a matter of discharging the responsibilities of our competence as well as dealing with the capriciousness of our circumstances. Having in mind those who tend toward the fortunate end of the circumstantial spectrum and who are situated in industrialized economies, Austrian-British economist Friedrich Hayek believed that one's choice of employment was a veritable burden. "The necessity of finding a sphere of usefulness, an appropriate job [for] ourselves is the hardest discipline that a free society imposes on us." Yet "it is inseparable from freedom," he added.[19] The key word here is "appropriate," for while we may theoretically be free to choose, what we can and should do in actual practice depends on our skills or capabilities and, vitally, their suitable application.

Consider the relative suitability of jobs to individual skills and capacity of the brick kiln workers on one hand, and the holders of any one of the "bullshit jobs" we encountered earlier on the other. Is there any reason to believe that the latter are any less suitably matched? Indeed, the reverse is likely true. The brick kiln workers are in fact very good at their job—watching them at close quarters is truly to marvel at their skill, strength, balance, and fortitude—and the bricks are indubitably an essential building material. But it is the atrocious conditions under which they work that is shameful, alongside the question of why bricks need to be manufactured in this way at all these days (to which the answer is simple: labor is so cheap in South Asia). In contrast, the abiding feature of Graeber's bullshit jobs the world over is not so much their conditions—many were in fact remarkably well paid, albeit soul destroying to undertake—but their social and economic worthlessness.

Though manifestly different in nature and consequence, the existential feelings of being trapped, used, and insignificant are present in both bullshit and just plain shit jobs, whereas the miserable corporate lawyer Graeber introduced us to lamented that their choice of job was the only way they could afford the greed-inflated prices of life's "necessities," which for that particular lawyer included buying property in Sydney.[20] Now this may sound like the very definition of a First World problem, but it is one, alas, that is showing no signs of abatement. Certainly, in my tridecadal experience teaching future generations of lawyers worldwide, I have seen too many students who are intellectually, emotionally, and pathologically ill-suited to the demands of the profession. Which, depending on your view of lawyers—and here I pause to acknowledge that for many of you that might be less than charitable—may be to a student's credit or shame.

In any event, what choice do any of us *really* have? For what it's worth, I certainly didn't feel I had many work choices—deservedly so, as I meandered through high school and my initial university years with a head full of notions about turning my meager experiences on stage into a profession (I kept a filled-out application for drama school in my desk for years) and a body being steadily disassembled by sports injuries. In the end I sort of fell into the law and academe (it helped that at the time the two were not seen as close companions), both of which, it must be said, do have thespian tendencies.

But in my (and your) quest to understand what freedom any of us has in our choice of work, a telling indicator is to be found in the reasons behind the choices that we *do* make. Given what we saw earlier about what motivates people at work, let me suggest that for those of us who have at one time or another made some sort of conscious decision about the work we do, it boils down to a calculus of balancing passion, pay, and perks. The weighting we apportion to each depends on a whole host of variables too numerous to list here, but insofar as we are able to choose a job or pursue a particular line of work, we consider all three of these factors, even if to dismiss one or two of them. Weightings could, of course, range between 0 percent and 100 percent, but for most of us they are less extreme. "Passion" may seem an overly strong word to use here, though certainly there are those who passionately love their work. And yet the degree to which you choose a job *for the sake of doing the job* must be the surest indication of an exercise of free will.

Perhaps all too few of us put enough store in our desire to do a job as distinguished from our willingness to do it merely to garner the pay and perks; too many of us are "leading lives of quiet desperation," as Henry David Thoreau poetically put it. This is not to suggest that pay and perks are unimportant—they are important, and they are to me—but given the various ways to get them, it is somewhere between sad and scandalous that more of us are not able to seek out and find jobs that satisfy or even exult. But here, you will see, is the nub of the problem—how and where are we to find these soul-satisfying, pocket-filling jobs, and further, how and to whom are they allocated?

There are two parts to addressing this problem, both of which involve the shouldering of responsibilities alongside the exercising of freedoms. One part stresses the need for each of us truly to search for what we want to do, as opposed to what is expected or thrust upon us, and the other focuses on how, as a community, we agree to allocate jobs when demand exceeds supply.

On the first part, illustrator, and the creator of the *Calvin and Hobbes* cartoon strip,[21] Bill Watterson's sage words in a college commencement speech in 1990 are worth heeding.[22] Reflecting on five years of finding rejection slips in his mailbox as he tried to get newspapers interested in his cartoons, Watterson admitted that while to continue pitching seemed delusional, the only reason he did so was that he loved the work: "Drawing comic strips for five years without pay drove home the point that the fun of cartooning wasn't in the money; it was in the work."

From this realization, Watterson drew inspiration to urge the graduating students to remember that just as there are many ways by which to measure success in life, there are many ways to measure success in work, and with both, how much money you have is but one counter. "Creating a life that reflects your values and satisfies your soul is a rare achievement," he continued, and the right job for you can play an important part in that quest. Here we should be casting the "right job for you" net very wide indeed. If your passions lie elsewhere, then you should feel free to take on any job that affords you the time and opportunity to pursue them. If you want to take leave from or abandon a career to raise children or care for elderly parents, that's fine, but so is staying in the job and making other arrangements. Or if you simply cannot abide working for others and you strike out on your own, then so be it. Whatever the consequences of these work choices—agreeable, unpleasant, or just awkward—they are yours to deal with.

What this idea points to is not just the freedom to choose labor that suits you but a personal responsibility to exploit whatever freedom you have to do so. It assumes or insists on a collective responsibility that we support such endeavors with, for example, maternity and paternity leave policies that don't consign parents to penury or shut their career doors forever. Or a guaranteed universal basic income that would both enable and encourage people to fulfill rather than just fill their workdays.[23] It also requires the active promotion of a wider suite of measures by which to gauge the worth of work—more, that is, than occupancy of a corner office, the possession of a grandiloquent job title, or a bulging pay package. The job you love, or at least find satisfying, can be unglamorous and humble or outrageously ambitious, but whatever its nature you should be free to chase it as best you can.

Job Selection

Which takes us to the second part of addressing the job choice problem. Demand for any job might outstrip its supply, thereby requiring some sort of selection process. The more specialized and demanding the position, the more selective the process. One's freedom to pursue any particular job or career, in other words, is curtailed by the need to be suitably qualified. Doctors and nurses must be medically trained, engineers need to know about physics, computer scientists about algorithms; plumbers, electricians, and carpenters all require apprenticeship training, lawyers need law degrees, professional athletes must have the requisite physical and mental attributes, singers must have a good voice, and politicians need to be prepared to do whatever it takes . . . and so on and so forth. Job applications are a fact of most people's lives; we all know the score. Our qualifications and character will be rolled out and picked over (if we are lucky), and, if they're deemed "better" than other applicants', the job will be ours. But equally we know that subjectivity inevitably plays some part in these processes, no matter how rigorously objective they claim to be. To be judged on your merits, without prejudice or bias, is supposedly the essence of the process. Unavoidably, however, two things stand in the way of this claim. First, the criteria on which "merit" is judged—how were they decided on and by whom? And second, who does the selecting and where do they come from?

You might respond to this conundrum by pointing out that there needs to be selection criteria that must come from somewhere and be settled by someone. You might add further that provided they are made known to all, we all get a fair go at show-ing how our merits meet or exceed the standards set. But to these points legal academic Daniel Markovits has a simple counterre-sponse: "Merit is a sham."[24] While most industrialized nations today have rafts of laws proscribing overt as well as (thinly) dis-guised discrimination on grounds of gender, race, religion, and sometimes age in employment settings, what remains is not a scorched earth of pure meritocracy. High school and university education—where and in what—are still hugely significant in de-termining people's suitability for many elite jobs, typically con-sisting of professions such as law, medicine, and engineering but in reality encompassing any high-powered, high-paying, and high-status job.

A skewed meritocratic system that rewards a privileged educa-tion inaccessible to those not already privileged stifles social mo-bility rather than opens it up.[25] The entrenchment of this system over the past forty years or so, argues Markovits, has critically di-vided societies between the (so-called) elite and everyone else in terms of jobs and all that comes with them. The subterfuge of meritocracy and its consequences may be especially grave in the United States, which is the focus of Markovits's study, but it is discernible elsewhere in the West, as well as more recently in places like China and Korea via their notoriously brutal and gameable final high school examinations (*gaokao* in China, and Suneung in Korea), which do so much to dictate the future of the young in those countries.

From the perspective of the individual, therefore, negotiating one's freedom to choose a job or work as one wishes is hedged in by social expectations as well as educational demands, one's psychological makeup, and even physical characteristics. But once in a job, whereof our freedom? Are we exploited or do we exploit?

Work and Exploitation

Exploitation need not be pejorative, of course. In the context of one's work and given what we have been discussing over the previous few pages, one might hope that we exploit both whatever opportunities we have to choose a line of work and, once engaged, the benefits of the work itself. But here we almost immediately run into definitional boundaries. For what exactly is exploitation in a nonpejorative sense—that is, in the sense of being both fair and justifiable? Who is exploiting whom or what, and with what consequences? Karl Marx believed that workers in capitalist economies were, by definition, exploited, as evidenced by the simple metric that they sell their labor to capitalists for less than the full value of the commodities produced by their labor. The part of the monetary value of the commodity when sold which exceeds the costs of production—namely the profit—represents, according to Marxist thought, the extent of expropriation of laborers by the owners of capital and means of production.[26] Precisely what level of worker exploitation is in fact tolerated by *both* sides of this relationship has been the frontier of abiding contestation throughout the history of work since the earliest days of the industrial revolution.

Coming to terms with the resilience, if not necessarily permanence, of capitalism, the International Labour Organization (which, uniquely, has represented workers, employers, and states for more than a century) reflects this tension in its definition of "decent work" as comprising "opportunities for work that is productive and delivers a fair income." To this tenet the ILO adds the need for workplace health and safety, and rights of association and nondiscrimination, to round out the parameters of what are considered minimally acceptable conditions of employment.[27] Theoretically, therefore, work that falls within these bounds could be considered a tolerable and negotiated compromise between the exploitation of workers and the nature and extent of their compensation.

When asked whether we are indeed happy in our work—happy, in other words, with the terms of this negotiated settlement—results are somewhat unclear. One survey of a wide cross section of 8,664 American workers by CNBC and SurveyMonkey, for example, revealed that 85 percent of respondents were either "somewhat" or "very satisfied" with their job, with "meaningfulness" being the single most important factor in determining people's views of their work.[28] Just a few years earlier, studies conducted in the United Kingdom and the Netherlands registered negative responses of 37 percent and 40 percent respectively, to the question, Does your job "make a meaningful contribution to the world?"[29] Supposed character traits of New World self-confidence versus Old World reserve may or may not explain these differences,[30] but whatever the reason, disputing levels of job satisfaction is a damn sight more appealing than suffering working conditions that threaten your life or livelihood.

In the pantheon of battles fought over what constitutes decent, fair, and above all safe work, a special role is reserved for laws and policies that seek to protect the rights and interests of workers. Since the earliest days of the industrial revolution the necessity of workplace protections for the most vulnerable was plain to see. Children, especially paupers and orphans, were so grotesquely exploited that public opinion forced the enactment of laws in Great Britain in the early 1800s to secure apprenticeships, provide adequate accommodation and clothing, impose age limits (no younger than nine years old!) and restrict working hours (no more than twelve per day). Slowly but surely, these were followed by further laws in Britain, across Europe, and eventually North America limiting working hours for adults, enhancing workplace health, safety, and accident insurance, and permitting and then protecting organized labor unions.[31] Major political parties were established on mandates to protect the rights and freedoms of workers: Germany's Social Democratic Workers' Party, Russia's Social Democratic Labor Party, the British Labour Party, and France's Socialist Party were all early examples of this trend.[32] Given the US Republican Party's foundational goal to combat slavery, you might also add it to the list, no matter its ignominious decline in recent times.[33]

Insofar as these labor reforms have lessened the burdens of work and increased its potential rewards, they represent the benefits of engagement with the freedoms and responsibilities of work, whether such engagement is wrought by protest, dispute, negotiation, or agreement. But, of course, not only does this enterprise remain unfinished in many places; elsewhere it has never or barely begun.

Cambodian author Vannak Anan Prum's vividly drawn graphic memoir of the depravity of his enslavement on a Thai fishing trawler for four years is remarkable in the way it brings to light the techniques used to control him and his fellow workers.[34] Tricked and trafficked on board (Prum was promised two months' work on good pay; he spent four years at sea before escaping and earned nothing), forced to work in all hours and weather conditions (with no more than two hours' sleep during the day and the same at night), shackled, starved, and beaten, the workers were drugged to keep them docile, and subjected to "demonstration killings" (in Prum's case the beheading of a coworker with a meat cleaver) to further cow them into submission. But while these details are shocking, Prum's story is not uncommon. It is shared by hundreds of thousands of slave or bonded laborers on fishing vessels across the seas and is also typical of the sorts of conditions endured by the tens of millions of people worldwide living in modern slavery.[35]

Slavery in its modern forms not only still exists; it exists everywhere. Instances of forced or bonded labor are found in the industrialized economies of Europe, North America, and the Asia-Pacific region, in the sex industry, domestic help, agriculture, and the retail sector.[36] And while the largest concentrations of modern slaves are to be found in developing, authoritarian, or dysfunctional states in sub-Saharan central Africa, Central Asia's so-called Stan countries, and Southeast Asia, the tentacles of the work they are forced to do reach into the lives of us all via the supply chains that produce the food we eat, the clothes we wear, and the technology we depend on. Of modern slavery's global total of 49.6 million people (including 12.3 million children), according to the Walk Free Foundation's latest estimates, slightly more than half are in forced labor, predominantly in the private economy (86 percent) and across all industry sectors. The remainder (22 million) are trapped in forced marriages and obliged to work for little or usually no pay; most are women or girls (14.9 million), but 7.1 million are men or boys.[37]

The work and life circumstances of all these people are such that they have no choice, no capacity to negotiate, and no freedom to leave. In the modern world of work, they represent its nadir. The sheer desperation of their situation and the breadth of the responsibilities of others to correct it have led to some surprisingly swift and even robust responses. The struggle to combat modern slavery has mobilized governments, corporations and employers, international organizations, civil society, workers, and consumers in campaigns for new and better-tailored laws criminalizing modern slavery, and for new legislation obliging corporations to seek out forced labor in their supply chains and publicize what they find and establishing governmental agencies to ensure that they do so.[38] Local and global organizations dedicated to exposing industries and individuals engaged in modern slavery and to rescuing and rehabilitating the workers they enslave (including LICADHO,[39] the Cambodian human rights body that secured Vannak Anan Prum's eventual release from slavery) have grown in number and impact.

Collectively, these anti–modern slavery initiatives represent an especially poignant feature, even an apotheosis, of a wider corporate social responsibility movement that has been gathering momentum over the past two decades, insofar as it encompasses the social (including human rights) responsibilities of corporations respecting their workers. While these responses have no doubt been spurred by the popular realization and outrage that so many are still enslaved more than twenty years into the twenty-first century (and more than 150 years since slavery was apparently abolished), they nonetheless demonstrate what can be done—and done across such a broad array of stakeholders—when minds are put to the task of defining the freedom and fairness of work.

A Working Future

For most of us our working lives are more mundane than demonic, more troubled by the insufficiency of rewards than by no rewards at all. We are concerned about how much work we have (none, too little, or too much) or are unhappy about how much time we devote to it rather than to our other interests and obligations. These are important, even life-defining, matters, and they continue to be the object of intense debate. Liberty's insistence that we attend to the ingredients of both freedom and responsibility in work's recipe does not wane even though the nature of work itself is certainly set to change. The politics of global migration from less to more developed economies and of internal migration from rural to urban centers; the demographics of shrinking birthrates in rich states, expanding populations in poor ones, and aging populations everywhere; and the menacing imperatives of combating climate change and preventing or containing pandemics, all will impact the shape of future work. But the most profound and immediate changes are likely to come from the accelerating march of artificial intelligence (AI) technologies.

A much-cited study by a pair of technology specialists from Oxford University estimated that in barely twenty years' time, 47 percent of all jobs in the United States will be drastically altered or usurped by machines.[40] When their methodology was applied to European economies, the figure was even higher, at 54 percent.[41] What challenges this shift will entail for work choices, working conditions, and work-related freedoms more generally will increasingly occupy our minds.

It is at least conceivable that such automation will lead to more leisure time for many or all of us, but a betting man or woman would get only long odds on it doing so. Neither the earlier revolutionary efficiencies of industrial mechanization nor the speed of the development of information technology have yielded any less work or more leisure (arguably they have achieved precisely the opposite). Indeed, self-proclaimed visionaries are telling us that the machine-learning revolution already upon us, together with the AI revolution yet to come, will not destroy jobs but "augment" them and increase "productivity."[42] So we'll all still be working, just differently. That seems a pretty safe bet,[43] especially when you consider our apparently ingrained *need* to work.

The West's prevailing work ethic—whether Protestant or peer pressured—has a lot to answer for in its seemingly unquenchable thirst to consume our lives. It is sobering to reflect on how we got to this point, eons after "the original affluent society," as noted ethnographer Marshall Sahlins once dubbed our hunter-gatherer forebears, managed to dedicate as much time as possible to the pursuit of cultural, social, recreational, and procreative interests, once they had satisfied the important task of fulfilling their individual and collective nutritional needs.[44] Philosopher Bertrand Russell's impassioned plea to attend to the neglected need for humans to work less—or rather to increase leisure time, as was Russell's concern—will likely have to wait a while longer.[45]

In the meantime, the age-old questions of whether to work and, if so, why, in what form, for how long, and with what rewards (including, all importantly, which rewards compared to others) continue to dominate our lives. The many stakeholders concerned to answer them—workers, employers, governments, and indeed everyone else—remain as keen as ever to have their say, whether on the freedoms of work or their associated responsibilities, or both. Understanding the value of work is central to these deliberations. Not just in terms of what it brings to the individual worker but also in terms of what their work contributes to society, whether by way of endeavors that are private, unpaid, and unsung or public, paid, and heralded.[46]

In times of crisis such questions are seen in sharper relief. The COVID-19 pandemic, for example, has not only underlined the critical importance of frontline workers (medical and hospital staff, caregivers, shopkeepers, bus drivers, delivery persons, and the police). It also revealed how some jobs have been largely sheltered from the economic consequences that followed (wealthier knowledge economy workers), while others were shuttered (poorer manual, mechanical, and face-to-face service workers).[47] One's freedom to, or in, work, therefore, can depend very much on the extent to which others shoulder their responsibilities at work or, exceptionally, their responsibilities not to work. The lessons afforded by such perspectives doubtlessly inform continuing debates on the inequities in divisions of labor within our societies, though it remains to be seen how well they are heeded.

7

Security
Freedom's Awkward Sibling

I'll tell you what freedom is to me: no fear.
I mean really, no fear!
—Nina Simone

He realized he'd been bitten only when he began to swim away from the shark: "As I took my first strokes," Paul de Gelder recounted, "I noticed my hand was gone." Paul was an elite Royal Australian Navy diver involved in an anti-terrorist training exercise in Sydney Harbor in February 2009. He'd been floating on his back when a bull shark attacked him from below. He felt "pressure" on his right leg, so he looked down to see what it was, "and there was a massive shark attached to me." The shark then shook him violently as its teeth sunk in and ripped out a huge chunk of his leg together with his right hand, which had been dangling by his thigh moments before. Paul managed to make it back to the safety boat, "swimming through a pool of my own blood" and holding "my [arm] stump above my heart to stem the bleeding." His two colleagues hauled him onto the boat and saved his life by staunching the hemorrhaging, one by pinching a severed artery in his leg. The shark attack had lasted eight seconds.[1]

In response to the flurry of media inquiries, and demonstrating impressive mastery of the art of understatement, the Australian

157

navy noted that the incident was a reminder of the hazards of the workplace, while Able Seaman de Gelder himself later described his ordeal as "a bad day at the office." However represented, the episode is a visceral illustration of why we are so preoccupied with concerns about safety and security.

Safe from What?

Besides needing to eat and finding a mate, seeking protection against predators and other dangers is one of humankind's constants, whether it is safeguarding ourselves against apex killers in the sea or on land, or ensuring safety in the workplace, on the streets, or at home, or whether it is national or global security concerns over poverty, war, dictatorship, corruption, and climate change. While nature itself presents dangers and predators aplenty, by far the greatest threats to our individual and collective safety and security are posed by our own actions. "Man's inhumanity to man/makes countless thousands mourn," lamented the great Scots poet Robert "Rabbie" Burns.[2]

De Gelder found himself in the water that morning because he was taking part in a coordinated exercise between security forces worldwide to protect populations from terrorist attacks by focusing on the particular vulnerabilities of high-profile public places or events in major conurbations, or of major transport and telecommunication routes such as roads, railroads, sea lanes, air corridors, and technology hubs. So, while de Gelder was a self-declared "wild man" who courted the thrill of physical risks, not only did he do so in a calculated fashion, but his chosen career was predicated on protecting the security of others.

Here we get a glimpse of the complicated layers of dilemma that security poses for freedom. At one level, while generally we may be free to choose how much regard we have for our own security or safety (whether to migrate to another country, overtake the car in front of us, have another slice of cake, or change jobs), our choices can nonetheless be limited insofar as they innocently or inadvertently threaten the safety of others. The scope of such "unintended" safety threats is very wide as shown by the variety of regulatory responses they elicit. These range from rules on road safety, bans on smoking in public places, pill testing at music festivals, and safe sex guidelines, to vaccination policies, health quarantine and social-distancing rules, safety regulations for sports, crowd control rules, and laws on gun ownership. The dangers such rules seek to avoid or mitigate are very real both for the instigating actor and for those they engage with, regardless of how careful or reckless the actor is with their own safety.

But then there is a whole other level of safety and security concerns posed by people's actions that are *intended* to endanger or hurt others, or that are so reckless as to amount to something approximating intent. Here we might agree that the freedom of actors behaving in this way ought to be actively restricted. Absent the narrow exceptions in which all parties involved fully and freely consent to the dangers (contact sports, for example), most, if not all, of our criminal laws and policies are designed precisely to curb such behavior. The variety of such regulated actions is legion, ranging from proscriptions on murder and assault, theft, and fraud to prohibitions on invasions of property or privacy, despoiling the environment, and the broadcast or incitement of hatred or violence. All in the name of protecting and promoting the safety and security of individuals, communities, and nations.

It goes without saying that such laws and policies are expressly intended to restrict the freedoms of those who engage in the impugned actions or are contemplating doing so. No reasonable person would disagree with the need to combat torture, terrorism, murder, rape, and slavery or, indeed, corruption, fraud, or theft. Neither would many quibble with the argument that the need justifies restricting freedoms that would otherwise permit such atrocities or offenses. Nor, equally, are we likely to object to the principle that these restrictions should be more extensive and severe for acts designed to hurt, damage, dispossess, or terrorize, as distinct from inadvertent incursions on people's safety.

This last point is an important one when it comes to our concern over how we negotiate the boundaries between freedom and security, for it constitutes the very essence of criminal law, and of all negotiating tools in this field, criminal law is the most powerful. A defining feature of criminal law is that it requires compelling evidence both of the accused's commission of the illegal act itself *and* their intention to commit the act (*actus rea* and *mens rea*, respectively). It is this added ingredient of deliberation (or sufficient recklessness) that distinguishes harmful acts that are criminal from those that are not, no matter that harm caused innocently or inadvertently can sometimes be equally grave.[3] Thus, although accidents caused by momentary lapses in concentration while, for example, supervising children in swimming pools or operating heavy machinery may be tragic, they are much more likely to be characterized as negligent than criminal.

That said, by increasingly adopting the perspective of victims of harmful acts or safety-threatening conduct, criminal law has shown itself to be responsive to changing views on the nature of people's culpability for the consequences of their actions. Thus, for example, where once the forceful claiming of conjugal rights within marriage excused what was in fact rape, most countries have now criminalized rape within marriage and de facto relationships.[4] Similarly, the recklessness of leaving firearms within reach of children or texting while driving have both been elevated above "mere" negligence to criminal offenses because of the gravity and foreseeability of the "accidents" they can cause.[5]

Alongside the critical question of the severity of harmful consequences caused by a person's or persons' behavior, these reforms and many like them are part of wider, perennial debates in and around criminal law circles about *levels* of intent or recklessness and the appropriate attribution of responsibility that should accompany them. Put simply, the greater the intent to harm, the greater the responsibility, and with that, the greater the sanctions, including the loss or limitation of one's freedoms.[6] Premeditated murder, assault, or torture; war crimes and acts of terrorism; and all sorts of organized and violent crimes occupy the highest levels of intent, whereas parking illegally, graffitiing public buildings, or begging in the subway or metro are at the lower end. The texting-while-driving and unlocked-firearms examples above are somewhere in between—neither innocent (because they are so foolish) nor premediated (which is of a higher order than "foreseeable").

The Trade-off

One of the most significant trade-offs between freedom and security in our lifetime unfolded while I was writing this book, though it will be some time before we understand its full consequences. The restrictions on people's movements and socializing triggered by COVID-19 have been profound, causing grief (geographically separated relatives dying alone) and pain (the mental health problems of isolation and loneliness), as well as shattering dreams and disrupting just about every aspect of daily life. But perhaps the most significant consequence of these restrictions—at least in the long term—has been their impact on the economy.[7] Throughout 2020 and 2021 and well into 2022 they spawned widespread losses of people's jobs and incomes, the destruction of small businesses and the evisceration of larger ones, the dislocation of global trade, and the drying up of international travel and investment, and they squeezed tax returns at the same time as public expenditure on stimulus packages and health and social welfare were skyrocketing.[8] During the earlier, prevaccine days of the pandemic, when fear and lockdowns spread rapidly, the shuttering of businesses generated mountains of public and private debt and precipitated a collapse and then rollercoaster ride of stock prices across the globe. And while initial fears for the very financial security of nations were gradually replaced by optimism among the well-heeled in advanced economies,[9] the same cannot be said for poorer states, or for tens of millions of less well-off individuals worldwide.[10]

The economic security question is a valid and necessary one to ask, even (indeed especially) in the context of trying to protect people's health security. China completely locked down Wuhan and all other major conurbations in Hubei province (some 60 million people in total) for two months and imposed strict travel restrictions across the country. The measures were brutal and the economic costs enormous, and while initially China appeared able to absorb the political and financial consequences through a combination of authoritarian suppression and its effective control or ownership of much of the country's economy, the longer-term social and economic ramifications of continuing such draconian measures across the country through 2021 and 2022 were far less promising.[11] In Western and many other states, the political and economic landscapes have been somewhat different, and the cost-benefit equations differently and variously weighted, even if the scourge has been the same.

In an editorial published at the very outset of the pandemic, the *Wall Street Journal* warned of the need to take seriously the "tsunami of economic destruction" that would swamp the United States in the event of any national shutdown beyond a handful of weeks.[12] It was a sobering read at the time, highlighting the mis-

ery in store for small- and medium-sized businesses, ordinary individuals, and whole communities alike, and it dismissed then–
treasury secretary Steven Mnuchin's bizarrely upbeat economic
projections as "happy talk." It also bore down on the dreadful security question at the heart of the dilemma. The matter "should
not become a debate over how many lives to sacrifice against how
many lost jobs we can tolerate," the *Journal*'s editorial board pronounced, before adding, "But no society can safeguard public
health for long at the cost of its overall economic health." Which
seems to veer pretty close to a trade-off between jobs and lives.

In truth, the equation is as complicated as it is unenviable,
whichever way to approach it.[13] Jobs and freedom of movement
and of assembly overlap of course, with personal, financial, and
even national securities sandwiched between them. The way
through such a maze of legitimate yet potentially conflicting
concerns requires strong leadership that relies on evidence-based
argument, long-term vision, and above all, the willingness and
capacity to put public concerns above private interests. Donald
Trump's egomaniacal projections in early 2020 for getting Americans back to work and worship in a time frame that suited his
reelection aspirations rather than a course dictated by the rates of
infection, hospital admission, and death failed spectacularly on
all these counts.[14]

Accepting that restrictions on freedom are necessary to preserve
the health, safety, and security of others (whether the harm or
safety threat is intended or not) is certainly important, but it is
not definitive. It leaves open the fundamental question of whether
the restrictions are proportionate. Proportionate, that is, to the
gravity of the harm or wrong they seek to correct and in terms of
their scope. What is the trade-off, in other words, between the
security gained and the freedoms lost? Such cost-benefit analyses
are not restricted to exceptional circumstances like those prevailing

during a pandemic. They are being undertaken all the time, everywhere, and in all sorts of situations where freedom and safety and security intersect. Examples include acceptable and unacceptable expressions of anger, prejudice, or discontent; wearing safety helmets when riding a bike; tax laws and their evasion and avoidance; the regulation of pornography, alcohol consumption, and drug use; and the appropriate levels of penalty for crimes committed. What is more, these calculations are being made by a wide array of players—governments, lawmakers, and social groups, by and between ourselves, and even within ourselves (to lie or not; to pursue a career or rear children, or both; how much to back up one's commitment to environmental protection with practice).

Security is freedom's awkward sibling not because it is often to be found in apparent opposition to freedom—setting limits and imposing restraints, the prudent parent to the boundary-pushing child, as it were—but because security's underlying motive is or should be to protect everyone's freedom. Order enables freedom, so this reasoning goes. Indeed, when freedoms are curtailed by reason of concerns for safety and security, the justification typically given is that the limitations are themselves necessary to protect freedoms that would otherwise be jeopardized in ways that are especially grave or widespread, or both. It is, in effect, a judgment call on what level of security intervention will safeguard a community's freedom *overall.*

Many instances of such reasoning may be found across almost all the domains of life discussed in this book: restrictions on hate speech; compulsory vaccination programs and pandemic stay-at-home orders; the regulation of euthanasia (if permitted at all); and age limitations regarding a host of activities from driving, drinking alcohol, and working to consensual sex, marriage, and voting. Security and safety concerns lie behind each of these examples of liberty in action, of freedoms limited and responsibilities assigned. What each of these security-freedom trade-offs illustrates is the importance of interrogating the reasoning advanced by all the participants in every debate as to what trade-offs are to be made and why.

This chapter looks at three talismanic examples of what's at stake in such debates. First, terrorism and the responses to it; second, the rights, responsibilities, and regulation of gun ownership and use; and third, how to address the impacts of climate change. Each represents a particular perspective on the often-paradoxical demands security makes of our freedoms: terrorism's strategic use of violence against civilian populations to achieve political ends including notions of "freedom"; the contradictions of gun ownership arguments that claim rights to individual freedom and security, no matter the consequences for collective freedom and security; and the existential question of how to balance present freedoms with the future security of life on Earth.

Terrorists and Freedom Fighters

I grew up amid terrorism in Northern Ireland during the 1970s and '80s. It was a sort of constant background thrum accompanying my childhood and teenage years, punctuated by occasional symphonic blasts. We were evacuated from our home several times when the neighboring hotel was bombed. I recall the swarm-like reaction of everyone in a packed pedestrian street when a car bomb exploded in the adjoining street and—as one—we all ducked. The police and army open-topped armored vehicles fitted with wire mesh skirts to stop petrol bombs being thrown under them and a tall steel rod bolted to their front to snap cheese wire strung across roads at head height. My physician father telling me of one patient whose femur had been shattered by a heavy iron door key blown into her leg by an explosion in a pub, and of another who had been "knee-capped" in a punishment shooting. My shell-shocked mother emptying pixels of shattered glass out of her boots after the windows of the bus she was riding were caved in by yet another exploding bomb (this one hidden in a nearby dumpster). In the lane beside one school I attended, we used lunch breaks to forage for rubber bullets fired by security forces during riots the night before; at another school perched on a hill, we were awakened one night (I was then boarding) to witness a controlled explosion of a massive bomb planted in the town's tax office below. And perhaps most of all I remember many long hours "carsitting" in Belfast city center's so-called control zones when my father was working there—the theory then being that occupied parked cars were safe because terrorists would never detonate a car bomb with one of their own sitting in it![15]

While the more recent predilection for suicide bombers as practiced especially by Islamic fundamentalist terrorists has thoroughly dispelled quaint notions of terrorist restraint in sacrificing their own, the challenge facing authorities charged with responding to terrorism remains the same today as before. Namely, how to balance the trade-off that such responses unavoidably entail between freedom and security for individuals and groups and for the community at large.

The terms of this equation are formidably complex and serious. For while there can be no mistaking the grotesque enormity of terrorism's destructive toll on people's lives and livelihoods, understanding, defining, and above all, effectively containing terrorism are tasks fraught with difficulty. Aside from the etymologically necessary condition of broadcasting terror, the sheer scope of actions or behavior that fall under the banner of terrorism makes defining the term an almost impossible task.[16] Terrorist agendas vary enormously from racial or religious hatred to constitutional independence; their intimidatory methods are predictably unpredictable; their organizational size and format can range between a lone wolf to quasi- or actual states (the Taliban in Afghanistan today, or the ISIS "caliphate" in Syria, or Pol Pot's Cambodia in yesteryears); and their targets can be public, private, civilian, or military. The line between a terrorist and a freedom fighter depends on the stated cause, who you ask, and ultimately, one's tolerance for the argument that ends justify means.[17]

The upshot of all this is that terrorism is decidedly elastic in nature and practice. From the earliest studies of the phenomenon in its modern form, its hydra-headed inscrutability was evident. Pioneering terrorist researcher Walter Laqueur admitted that the best he could do was to say that we know it when we see it! That was back in the mid-1970s. But even today, and despite all that has been written and said about these and other features of terrorism, the term eludes precise classification, there being no universally accepted definition.[18] This is no mere academic headache, as adequately defining terrorism is a necessary first step toward combatting it.

Anti-terrorism's Freedom Dilemma

What makes terrorism an especially difficult problem to deal with in terms of drawing freedom's boundaries is the question of what distinguishes acts of terrorism from other types of criminal behavior. It is not so much the avowed intent to terrorize and to do so often with extreme violence—though these are hardly trifling matters—but the indiscriminate use of such tactics that is so problematic. Innocents, even those only nominally associated with terrorist causes, are typically seen as fair game or collateral damage, the indiscriminateness of terrorism's victims being a vital ingredient in the recipe of spreading terror. Here both the intent and the consequence of terrorism present special problems for security responses. Being tough on terrorism may or may not work, but either way it might compound terrorism's damage to a community by being so draconian as to endanger the principles of freedom and equality on which that community is built. This is the dilemma that security poses for freedom. When is an anti-terrorism policy *too* "draconian"? Where should the line be drawn between acceptable and unacceptable restrictions on freedom? These are key questions in security debates today.

Many of us may be adamant that the torture of suspected terrorists is always unconscionable, being both morally and legally wrong. Detention without trial is likewise unacceptable, being a fundamental violation of the rule of law. Yet others will disagree. The barbarism of the 9/11 terrorist attacks on the United States was such that J. Cofer Black, for example, then the director of the CIA's Counterterrorism Center, was comfortable testifying publicly that his organization was now pursuing a "No Limits" anti-terrorism policy. "After 9/11," as he put it, "the gloves come off."[19] Waterboarding; sound, sensory, and sleep deprivation; and ritualistic humiliation of terror suspects followed in places like US-controlled Abu Ghraib prison in Iraq, as did the "rendering" of some suspects to friendly nations such as Egypt where torture is routine.[20] Government lawyers even drafted "Torture Memos" detailing what sorts of cruel, inhumane, and degrading treatment they believed fell short of torture and therefore were permissible under American law.[21]

Detention of terrorist suspects without trial, which had been such a controversial feature of the UK government's response to "The Troubles" in Northern Ireland, became a fixture of responses to 9/11. The United States detained more than seven hundred suspects at Camp X-ray and Camp Delta in Guantanamo Bay, few of whom were tried, let alone convicted. At the same time, the United Kingdom introduced legislation immediately after the attacks to permit the indefinite detention of non-British (or "international") terror suspects.

The nature and extent of these responses rightly attracted intense debate over their morality, legality, political expediency, proportionality, and effectiveness. The trade-offs between responsibilities for security and the freedom of individuals focus not just on the specific consequences for detainees but also on the more diffuse ramifications for societies and nations. For example, many lamented post-9/11 torture tactics that stooped to the level of the terrorists themselves, thereby "violat[ing] our core values as a nation," as forty-two retired US generals and admirals put it in an open letter to the 2016 presidential candidates.[22] In a similar vein, the United Kingdom's House of Lords lambasted as entirely wrongheaded the British government's claims that post-9/11 laws authorizing indefinite detention were necessary to combat terrorism's existential threat to the nation. "The real threat to the life of the nation, in the sense of a people living in accordance with its traditional laws and political values, comes not from terrorism but from laws such as these," said Lord Hoffman, hammering home the point in a case challenging the legality of indefinite detention.[23]

Since terrorism became a truly global affair after September 11, 2001, many security responses to it have become part of everyday life. No longer restricted to terrorism hotspots, bag searches, pat-downs, security scanners, identification checks, and restrictions on liquids, gels, and sharp objects on airplanes are today familiar inconveniences. More ominous, however, are the incursions on our privacy made possible by the exponentially increasing capacities of technology. Wherever we go, physically or online, whatever we do or say, when, with whom or what, and how often—all of this is now open to surveillance by official and unofficial agencies screening for supposed signs of terrorist activity or sympathies (among many other proclivities or traits), at staggering levels of detail. Many of these intrusions may be relatively inconsequential, but some are extraordinarily invasive, whether with or without good reason.[24] The surveillance state is well and truly with us.

Side Effects

The temptation to use this enhanced capacity to snoop on people's lives under the broad license afforded by the label of anti-terrorism security is great indeed, and such data drag-netting yields all sorts of privacy-invading and freedom-crimping potential for private as well as public sector abuse. China, for example, has created a system of state surveillance that is unparalleled in terms of its reach and suppressive control by exploiting both the authority of autocracy and what Chinese author Jianan Qian calls a national "mindset . . . wired to see safety and freedom as an either/or choice."[25] In Western democracies, despite the absence of such accommodating circumstances, the private sector's exploitation of the profit potential of data collected under the guise of security also presents serious problems for privacy and freedom. The purpose of *surveillance capitalism*, as Shoshana Zuboff argues, is to use (and abuse) data collected from any source or for whatever reason, including security, by storing it, reconfiguring it, or selling it in ways that yield profitable returns.[26]

Given the enormity of what's at stake, therefore, we might expect that the terrorism dimensions of the security-freedom transaction would not only be widely debated (which they are) but tightly policed (which there are not). The reason is that while the responsibilities of freedom associated with protecting people from the fear and harm of terrorism are certainly daunting, they are also very peculiar. Effective security, it is argued, demands discretion and often secrecy, which when paired with the extraordinary technological capacity of surveillance today, means that many (or even all) details of the resultant compromises of people's freedoms are unknown. Quality controls are missing from nearly all security apparatuses. Assessments of whether surveillance mechanisms "have brought us any closer to achieving the declared goal of greater and lasting security" are either absent or platitudinous,[27] relying on what are in effect "false positive" claims of the clandestine thwarting of terrorist attacks. It may be true that many attacks have been thwarted, but we cannot know for certain, having to rely on the assurances of the self-proclaimed thwarters themselves or occasional incomplete or inchoate leaks by whistle-blowers.[28] If we do not or cannot know the security gains, how can we assess whether the restrictions on freedom taken in security's name are worth it?

To be sure, the potentially existential threat posed by terrorism touches the raw nerve that connects a state's authority to protect its citizens and its responsibility to promote their freedoms. The nerve is raw because the demands of liberty require a balance to be struck between these two duties, no matter how difficult that may be. At times they may complement each other—as when terrorist threats are minimized by security forces that are well trained and held accountable and by terrorist "watch lists" that are adequately maintained and implemented. But at other times, as we've seen, they do not. Liberty's task—our task—is a matter of not just making more security information available (mindful that there are some legitimate reasons for secrecy classifications) but also maintaining or regaining trust in our institutions of government. Trust, that is, in their formulation of legitimate reasons as openly as possible and with due regard to alternative and counterarguments, rather than shamelessly exploiting the cover that "security concerns" provides them. This is the essence of an open society. One in which even freedoms compromised on grounds that are highly or somewhat opaque are nevertheless still challenged, and safeguards still demanded.

Terrorism and the history of responses to it vividly illustrate how imperiled that trust can be. But rather than undermining the role of political trust and responsibility, such problems serve to underline their significance.[29]

Bearing Arms

For philosopher and father of modern sociology Max Weber, one of the defining features of a state is what he referred to as its "monopoly of the legitimate use of violence" within its territory.[30] Like so many intellectuals before and after him, Weber was especially concerned with the *legitimate* use of such power. How do we justify the state's power to arrest, incarcerate, fine, deny rights and freedoms to, and even kill its citizens? Among the many answers to this question, "to provide security and protect the rights and freedoms of citizens as a whole" occupies a central position. Depending on the nature and extent of the protection thus afforded us, the citizenry, we might be content to cede to the state the authority of violence. Or we might not be.

Possessing a weapon, for defense or attack, has been a feature of human existence for as long as our ancestors have been able to fashion one. While the use of lethal weapons remains a part of all societies today, one of the beneficial consequences of socialization and the development of states in their modern form has been to mitigate or even eliminate the *need* for individuals to possess weapons. The violence associated with weapons is instead to be wielded and controlled by the state in its quest to keep us all secure and free. The better governed the state—that is, freer and safer life under it is—the less call there is for individuals to arm themselves. Where states are badly or barely governed, as in Afghanistan, Syria, Venezuela, or Yemen today, where people are neither safe nor free, weapons, and especially firearms, will be abundant and in open circulation. By and large this theory is borne out in practice. The rich democracies of the West are nearly all free of guns among civilians in day-to-day life. Police forces may be armed and criminals may use guns and other weapons, but among ordinary folk guns are rarely seen, still less owned and openly brandished.

Civilian gun ownership worldwide is in fact relatively low and is concentrated in groups such as hunters, farmers, enthusiasts, collectors, and gun club members, who tend to possess multiple firearms. The vast majority of people in all countries do not own guns. Except, that is, for the United States, where 32 percent of all Americans own guns and 44 percent report living in a gun household.[31] There are nearly 400 million civilian-owned guns in the United States, which equates to 1.2 firearms for every American man, woman, and child, and accounts for a truly staggering 46 percent of all civilian-owned guns worldwide.[32] In the global league of gun ownership, Canada is the closest major Western state to the United States with 5.7 percent of its population possessing one or more firearm (Canadians own 12.7 million guns in total, which still seems like a lot of firepower).[33] The United Kingdom, which has nearly twice Canada's population, has only 2.7 million guns in private hands, and Japan has a meager 370,000 guns across a population of 126 million. Even Australia, which alongside Canada might be considered closest to the rugged individualism image of the United States, has a relatively modest 3.6 million guns in circulation, owned by some 3.4 percent of the population.[34]

What are the security implications of these levels of gun ownership and possession? Could it be, for instance, that the United States' outlier status is in fact an indication of especially effective democratic governance that manages to balance high degrees of freedom and security. After all, notably unfree, authoritarian states like China, Vietnam, and Singapore are among the countries with the lowest levels of private gun ownership. Here again statistics are instructive. Although overall crime rates in the United States are similar to, if not significantly lower than, comparable rich-world states, the number of gun homicides in the United States far exceeds the rate in those other countries—7.7 times more than in Canada, 23.3 times more than in Australia or Sweden, and 70 times more that than in France, Germany, or the United Kingdom. The US gun death rate keeps company with those in the Dominican Republic (the same), Haiti and Libya (which are slightly more), and Iraq, the Philippines, and South Africa (slightly less).[35] Gun homicide rates for China, Vietnam, and Singapore are on par (or, in China's case, much lower) with most Western European nations, but without the added benefits of the civil and political freedoms enjoyed by the latter.

What makes the prevalence of gun ownership and gun deaths such a trigger issue for the relationship between security and freedom in the United States is that bearing arms is a right or freedom as well as a security concern. The United States is one of only three countries that constitutionally enshrine the right to bear arms (Mexico and Guatemala are the other two), which in the case of the US Constitution's Second Amendment is conditional on the right being exercised to uphold the "security of a free state." This constitutional embodiment has had important implications. First and foremost, the right to bear arms is today regarded with something close to religious reverence by its many supporters in the United States, no matter that the country's peculiar war-torn circumstances in the late 1700s that gave rise to the Second Amendment, and even the Civil War that followed seventy years later, have long since evaporated. The right's claimed inalienability has attracted serious political and financial backing, and accommodating (that is to say, lenient) regulatory oversight of the sale, possession, and use of guns in many states has permitted the creation of a veritable civilian arsenal.

The intransigence of the debate of whether the right is worth the death toll is truly flabbergasting: more Americans—some 1.5 million—have died in gun-related incidents over the past fifty years than have died as servicemen and servicewomen in all wars combined in US history.[36] After every school shooting, mass murder, or horrific firearms accident involving children or infants,[37] the same lamentations and counterassertions are voiced ("people kill people, not guns"),[38] and little changes. The very fact that US government deems it necessary to fund a "K–12 School Shooting Database" to record "the full scope of gun violence on school campuses" from 1970 to the present day is a numbing indictment of the state of American civil society.[39] In terms of repair, it is not so much that the Second Amendment itself needs to be amended or removed as it is that its alternative, more restrictive interpretation and implementation at federal and state levels need to be promoted. Thus, for example, while the watershed 2008 Supreme Court case of *District of Columbia v. Heller* affirmed an individual's right to bear arms, it did so conditionally. The right is inalienable only to the extent that it is exercised in self-defense in one's home, and further, the Court underscored the validity of existing restrictions relating to possession by felons and the mentally ill, as well as "the carrying of dangerous or unusual weapons"—the latter without any hint of irony.[40] Even this tiny glimmer of rational conservative reasoning, however, was extinguished by the Supreme Court in 2022 when it overturned a statutory requirement in New York State that citizens show "proper cause" when carrying a concealed handgun in public such as for "self-protection distinguishable from that of the general community." In so deciding, the majority of the Court bemoaned the imposition of any limits on Second Amendment freedoms, writing (in the words of Justice Clarence Thomas): "We know of no other constitutional right that an individual may exercise only after demonstrating to government officers some special need."[41] The gauche absurdity of such reasoning beggars belief when you consider that it is precisely to try to limit the appalling levels of destruction of human lives caused by guns in the United States that the special-need requirement to carry a concealed firearm is designed to achieve.

As a matter of fact, the door remains open for Americans, through their elected lawmakers, to negotiate a more secure, less lethal balance between the freedom and security to arm oneself and one's freedom and security to live without gun-related violence. Data compiled by Giffords Law Center to Prevent Gun Violence shows a clear correlation between the strength of a state's gun regulations and the number of gun-related deaths in that state.[42] It's not hard to comprehend. Some US states and nearly all other Western nations strictly regulate who owns guns, what sort, how many, and when and how they use them. As a result, they have markedly lower levels of gun violence.[43] American exceptionalism regarding gun ownership may continue to resonate loudly within domestic politics, but it cannot alter the evidence of its dire consequences. The right to bear arms is a freedom like any other, limited and accompanied by responsibilities, including and especially respecting the safety of others. Not only is it perverse to suppose and act otherwise in the face of such overwhelming evidence of lethal consequences, but such obstinance undermines the wider notion of a community founded on the principles of liberty and rationality.

A Safe Environment

Compared to terrorism or gun violence, human degradation of the environment seems a slow burn security problem. Its impact is often discussed in generational or multigenerational terms.

What we do (or do not do) today to address the issue will be inherited by our children tomorrow. That said, the full significance of the problem cannot be grasped when viewed across a time span of mere generations. To truly understand the speed and gravity of our impact on our environment, we must use a time frame that stretches back to when Earth became an animal-inhabitable planet (approximately 600 million years ago), in which case we see that the changes humankind has wrought on the environment have been achieved at hyperspeed. Even contracting the measurement period to the 200,000 years or so that *Homo sapiens* have lived on Earth, the fact that nearly all of humanity's major contributions to environmental change have occurred in the past 200 years (and most of them in the past 100 years) reflects a history of phenomenal and accelerating suddenness. In the context of the Earth's twelve-hour clock, we've done a whole lot in just a tiny portion of the human race's "one second to midnight" existence.[44]

Not all our human-generated changes to the environment need necessarily be detrimental to it or to our own safety and long-term security. Anthropogenic perspectives of the environment recognize that humans are themselves part of the environment, not separate from or superimposed on it, and so will play *some* part in the ever-changing nature of Earth's environment.[45] In this respect our species is like any other animal or plant genera. Environmental and climatic changes themselves are not necessarily the problem; rather, it is the extent and speed of change caused by humans that ring alarm bells. From an increasingly carbonated atmosphere, warming climate, shrinking ice caps, and rising sea levels, to deforestation, species extinctions, radically declining fish stocks, air particle and microplastic pollution, and the progressive nitrogenization of coastal seas, humanity's footprint on Earth has dramatically widened and deepened over the past century.[46]

What has precipitated these changes is our astonishing capacity and willingness to exploit the environment. Far more than any other living thing, past or present, humans have developed skills that enable us to bend the environment to our demands, to modify it locally and globally, and to do so with such efficient rapidity that we can see it, feel it, and measure it.[47] We certainly have the power effectively to destroy the planet. But we also have the power to preserve it.

The nature of our relationship with the environment today—how it protects and nurtures us, as well as the dangers it poses—is summed up by the notion of our quest to "master" it, to regard it as an instrument in our power. Whether that involves how we have learned to use plants and animals to feed ourselves and keep ourselves healthy, enabling the human population has grown exponentially, or how we have transformed Earth's elements and minerals in ways that provide us with shelter, transport, communication, comfort, and convenience, such instrumental use of the environment alters our perspective of it. No longer are we part of it; we are removed or separated from it. Yet this makes no sense. The Anthropocene *is* the human environment. True, it is an environment dominated by humans, but humans are nonetheless part of it.[48]

Our freedoms to explore and exploit the planet's resources have consequences for our security and safety, both individually and collectively. More especially still, they are certain to have even greater consequences for future generations. Managing those consequences boils down to the environmental responsibilities that attend these freedoms. Responsibilities that require recognition of and respect for the planet we live on, if only out of a sense of mutual self-preservation. In honoring these responsibilities, our paradoxical alienation from the environment in which we live and of which we form an indelible part has serious implications. An

"us and it" perspective tends to rob us of a sense of instinctive belonging to the environment, of a spiritual or even physical connection to it, and thereby makes care for it that much harder.

In recognizing the seriousness of this dilemma, environmental
philosopher Steven Vogel urges us to cast aside the "untenable"
distinction between what is "natural" and what is "artificial."[49] *All*
that is man-made is part of nature. Shopping malls constitute the
natural environment in which we live, he argues, and so "deserve
as much serious consideration from environmental thinkers as do
mountains." He's right. It's not that we must love (or hate) malls
as we do mountains but simply that we accept that both are part
of nature, as are we. By so doing, Vogel continues, we are forced
to recognize "that the problem of the environment is a political
matter,"[50] and being political, it is our responsibility to resolve it.

Innate responsibility is also at the heart of the intense and mutually self-sustaining, spiritual relationship that our forebears and
many Indigenous peoples today have with the environment. Aboriginal peoples of Australia, for example, consider their connection to "country"—by which they mean the environment of land,
water, and sky—as existential. They, their ancestors, and all who
follow them are *not* merely its caretakers or custodians—still less
its owners—but rather are part of its whole. "Country is loved,
needed, and cared for, and country loves, needs, and cares for her
peoples in turn. Country is family, culture, identity. Country is
self," is how Palyku woman Ambelin Kwaymullina explains it.[51]

By whatever means we reestablish a deep appreciation of the
role we play in our own environmental future and the security it
may or may not provide us, doing so will help us balance the freedoms and responsibilities associated with its care and use. The
science of climate change needs to be interpreted within the context of our visceral connection to and dependency on the environment.[52] These are the parameters of our assignment, whether

we are extinction rebels or climate change skeptics, and it is within them that together we must judge either viewpoint and all others in between.

Securing Freedom

We have our work cut out for us in using liberty to navigate the intersections between people's freedoms and their security. Whenever any of us feels threatened or unsafe—when we are truly fearful, as Nina Simone puts it in the quote at the head of this chapter—we have little thought for much beyond how to remove the treat and quell the fear. That is certainly true when we're faced with someone brandishing a gun in our direction, and it is also true when we live in circumstances where terrorism is a quotidian experience. A pandemic like COVID-19 excites both instant and long-term responses in an uneasy alliance. Climate change, however, is more diffuse, less obviously immediate in its impact, even if the threat is very real and very great. It is therefore easier—at least in theory—to understand, identify, and possibly even agree on what freedom restrictions are necessary to curb the violence rent by guns and terrorism than it is to do the same for the insecurities we create by degrading the environment or locking down communities to combat disease.

As our individual and collective histories bear witness, environmental insecurities are prone to being ignored or delayed, while threats of violence attract swift responses, even if they too can be ineffective (as with the remarkable resilience of US gun laws) or damagingly overreactive (as with draconian anti-terrorist measures). Our reactions to a new and highly contagious pathogen are also typically swift and tumultuous, lasting until a combination of natural and vaccine-induced immunity reaches herd levels, which can take years or even decades.

The whole wide gamut of our everyday security concerns as well as our freedom-related responses to them falls between these two poles. The immediate needs—shelter, enough to eat, sanitation, physical safety, and sufficient money to live on—and the distant—long-term health, psychological fortitude, financial security, and what sort of future we bequeath our children. The realization of each of these depends on all of us shouldering certain responsibilities by conceding not only that our freedoms may be limited insofar as they endanger the security of others but also that the balance struck between security and freedom is an unending negotiation, as often gray as it is black-and-white. With so many freedoms themselves providing security—being free from oppression or discrimination, for example, as well as being free to believe and speak one's mind—the task is unavoidably communal and mutually supportive, demanding respect and compassion for one another.[53] For the succor of security is not just a matter of individual self-preservation; it is a cohesive force that keeps society together. So much so that, as neuroscientists tell us, our brains actively inhibit our compassion for others until we ourselves feel safe.[54] It's in all our best interests, therefore, that we look after one another.

8

Voice

Free to Offend or an Offensive Freedom?

If liberty means anything at all, it means the right to tell
people what they do not want to hear.
—George Orwell

It was the height of summer in 1794 in Paris, and Tom knew he was going to die the next day under the blade of a guillotine. The prison guards had already chalked his cell door, signaling his fate as one of 168 prisoners destined for execution in the morning. But when dawn broke, his cell door remained closed; no one came to haul him out to the waiting scaffold. Incredibly, the jailors had absent-mindedly marked his door on its *inside*, as the door happened to be open (it opened outward) at the time they were doing their "death rounds" the day before. After the cell door was closed and locked that night, the chalk mark simply disappeared from sight, and "the destroying angel passed by," as Tom later said of his good fortune.[1] This first stroke of extraordinary luck was then followed by a second, equally fortuitous. Tom would certainly have been executed in the days that followed, once the error was discovered, had it not been for the fact that at the very same time, Maximilien Robespierre, the architect of the French Revolution's Reign of Terror and the man responsible for Tom's incarceration and death sentence as an "enemy of the Revolution," was deposed and himself promptly guillotined.[2] As a result, thousands of prisoners, including Tom, were pardoned and immediately released.

This is how Thomas Paine—philosopher, activist, and one of history's greatest advocates of freedom and free speech—escaped death not once but twice in the same week.

In searching for someone prepared to sacrifice everything for the sake of speaking their mind, it is hard to go past Paine. Having been exiled from Great Britain for being too revolutionary (he was a vocal supporter of America's war of independence) and ostracized in America for being too radical (he despised slavery and defended women's rights), he had found himself sentenced to death in France for being insufficiently bloodthirsty in his postrevolutionary inclinations (he opposed the death penalty and argued against the execution of Louis XVI, preferring banishment instead).

In each country where he lived, he was at first, praised, and feted, but when he stuck to his principles by saying and publishing what he believed in, he soon made enemies. Even when he returned once again to America some years later, his reputation as a free thinker and, more especially, a free speaker attracted more negative than positive attention. He continued to rail against the evils of slavery and the injustices borne by women, to which he added criticisms of church and state, and his championing of ordinary people against decadent, self-satisfied elites.[3] In the end, he died in New York City, penniless and alone, "maligned on every side, execrated, shunned and abhorred, his virtues denounced as vices, his services forgotten, his character blackened," as historian Robert Ingersoll put it. The funeral of the man founding father John Adams once credited as being a decisive inspiration for the US war of independence was attended by only five mourners.[4]

Free Speech Consequences

Freedom of speech has consequences, both for speakers and those who hear them. Indeed, we might say that such consequences are the very point of speech: to be heard and to have an impact, to hear and to be affected. Very often such exchanges are unremarkable affairs. Information, instruction, opinion, and passions are conveyed constantly and with little or no complication. Think of all the times and ways you have expressed yourself in interactions with others today. Whether physically or electronically, in speech, writing, or visually, or even surreally (like conversing with God or texting teenagers). Conveyed with conviction or tenderness, in anger or jest, loudly or whispered. Most of it has, I hope, been free and unhindered (at least in any obvious sense), and the messages conveyed have been more prosaic than profound.

Sometimes, however, what is said and heard is truly remarkable and the impact significant. Insights, inspiration, praise, and empathy can bring great elation, just as ignorance, malice, and selfishness can damn and denigrate terribly. For Tom Paine, the consequences of speaking his mind often ranged across all these emotions and outcomes, as apparently was also the case for many who heard him and read his words. George Washington, for example, recited lines from Paine to inspire his troops before battle, and Robespierre initially embraced Paine's stirring support for the overthrow of monarchies and aristocracies in his iconic *Rights of Man*. Yet, subsequently, Paine spectacularly fell out of favor with both men. The dire consequences of which, alongside his banishment from his native England after he was tried and convicted of treason in absentia for writing his *Rights of Man*, represented his life's nadir. All on account of his determination to stand up for what he believed in. Still, in America he was at least free to express his opinions, no matter who he offended and how he offended them. For Paine lived the last years of his life under the protection of what was and is rightly seen as the most powerfully protective statement of free speech the world has ever known.

The First Amendment to the US Constitution, adopted in 1791, prohibits Congress from "abridging the freedom of speech, or of the press." Since its adoption the First Amendment has been held to protect all sorts of speech and expression from governmental interference.[5] Political dissent, criticism, and opinion are vigorously protected whether conveyed via usual or unusual means (such as flag burning, kneeling during the national anthem, or photographing police officers on duty), as are artistic and religious (and anti-religious) expressions, as well as most pornography and depictions of graphic violence. Many laws that compel speech or expression have been proscribed, such as compulsory school prayers, obligations to show ultrasound fetal images to women contemplating abortion, and mandatory political statements on vehicle license plates (like New Hampshire's state motto, "Live Free or Die"). Authors' right to anonymity has also been preserved, which right also extends to journalists protecting their sources under so-called shield laws in most states.[6]

The baseline for the interpretation of the right to free speech in the United States is that it be read widely. It is no "mere shadow of freedom," the US Supreme Court held in the landmark case of *West Virginia State Board of Education v. Barnette*,[7] involving Jehovah's Witness children refusing to salute the national flag on religious grounds. "Freedom to differ is not limited to things that do not matter much," continued the Court; "the test of its substance is the right to differ as to things that touch the heart of the existing order." This robust defense of the freedom of expression is all the more remarkable given it was delivered in June 1943 at the height of the US involvement in a world war, when nationalist sentiments did indeed matter greatly.

A Freedom "Squared"

That the right to free speech is jealously guarded is as it should be. It promotes the benefits of liberty more generally by elevating the value of such important social virtues as our practices in learning, sharing, respecting, and disagreeing with one another. As author, provocateur, and unapologetic champion of free speech, Christopher Hitchens was keen to say, "I could make the case that it [free speech] is the essential liberty, without which all other freedoms are either impossible to imagine or impossible to put into practice."[8] For without freely expressed points of view, passions, prejudices, and all else that makes up social intercourse, we could never know what we all truly think, want, and need. And without knowing these things, how could we ever deliver a society in which we might thrive, or even survive? Free speech, in other words, is not only significant in its own right but also critical to the creation and maintenance of our civil and political freedoms as well as our economic, social, and cultural welfare. It is the freedom of freedoms, or freedom "squared." Such is the importance of free speech as "a principal pillar of a free government," as Benjamin Franklin wrote almost sixty years before the First Amendment came into being, that when it is forsaken, "the constitution of a free society is dissolved, and tyranny is erected on its ruins."[9]

In the context of this book's central argument, moreover, the guarantee of free speech is essential to negotiating the very nature of our liberty—the extent of our freedoms and reciprocal responsibilities across the full sweep of activities and thoughts that occupy our days. Yet in practice the protection of free speech raises the very same questions of itself as it helps to provide answers in all life's domains of health, happiness, work, wealth, security, love, death, respect, and trust: what are its justifiable limitations, and how are they decided and enforced?

A Freedom Limited

Our voices, however sounded, are always limited to some extent. They are never truly free. Speech is always situational, colored by the circumstances in which it occurs and by the predispositions of the person speaking. Such circumscriptions are unavoidable, as speech is not to be valued in and of itself. Speech, for example, would be of no value whatever to the hypothetical last person on Earth. Rather, speech "is always produced within the precincts of some assumed conception of the good," as law and literary theorist Stanley Fish argues. Otherwise, he adds, "there could be no assertion [of what is good or bad] and no reason for asserting it."[10] Our search for the answer to the question of what limitations might justifiably be imposed on speech shifts to our perceptions—individually and collectively—of what is "good."

Deciding what is good is a fraught task for any community as there will nearly always be differences of opinion between the individuals and coalitions it comprises. Collective deliberations inevitably reach what Stanley Fish calls the "pinch" point, where on some matter or other there is serious disagreement. What do we do then? Whose opinion prevails and how do we decide?

For as long as humans have lived in social groups, some form of governance or authority has made these sorts of decisions. Whose voices are to be heard? What content or beliefs are to hold sway? Which assumed or accepted conception of good will prevail? Speech is such a powerful instrument, used both by and against governments, that it is unsurprising to see its control so often the subject of intense debate and dispute. Governments and states can have very different views on what good is and therefore what the corresponding regulation should entail. If we are lucky, oversight should more or less reflect the community's prevailing sentiments on what is acceptable speech, and even if it does not, the official views are open to challenge and change. The less fortunate of us may find we are obliged to submit to views and rules on speech we don't believe in and have little hope of altering, precisely because avenues and opportunities for dissent have been restricted or removed altogether.

Some years ago, when I was working in Myanmar, the then-ruling military dictatorship believed that "law and order" was *the* defining imperative of government and so no speech or expression of any kind that threatened the military's control of civilian life was tolerated. Self-proclaimed as the "State Law and Order Council" (or SLORC, its fittingly dystopian acronym), such emphasis was perhaps not surprising.[11] China today also stresses the importance of law and order in its stringent limitations on any political communications that challenge the authority of government generally and the Chinese Communist Party in particular.[12] Theocracies and strongly religious states often restrict the voices of women, apostates, and homosexual and transgender persons, and history is littered with examples of governments silencing people based on their ethnicity or race. Political and philosophical convictions, whether too far Left or Right, or not sufficiently so in either direction, also regularly attract fierce censorship and sanction.

These radical restrictions on speech, backed by dire consequences for their breach, mark one end of the spectrum of (un)-free speech across the ages and as we know it today. Yet it is at, or near, that end that most peoples on Earth have long lived, and still do. According to watchdog Freedom House, significant restrictions on a free, independent media—as clear a barometer of free speech as one can get—are the norm for most countries, substantially free media existing only in North America, Europe, Australia, and New Zealand. And the situation is getting worse, with repression of media everywhere—in open societies and authoritarian states alike—rising sharply over the past decade.[13] Reporters without Borders agrees, noting in its 2021 World Press Freedom Index that journalism was "completely or partly blocked in 73% of the 180 countries ranked." This included the United States: the organization reports that "President Donald J. Trump's final year in the White House [2020] was marked by a record number of assaults against journalists (around 400) and arrests of members of the media (130)."[14]

Unprecedented though that level of harassment might be for the United States, it pales beside the uncompromising suppression of press and people by dictatorships in the Middle East, Eurasia, Africa, and East Asia, and now, increasingly, in Eastern Europe (Belarus, Hungary, Poland, Russia, Serbia, and Turkey), South and Southeast Asia (India, Pakistan and Myanmar [again]), Central and South America (Nicaragua and Venezuela). Verisk Maplecroft, another global free speech monitor, estimates that some 3.4 billion people worldwide (or 45 percent of the world's population) live in countries rated as "extreme risk" according to the organization's "Freedom of Expression and Right to Privacy Indices."[15]

The methods of censorship can be subtle or crude.[16] Journalists and their families are intimidated, assaulted, jailed, or murdered.[17] The internet and social media are screened for "undesirable" content and suspect individuals and organizations are harassed, fined, or bankrupted; increasingly, whole national networks are simply shut down. Indian authorities are particularly prone to hit the internet kill switch, having done so on no fewer than 106 occasions in 2021 alone (more than the rest of the world combined), nearly always in response to civil unrest such as in Jammu and Kashmir.[18] Bangladesh, Cuba, Iran, Myanmar, Pakistan, and South Sudan have all used the same tactic when facing internal protests, opting to shut down the internet either for lengthy periods or every night (as was regularly the case in Myanmar following the February 2021 coup), thus enabling authorities to terrorize communities under cover of both physical and electronic darkness.[19]

Media outlets are also closed down, bought out by regime-friendly competitors, or bribed to toe the government line, enabling state-controlled media to become the dominant or only voice while giving the impression of being independent and fair-minded. China and Russia are global leaders in this regard, but a raft of other nations, including Hungary, Turkey, Kyrgyzstan, Somalia, Papua New Guinea, Qatar, Uganda, and Kenya, have followed suit in recent years.[20] The interpretive elasticity of "hate speech" and anti-terrorism laws is also routinely exploited such that just about any speech criticizing a ruling regime can be deemed to be inciting hate or terrorism and therefore banned and speakers punished. The governments and courts of Belarus, Kazakhstan, Rwanda, Egypt, and Saudi Arabia, for example, have all employed such creative interpretations to protect themselves and silence their critics.[21]

Power and Legitimacy

Such repressive restrictions on free speech are all about power. Its exercise, preservation, and almost invariably, expansion. The more you can control what is said and not said, the more the agenda is yours to set. And the more you set the agenda, the more entrenched your power and authority becomes over what is said and by whom.

This same narrative of power is found in open societies as well as tyrannies. There too people jockey for control and influence; there too they spar over what can and cannot be said and what should and should not be heard. Free speech restrictions in liberal democracies not only exist but can also take the same form as some of those deployed in repressive states. The ownership and control of media outlets is perennially questioned, and while antitrust laws exist in many jurisdictions, seeking to prevent concentrated or monopoly ownership, private sector media behemoths with distinct political agendas continue to operate in all Western states.[22] Public media outlets are also often the subject of heated debate about political bias, especially when they criticize incumbent governments, at which times the fragility of their reliance on state funding becomes readily apparent.[23] Anti-terrorism laws and hate speech laws are now features in the statute books of all democracies, with debates raging over their reach and application. For while nearly everyone agrees that there is some point at which speech inciting hate and violence ought to be banned, opinions differ widely about *where* that point is or should be.

What distinguishes the power battle over free speech restrictions in democracies from that in autocracies, however, is that speech about the restrictions *themselves* is not only expected but permitted and even encouraged. They are open to debate, they are queried, criticized, or praised, and they are subject to change or removal when the weight of freely expressed opinion so demands. Or at least that's the theory.

Debates about freedom of expression and what, if any, limits it should obey are inherent to free societies—the so-called freedom squared that was described earlier. Such freedom necessarily includes a right to express the view that certain speech or certain speakers should not be heard at all.[24] Contradictory though this seems, those who hold such views argue that without silencing some speech and speakers, others will be or will remain silenced, or will otherwise suffer in ways that far outweigh any benefit gained by letting the original speaker be heard.

Religion has long been a lightning rod topic in this regard. Expressions of religious belief may be protected, permitted, or proscribed, depending on the country and the religion. Similarly, anti-theist opinion can be subject to the very same boundaries and conditions. Across Europe, for example, blasphemy laws have been upheld by the European Court of Human Rights as complying with the rights to free speech and religious freedom. At the very same time, the Court has condoned greater tolerance of blasphemous speech as states increasingly ax such laws. Thus, the Court has declined to overturn a woman's conviction in Austria for disparaging the Prophet Muḥammad in a public meeting (she labeled as pedophilia Muhammad's marriage to the six-year-old Aisha), while acknowledging that in other states such remarks would escape sanction altogether.[25] This is not necessarily inconsistent but rather reflects the application of jurisprudential pragmatism. The Court frequently uses the elastic notion of a "margin of appreciation" to permit some differences in interpretations between European states over where human rights boundaries can be drawn.[26]

All such boundary debates regarding free speech, wherever they occur, center on balancing competing views not only of the impact of speech on individuals or groups but also of their effect on society as a whole. Such balancing requires both quantitative measurement (how many winners and losers, if they can be clearly identified at all) and qualitative analysis—whose voice or what harm carries more weight and why. These are incredibly difficult calculations to make, especially when the circumstances are highly charged, as they often are when societies are deeply divided on particular issues.

Hate Speech

Take, for instance, the impassioned debates over what, if anything, one should do about "hate speech." Groundwork for the dilemma such speech poses is to be found throughout international human rights law. Both the 1948 Universal Declaration of Human Rights and the United Nations' 1966 International Covenant on Civil and Political Rights (ICCPR) recognize the two sides of the problem by first proclaiming the right to freedom of expression (which includes "freedom to seek, receive and impart information and ideas of all kinds") and following that with an equal insistence that "advocacy of national, racial or religious hatred that constitutes incitement to discrimination, hostility or violence shall be prohibited by law."[27] Neither instrument provides instructions as to how precisely to settle the disputes that unavoidably arise out of these competing ideals. Nor have any been forthcoming in their interpretation since. This is not because of neglect or want of trying by the now-many international human rights instruments and institutions that concern themselves with freedom of expression,[28] but because no such clear, definitive direction is in fact possible.[29] Negotiating free speech is "an experiment," as the great American jurist Oliver Wendell Holmes put it, ongoing and never ending. And that includes negotiating its boundaries in the face of virulence and hatred.

The bottom line is that responsibilities (and "special duties" as the ICCPR adds) must be shouldered by everyone who voices an opinion. All of us ought to be accountable for the consequences of what we say, including—indeed especially—what we say about the rights of others to speak. Whether you want to promote speech or shut it down, a knee-jerk invocation of the mantra of "protecting free speech" without backup reasoning or evidence of consideration of others simply doesn't wash. *How* we are to be held accountable, against *what* measure of permissible speech, and, perhaps above all, by *whom* are the critical questions.

Laws restricting hate speech are in fact the norm in Western states; the United States is the only major jurisdiction among liberal democracies not to have them. In Europe, for example, such laws typically proscribe expressions of any kind that incite hatred or violence against persons based on their race, religion, ethnicity, gender, disability, or sexual orientation.[30] Language that is inflammatory or offensive but that otherwise fails to reach this threshold of incitement is generally permitted, at least in legal terms. On the whole, Europeans and their governments seem to be content with the existence of such limitations in principle, even if their implementation in practice is riven with compromises and apparent inconsistencies.

In Germany and Austria, broadcasting Nazi propaganda and Holocaust denials is criminalized, but burning the Israeli flag is tolerated.[31] In France, 1960s icon and animal rights activist Brigitte Bardot has been repeatedly convicted on charges of inciting racial hatred for her Islamophobic outbursts bemoaning the Muslim community "destroying our country by imposing their ways."[32] At the same time in France, Charlie Hebdo's cartoons satirizing Muhammad escaped censure and Muslim women have been prohibited from expressing their faith by wearing a burqa or niqab in public, or even a burkini in public swimming pools.[33] In the Netherlands, opposing but equally trenchant views on immigrants appear to have been treated differently. Right-wing politician Geert Wilders was let off with a warning for potentially ominous threats toward Moroccan migrants, while under the same hate speech provisions refugee activist Joke Kaviaar was given a suspended (later imposed) custodial sentence for suggesting that people should storm the Dutch immigration authority and destroy its records.[34]

Hate speech laws are also often tied up with defamation claims, which may be deployed by either side in free speech disputes. American historian Deborah Lipstadt, for example, was sued by renowned Holocaust denier David Irving in the UK courts in 2000 for claiming in her book *Denying the Holocaust* that Irving was profoundly anti-Semitic.[35] Not only did Irving lose this civil case (Lipstadt's account was considered fair and accurate), but shortly thereafter he lost a criminal case brought against him in Austria for violating that country's Holocaust denial prohibitions. While Lipstadt had nothing to do with the second case, her response upon hearing the news of Irving's conviction and sentencing by the Austrian court to three years in jail was intriguing. "I am not happy when censorship wins," she told the BBC, "and I don't believe in winning battles via censorship. . . . The way of fighting Holocaust deniers is with history and with truth."[36]

Christopher Hitchens, as we saw earlier, was similarly committed to unhindered speech. Throughout his career, Hitchens, whose mother was Jewish, wrote a number of essays defending the right of Holocaust deniers and other Nazi sympathizers to publish their views, not because he believed in their arguments but because he believed in his right to hear (and denounce) them.[37] Moreover, as he was fond of saying, "I have never met or heard of anybody I would trust with the job of deciding in advance what it might be permissible for me or anyone else to say or read." So compelling is this statement that I must confess it is a favorite of mine to put to students along with the rider: "Have you?" At which point, and after a brief pause, a torrent of debate flows across the classroom.

Shifting Boundaries

Such openness even to vituperative speech, it is often supposed, sits more comfortably in the United States (where Hitchens lived much of his adult life) despite evidence, both historical and contemporary, to the contrary. It is true that European-style hate speech laws do not exist in the United States today, but that was not always the case. First Amendment *in*tolerance of hate speech (especially that promoting fascism or communism) was prevalent in the United States throughout the 1940s and 1950s.[38] So-called group libel laws, that limited free speech were upheld by the US Supreme Court, including a law in Illinois that protected racial and religious groups from vilification. In the landmark case of *Beauharnais v. Illinois* in 1952, the Court found that the distribution of leaflets disparaging "negros" for the "encroachment, harassment and invasion of white people" was libelous and did not fall within the protection of the First Amendment.[39]

As America moved into the 1960s and as society, including the young and students in particular, became more vocal and even radicalized, the restrictions on free speech fell away. Malcolm X's "college debates" between 1960 and 1963 on whether races should integrate or segregate were as eye-opening and inflammatory as they sound, and yet he was allowed to speak.[40] Feminist, gay, and civil rights voices were heard loud and strong, even if they too antagonized establishment figures and institutions. The free speech beneficiaries, however, were not all from the counterculture Left. The voices of anti-abortionists, Christian fundamentalists, and white supremacists were also given freer rein. Indeed, it was a Supreme Court case involving the Ku Klux Klan in 1969 that cemented this liberalized interpretation of the First Amendment. In *Brandenburg v. Ohio* the Court determined that local Klan leader Charles Brandenburg's suggestions of racist violence and armed insurrection retained protection under the First Amendment so long as they did not incite or produce "imminent lawless action."[41] This constitutional high-water mark for free speech has since paved the way for a flourishing of protected dissident speech of all stripes, from the Black Panthers to Black Lives Matter, feminists and LGBTQI rights advocates to anti-feminists and homophobic groups, pro- and anti-gun lobbies, and wide a range of religious zealotry.

The point of this potted history of extreme free speech is to show how its boundaries can and do change. Political contexts, social trends, and preexisting legal structures all play their part in this perpetual "experiment." Good and harm can come from *both* free and restricted speech. That cannot be denied. However much we might wish it otherwise, there is no "invisible hand" guiding the open market of free speech, no mechanism to ensure that on balance the outcome is always, or even mostly, positive.[42] So the boundaries of free speech must be proactively policed, by legislatures and courts, as well as by all of us as participants as best we can. The demands of liberty require us, individually and collectively, to take responsibility for the consequences of our words and actions, to try to understand the impacts and implications of speech and of its restriction, and to attempt to balance the one against the other. On which point, the sanctioning of sadistically perverted speech, such as alt-right American radio host Alex Jones's vile claim that the Sandy Hook Elementary School massacre of twenty-six children and adults in 2012 was a hoax, is to be welcomed as a means to hold accountable those whose hateful words cause grave, tangible harm to others.[43]

A collectivity of voices is certainly desirable, not least because of the democratic ethos it reflects. But it also invites a host of problems. Voices differ not just in content but also in volume. The loudest voices may or may not represent most people's views. It is often hard to tell. Even if they do not, but represent minority interests instead, how do we decide whether they ought nonetheless to be heard? What about quieter voices; "silent" voices, lone voices, dissenting voices, or anti-dissenting voices? These are not just legal problems. In fact, more often than not, these questions arise in everyday encounters where the law is, at most, a shadow in the proceedings.

College campuses are in many ways ideal laboratories for examining how these encounters play out in daily practice. They are educational environments designed to promote learning by encouraging exchanges of knowledge as well as opinions. Places to speak one's mind, but also to listen and learn, to have one's own views confirmed or confounded. In short, arenas in which to test oneself, to establish some solid, thought-through foundations for believing in what one believes in. Conventional wisdom as well as contrary and controversial viewpoints should all find space here. For, if not here, where? And if your answer to *that* question is "nowhere, and never," then I think you've misunderstood the question, or least what the question implies. Because insofar as any opinion or belief is *held* by someone, somewhere that viewpoint will be *expressed* in one form or another. Of course, this does not mean that university lecture theaters, still less public halls or private rooms, should be obliged to host any voice no matter how ludicrous or vile, but rather that in the decision of which voices deserve hearing and which do not, good reasons need to be given. Engagement at some level with controversial viewpoints is essential even if only to enable the broadcasting of more powerful arguments mounted against them. Outright rejection without reasons and with no engagement is always undesirable and often counterproductive.[44]

Debates over free speech in US universities and colleges often take on a heightened intensity, reflecting, no doubt, the broader context of the special place free speech occupies in the US Constitution and polity.[45] With fewer legal impediments (but not none—incitement to violence, if proven, is always prohibited), the job of setting and policing boundaries of "acceptable" speech falls to social forces. In practice, this challenge is taken up jointly by students, professors, and the administrations of universities. They don't always agree, of course, but even in their disagreement a plurality of opinions prevails. Sometimes tough decisions have to be made in the face of implacable opposition—whether, for example, to permit white nationalist Richard Spencer to speak (as did the University of Florida) or deny him a platform (as did the state universities of Ohio, Pennsylvania, and Michigan). Safety and security must always be considered, as must personal health and welfare when facing aggressive or exclusionary speech. But overall, not only are heated clashes relatively rare, but those that do arise are fairly evenly spread across the political and social spectrums.

As *Vox* media journalist Zack Beauchamp convincingly argues, multiple data sources tell the same story: "There are several dozen incidents of speech being suppressed on [US] college campuses per year," which, he says, may be considered unfortunate. But given that there are 4,583 colleges and universities across the United States, and that the speakers targeted were "liberals and leftists" just as often as "conservatives," such a number does not amount to a national crisis; still less is the cancel culture movement an existential threat to free speech.[46] The principle, therefore, that for universities to fulfill their "modern missions of knowledge creation and dissemination," students and scholars must be free to think, hear, and express ideas that challenge as well as promote conventional wisdom appears not only to remain intact, but the strength of debate over what that means in practice reflects its continuing vigor.[47]

Voice Control

Negotiating the boundaries of free speech is most effective when the process, whether legal or social (or both), is as inclusive as possible. This should and usually does mean that all sorts of weirdness and wackiness gets to stay inside the tent, from flat-earthers and creationists to mega–conspiracy theorists and reality

TV stars. However, by their very outré nature they nearly always remain curiosities, commanding peripheral rather than mainstream attention (OK, so maybe not reality TV stars, on which more below). But what happens when the truly bizarre or malevolent or just plain delusional veers toward the center? When conventional voices embrace or even propagate dishonesty and deception, or when new platforms for expression fundamentally change the ways we communicate with one another and with those who govern us?[48]

Donald Trump was hardly the first leader to lie, though his propensity to do so was truly astonishing. It was and is so entrenched that the line between what he sees as fact and what as fiction is not so much blurred as nonexistent. According to the Poynter Institute's *Politifact*—an agency dedicated to fact-checking statements made by leading politicians—Mr. Trump spoke the truth just 3 percent of the time during his presidency (at which level he has remained postpresidency). Seventy-three percent of his statements were categorized as "mostly false," "false," or "pants on fire."[49] At the conclusion of his presidency in January 2021, the *Washington Post* reported that throughout his four years in office Trump made a total of 30,573 false or misleading claims, with an average daily rate of lies that accelerated year on year.[50] In his first year as president, he was trotting out around 6 lies per day, which, studies show, even then far exceeded the average rate of lying in the general community (at 1.65 lies per day).[51] During his second year the rate jumped to 16 lies per day, then to 22 lies per day in his third year, and finally to 39 lies per day in his fourth year. Incredibly, on November 2, 2020, alone, the day before the presidential election, Trump made 503 false or misleading claims.[52] And all these were just the lies he told in public. It was Humpty Dumpty who said, "When *I* use a word . . . it means just what I choose it to mean—neither more nor less," in

Lewis Carroll's *Through the Looking-Glass*, but you would be forgiven believing that the statement's provenance lay in the Wonderland of the Trump White House.

Whether this pathological condition represents personal predilection or, as some argue, an evolving art form,[53] the result is a concerted and systematic assault on truth, the implications of which cannot be underestimated. When fact-based discussion is so debased and reasoned argument so distorted, "freedom of opinion becomes a cruel hoax," as author and peerless scholar of totalitarianism Hannah Arendt warned us.[54] For the free speech problem with fictitious propaganda is not so much the message as how it is received.

Not only have many Americans apparently warmed to Trump's inchoate message—either not caring or not understanding the lies—but so have influential media outlets as well as populist leaders elsewhere. "Facts be damned is Trump's approach, and it's working," wrote Susan Glasser in *The New Yorker* in November 2019.[55] The kicker in Glasser's remark is contained in the last three words. During his time in office, Trump's presidential approval ratings among voters remained steady at around 40 percent,[56] even during his impeachment hearings in 2019 and 2021 and throughout the calamity of the COVID-19 crisis (during which his mendacity reached new and deadly heights),[57] and he has since retained the almost unwavering support of Republican Party members. For politicians of all persuasions well used to playing fast and loose with facts, the supplication of Republicans to Trump's fact-free narrative, even after he lost the presidency (but asserts he didn't) and the party lost control of the Senate, has been spectacularly gutless and will surely haunt them when the hindsight of history reviews these years.[58] In the meantime, however, the institutions of democratic and responsible governance are enfeebled, the citizenry is infantilized, truth is twisted, and logic abandoned or reversed.

Without respect for these standard rules of communication, argument is replaced by assertion, accountability withers, and authoritarianism thrives.[59]

Autocrats everywhere, past and present, know this only too well, which is why their control of speech is always so uncompromisingly guarded. Vladimir Putin, for example, so thoroughly controls Russian media today that he is able to feed Russians what is essentially an alternative reality of the war in Ukraine (or the "special military operation," as it is invariably labeled inside Russia). The whole narrative is not just warped but entirely inverted: Russia is on a peacekeeping mission to liberate Ukraine from a Nazi regime led by (Jewish) President Volodymyr Zelenskyy; the Ukrainian army is preparing to use a "dirty bomb"; Ukraine's military casualties are enormous and Russia's are negligible or nonexistent; Ukrainian and Western reporting on the war is all fake news.[60] The Kremlin has so perfected the art of Orwellian "doublespeak" that, as Orwell put it himself, one gets "the feeling that the very concept of objective truth is fading out of the world."[61]

Aspirant authoritarians, unable to enlist quite the same brutal forces of censorship as employed by established despots like Putin, are, however, learning from Trump's wrecking-ball assault on democracy. In Poland, the ruling right-wing Law and Justice Party (PiS) has throttled the free press and denounced its critics as fake news propogandists, including my Sydney Law School colleague the internationally acclaimed jurisprudence and constitutional lawyer Wojciech Sadurski, who since mid-2019 has been facing one criminal charge and two civil (libel) suits for likening the Polish government to an "organised criminal group."[62] Meanwhile, Brazil's Jair Bolsonaro has preferred to generate his own fake news, as when he orchestrated waves of bogus stories about rival contenders during his successful campaign for the presidency in

2018,[63] and then ludicrously dismissed COVID-19 as a just "a little cold" that everyone is going to catch so "what are you afraid of?" The imbecilic tenor of these remarks must surely have grated on the families of the one thousand Brazilians per day who were dying of the disease at the time.[64]

It is no mere coincidence that today communication technologies lie at the heart of voice control. While technology has massively inflated our capacities to broadcast and to access information, it has also expanded the opportunities and means for the manipulation and control of information. Now everyone is an author, photographer, filmmaker, or artist. Internet influencers don't just persuade you to buy whatever will make your life whole. They also tell you what to think, how to vote, what to say, and how to say it. And they can be presidents or profiteers (or both). Most of all they tell you what you *want* to hear. Sure, you can do some filtering yourself, and some of us are adept at using IT as a tool. But we are all, increasingly, passive rather than active users, gatherers rather than hunters, with our newsfeeds and online movie choices now autoselected by algorithmic predictors based on our previous choices (or passive acceptances).[65] More than anything, we are now the unwitting objects of the technology corporations and government agencies that control cyberspace.

In our overwhelming subscription to and reliance on online platforms of all sorts, we engage not just in accessing and disseminating images, information, and opinion but also in submitting ourselves by our keystrokes to rafts of back office psychoanalysis and exploitation. Information for or from us is forensically filtered, customized, and preferenced or blocked, and information about us is compiled, enriched, categorized, stored, and onsold almost always without our knowledge, still less our permission.

In terms of controlling what people seek, say, and share online, nowhere on Earth is that power as suffocatingly complete as it is in China. The Communist Party there has in effect weaponized the internet, turning it into a sophisticated tool of social surveillance and political manipulation. Moving far beyond its fabled "Great Firewall," the government has constructed what John Lanchester calls a "Giant Onion" that selectively nurtures and cocoons the citizenry at its center.[66] Comprising layer upon layer of word-sensitive filtration ("democracy," "Tiananmen," "free speech," "coronavirus coverup," and "Winnie the Pooh" [as a metonym for President Xi Jinping]),[67] all of which attract censure, armies of censors, harsh criminal sanctions, state media monopolies, and legions of flag-waving sycophants who flood social media with fake good news stories and jingoistic claptrap,[68] the system is truly formidable. No politically charged dissent of any kind is tolerated, whether from within or from outside the country, with Beijing's speedy erasure from Weibo and WeChat of WHO's May 2022 statement questioning the sustainability of China's "zero-tolerance" policy on COVID-19 being but one more example of the leadership's techno-totalitarianism.[69]

Such uncompromising control of political discourse flies in the face of John Milton's passionate counsel nearly four hundred years ago: "When complaints [against the state] are freely heard, deeply considered, and speedily reform'd then is the utmost bound of civil liberty attained,"[70] and it also stands against history, which records all such despotic efforts as eventually ending in failure. But these are cold comforts for those who must presently endure such corrupted civil liberty where the freedom to complain or contest is displaced by a tyrannical duty of political fealty.

While not without their own concerns over increasing levels of state surveillance, citizens in Western states are also focused on the free speech responsibilities of the corporations that own and control social media platforms.[71] Few deny that screening social media for violent, abusive, or exploitive content is necessary, but the questions still remain, How well and against what criteria are the media giants like Google, Facebook, and Twitter doing it, and what else are they—or should they be—screening?[72] The deplatforming (and subsequent replatforming) of Donald Trump (among others) by Twitter and Facebook, as well as the latter's much-vaunted and -criticized establishment of an independent "Oversight Board,"[73] signals how seriously these questions are being taken and that the possible answers are a moving feast.[74]

As the handwringing of media corporations, lawmakers, and the rest of us clearly shows, we are only beginning to think about speech in complicated ways befitting an era of information flows driven by online social media juggernauts.[75] The "vast democratic forums of the internet," as the US Supreme Court has labeled them,[76] together with preexisting physical forums, offer opportunities as well as challenges for all of us concerned with liberty's task of hammering out the boundaries of free speech and the responsibilities that come with them.

Love

What's the State Doing in Your Bedroom?

Their Land of Heart's Desire,
Where beauty has no ebb, decay no flood,
But joy is wisdom, time an endless song.
—W. B. Yeats

The last time she had laid eyes on her husband she was nineteen years old and six months pregnant. Sixty-five years later he was still square-jawed and nuggety; she, still a wisp of a thing with dancing eyes and a winsome smile. They held each other at arm's length for an age, trying to take it all in, before she looped a simple gold watch engraved with both their names around his wrist, telling him, "I've always regretted not being able to give [you] a watch." South Korean Lee Soon-kyu and North Korean Oh In-se (as they are today) had become separated one day in September 1950 during the initial months of the Korean War. Their house ended up on the South Korean side of the border after the war ended in 1953. Lee made it to her home, in which she brought up their son, never moving out and never remarrying, hoping against hope that one day Oh would return.[1]

The governments of the two countries into which their homeland was divided are still technically at war (fighting ended with an armistice, not a peace treaty), yet every few years or so, when relations between the two Koreas are sufficiently cordial, they agree to permit groups of such reunions to take place. The reunions are always held in the North and are closely supervised by its pathologically paranoid regime. Typically, the meetings last only a few hours, and there are never any second chances. Lee and Oh will die apart.

Does Love Conquer All?

The love between Lee and Oh certainly endured, but one can hardly say that it was free or that it conquered all. Love's power is nevertheless legendary. No matter the odds, it flourishes in the most challenging circumstances, at the strangest times, and between the unlikeliest protagonists. From Antony and Cleopatra, and Helen of Troy and Paris, to Romeo and Juliet, Heathcliff and Catherine. Gertrude Stein was devoted to Alice Toklas, declaring that in love "one must dare to be happy." Eleven-year-old Tom Buergenthal (later a judge on the International Court of Justice) survived both Sachsenhausen and Auschwitz, never losing faith that he would be reunited with his mother (he was, in 1947).[2] After twenty-four years a slave in Caroline County, Virginia, the first thing Hawkins Wilson did when he was freed was to begin searching for his sister from whom he had been separated when sold:—if "we do not meet on earth," he wrote, "we might indeed meet in heaven" (there is no record of either).[3] And so it goes on, tale after tale of ordinary as well as extraordinary love and case after case of remarkable fealty to its demands and responsibilities.

But are we really free to love? At the level of psychology there is certainly room to doubt it. We have, it is often said, little control over affairs of the heart. People love all manner of things—deities, ideas, fauna and flora, inanimate objects, machines and buildings, anime characters, and extraterrestrial beings, as well as one another (whether alive or dead) and, of course, themselves.[4] Brain scans of people who had recently fallen in love analyzed by social psychologist Arthur Aron show that new lovers have the same complex brain activity as occurs after taking cocaine.[5] A coup de foudre, as the French (well, yes, it would be, wouldn't it?) label the potency of this chemical and emotional rush. Though unlike a thunderbolt (its literal translation), such sudden and overwhelming elation often defies rational explanation. "Objective knowledge doesn't come into it," argues philosopher Alain de Botton; "what matters instead is intuition: a spontaneous feeling that seems all the more accurate and worthy of respect because it bypasses the normal processes of reason."[6] Or, as W. B. Yeats puts it rather more poetically in the lines at the head of this chapter, love's ethereal embrace can make us believe in a sublime fantasy world far removed from the flawed real one we actually inhabit.[7]

So, at the level of the inscrutable intricacies of our individual psychologies, a conscious *choice* of who, what, when, and how we love may not be much in play.[8] This is not to say, however, that choices are not made by ourselves and by others for us. Expectations, directions, requirements, and even proscriptions—some loud and demanding, but many others quietly imposed—surround matters of endearment. It is a fixture of the human condition that we can be foolish, unlucky, mistaken, and unhappy in love, but we can be the opposite of all of these as well. Indeed, it is often not quite knowing which end of the spectrum you're occupying (if not both at the same time) that makes love so confoundingly alluring. So exquisite is the emotion that the lines between adoration and destruction, bliss and misery—between love and hate, in fact—can be blurred to the point of abstraction. Few have expressed the character of this incongruity better than Oscar Wilde when reflecting on his catastrophic relationship with the vainglorious Lord Alfred Douglas:

Yet each man kills the thing he loves,
By each let this be heard,
Some do it with a bitter look,
Some with a flattering word,
The coward does it with a kiss,
The brave man with a sword!

Some kill their love when they are young,
And some when they are old;
Some strangle with the hands of Lust,
Some with the hands of Gold:
The kindest use a knife, because
The dead so soon grow cold.

Some love too little, some too long,
Some sell, and others buy;
Some do the deed with many tears,
And some without a sigh:
For each man kills the thing he loves,
Yet each man does not die.[9]

Love's cruel dark side, its capriciousness, our temperamental responses to its grip, and the searing consequences of its loss—it's all there in the rawness of Wilde's words.

Yet, despite—or perhaps because of—such dangers, we all seek it, often fervently, and some of us find it. Thus, for every Wildean tale of caution in love, there are many in which caution is thrown to the wind in the chase and its glorious embrace. Falling in love, writes Louis de Bernières, is like "a temporary madness. It erupts like volcanoes and then subsides."[10] Love's draw is irresistible, adds A. S. Byatt; "no mere human can stand in [its] fire and not be consumed."[11] At once both intoxicating and disturbing, love's enigma never wains.

Love Is in the Air

Insofar as our psychological predispositions do allow or demand, we are in fact generally free to love who or what we want. Our private infatuations, as it were, are all well and good, provided they remain private. It is once they enter the public domain, by way of how we *express* our love, that we run the risk of censure or interference. Not always, of course, but often enough, and often without us realizing it. No matter the fact that love is such an intensely personal affair for every one of us, how we choose to practice it attracts an inordinate amount of public attention. Family, friends, strangers, and the community at large, as well as the law, all have their say in one way or another.

In this regard one can see some similarity to the domain of health (explored in chapter 3). Certainly, the two are closely related, especially when thinking in terms of one's mental health. But in the context of their respective relations with freedom and its responsibilities, love is qualitatively different. Here it is more like happiness, in that both are peculiarly personal and compelling forces in our lives. Indeed, so closely aligned are they that for some, like veteran psychiatrist George Vaillant, the former director of the world's lengthiest longitudinal study of human development, they are one and the same. "Happiness *equals* love—full stop," says Vaillant.[12] Whatever the extent of their overlap, the pursuit of love, like the pursuit of happiness, ought to provide no significant practical reasons for interference or hindrance aside from obvious deleterious effects that the pursuit of either might have on others. Ideally, argued Simone de Beauvoir, we "should be . . . capable of loving a woman or a man; either, a human being, without feeling fear, restraint, or obligation."[13]

That, however, hardly settles the matter, because the concerns of love are far beneath the ideal and much more than the merely practical. Love is so tightly bound up in our social relations that its evocation of strong political emotions is an inevitability. At the most basic level, anthropologists tell us, love in all its various forms is a social glue critical to our survival and evolution as individuals and communities and as a species.[14] Romantic love between a man and a woman ("pair bonding"), for example, is seen as biologically significant because it secures mutual care and protection, nurturing, and a combined commitment toward raising any children they might have.[15] And as romantic love, in some form or other, is to be found in all cultures, so cultural mores, social expectations, political interference, and legal (and religious) prescriptions all make demands on how it manifests itself.[16] From the Kama Sutra and the poems of Sappho, to China's Butterfly Lovers and the Celts' Tristan and Isolde, tales of romance are found throughout the world's ancient literatures.

Romantic love is certainly not, as anthropologists now somewhat shamefacedly admit was once assumed, either a product of medieval European thought or confined to the ruling classes, which have the time and opportunity for such indulgence.[17] No matter how hard one's life or dire the circumstances, romance nonetheless blossoms. Even when fighting a war in the Vietnamese jungle.

One evening some years ago, during my time working with a team of scholars at the Vietnamese Institute of Human Rights in Hanoi, I found myself sitting beside the wife of the institute's then director at a celebratory dinner for the whole team. She was a strikingly elegant, beautifully dressed woman in her sixties, poised and very proper; a fitting contrast to her slightly disheveled, intellectually impish husband, with whom I had been working closely for many months. It was the first time I had met her, and as is often the way with casual conversations in Vietnam, banter around the table moved to relationships, past, present, and possible.

I politely inquired how my colleague and his wife had met, to which he responded with a wry grin and she with a shy cough.

It was during the war (the "American War," as the Vietnamese call it), my professorial friend explained, when North Vietnamese soldiers conscripted teams of villagers to dig trenches as the fighting raged across tracts of jungle. It was difficult and dangerous work. The teams were separated by gender in the belief that temptations of the flesh would thereby not hamper the task at hand, and rewards were offered to the teams that dug the fastest. "But the military had not counted on the ingenuity of the women," my colleague noted. "They stripped off all their clothes," he added with a chuckle, which not only made the women's work more comfortable in the stifling heat but also—they knew—created a major distraction for the male teams working nearby, whose digging speed and efficiency duly suffered. "That's how I first saw my wife!" he concluded with an animated flourish and a teasing wag of a finger. His wife just smiled and gently placed her hand on his. The mind boggled.

Love and Subversion

It is true that while romance may be universal, it nevertheless can "look very different in different places," according to social anthropologist Dredge Kang.[18] Exuberant or reticent, public or private, open or secret, mutual or unreciprocated, fulfilling or not, wherever and whenever love is found, commentary and interference from others, including the state, is seldom far away. Whichever the case, the very fact that falling in love can evoke such strong, uncompromising passions is reason enough that the condition is "seen by many peoples throughout the world as dangerous and subversive."[19] As a result, romantic love and how it is practiced may be restricted or repressed by economic exigencies or cultural mores (as through arranged marriages in many South

Asian countries), by laws (governing issues such as age of consent, bigamy, and sexuality), or by social or familial expectations (as demonstrated by the fact that in most countries "structural patterning" predominates with like still tending to partner with like).

Structural patterning is a remarkably powerful force precisely because it is self-imposed. Unlike either overt cultural norms or social expectations, and unlike express legal mandates, it appears to be the result of individuals making decisions of their own accord over whom, where, when, and how they bestow their affections. Love's social mosaic, in other words, is shaped by people's deeply held preferences that anticipate community expectations and thereby help perpetuate a particular social order. The patterning appears to evolve naturally, of its own volition, rather than by persuasion or coercion, and to reflect drivers that are both conscious and subconscious.

From his research on pairing, Dredge Kang sees socioeconomics and race as two of the most important defining features of this phenomenon. Relationships in most Western countries, he ventures, are "still very highly structured . . . there aren't so many marriages where people cross class, and then when they do, it's much rarer for the male to be of a lower status than the female." Crossing racial divisions is even rarer, especially when transnational and reflecting very different cultural traditions. Even in countries known for their tolerance of interracial relationships, social pressures can nevertheless prove decisive. Drawing on his work in Thailand, for example, Kang observes that nowadays the sight of a Thai (whether male or female) with a Caucasian male is so strongly associated with the country's somewhat notorious sex trade that many Thais are greatly disinclined to partner with a Caucasian man, no matter what their feelings might be for him.[20]

All sorts of love-related behavior are in fact regulated by our individual interpretations of love's limits and responsibilities, of its prescriptions and proscriptions, both formal and informal. Our interpretations of the "liberty of love," one might say. Who we deem suitable partners and how we show it; what levels of devotion and commitment we make to our families or to our friends, or creed, or country; and whether and how we might love all manner of other things, from pets and places to hobbies and heroes. Sometimes we flout these rules—by pairing with a tremendously unsuitable partner, by estranging families or friends, or by dedicating oneself to the patience-trying sporting team—but more often we follow them, whether consciously or not. But, however it manifests itself, it is our capacity for self-censorship that so appeals to those concerned to interfere with the balance between our freedoms and responsibility in love.

It is not without reason that the Ministry of Love in George Orwell's dystopian novel *1984* has responsibility for maintaining law and order, which it carries out by inculcating in people a sense of growing pride the deeper their abstinence from any sort of intimacy. "A real love affair was an almost unthinkable event," Orwell writes, emphasizing how successfully self-denial has been socialized throughout the citizenry of his Oceania and how much power Big Brother and The Party exert over everyone's lives.[21] In reality, we may not have any Ministries of Love—though Afghanistan, under the Taliban, once again has a Ministry for the Propagation of Virtue and the Prevention of Vice, and Spain, representing a very different interpretation of the issue, has a so-called minister of sex[22]—but everywhere there are government agencies aplenty concerned with law and order, censorship, and family planning.

It is here that we are getting to the nub of what so often exercises the interests of others in our love lives. For the stark fact of the matter is that who or what we love is often far less important than how we love. Or, more specifically, whether and how sex is involved.

What's Sex Got to Do with It?

Regarding love's freedoms and responsibilities there seems to be no more compelling a matter for others to get bothered about than the extent to which lust accompanies our love and leads to sexual relations of some kind or other.

If the proverbial Martian were to pay us a terrestrial visit on almost any occasion when sex is on the table (the subject matter, that is)—and it's seldom far from any agenda—they would be forgiven for believing that perhaps we overthink the matter. Sure, it is the biological sine qua non of our species' survival, and certainly it is an integral component of our individual mental health and physical well-being, but, really, the Martian might ask with a raise of whatever goes for eyebrows on Mars, is it the root (sorry) of everything in human society? Well, "yes, just about," might be a fair answer. Of all modes of love's expression—acts of devotion and dedication, proclamations and declarations, sacrifices and supplication made in its name, signs of its fevered appropriation of our lives, and the all-consuming chasms it creates when lost—there is nothing quite like sex for attracting attention.[23] Obviously, the sexual intimacy of "making love" is not part of all loving relationships and not even necessarily the most important part in those relationships where it is, but our collective obsession with its realization—past, present, or possible—is matched only by the zeal of our leaders and many others to have their say on its propriety.[24]

Priests and politicians try to tell us what we can do, where we can do it, and with whom, even if they don't always follow the same rules themselves. Scientists and sexologists show us how it works, when it doesn't, and what we can do to make it better.

Storytellers and poets weave it into our dreams and remind us of its realities, and not a day passes without the sexual activities of someone or another being held up as an example of what, or what not, to do. You may not like or want any of this—though the odds are that at least some of it appeals—but you'd be hard-pressed to avoid it.[25]

Whenever sex, or the prospect of sex, forms part of any human encounter, it often exerts a disproportionate influence on the encounter's scope and outcome. Sometimes this is warranted, such as taboos regarding incest or bestiality, prohibitions of sex with minors or with anyone when consent is absent, and regulatory controls to protect sex workers, for example. Sometimes its high profile is debatable, such as whether and what to provide children by way of sex education, or to what extent the law should take account of adultery. At other times the hold sex has over matters ostensibly of much wider concern is simply astounding or ridiculous or dangerous (or all three).

The free market economy, for instance, would be crippled if the allure of sex was stripped out of selling what we all buy. Given the prescriptions of Catholic priesthood, it seems odd, to say the least, that sex occupies any part of the Church's teachings. Or, as George Bernard Shaw chose to put it: "Why should we take advice on sex from the Pope? If he knows anything about it, he shouldn't!"[26] And where consensual sexual relations are deemed to step outside presupposed norms, there is a public tendency to define the totality of the lives of those concerned as abnormal, if not immoral, deviant, unnatural, or some such. It is hard to think of any other single attribute of a person's existence that exerts such definitive power over how others see them.[27]

To the extent that sex forms a part of any of our relationships, when it is pursued in private between consenting adults, the question must be asked whether it is anyone else's business. Now, there may be good reasons why it is—a jilted lover or rudely awoken neighbor spring to mind—but, generally speaking, surely the matter should be free from interference, including and especially from state authorities. As defense counsel in one of America's most famous sexual privacy cases chose to frame it, the appropriate question should not be what we are doing in the privacy of our own bedrooms but what the state is doing in there with us. In *Bowers v. Hardwick* (1986) Michael Hardwick asked the US Supreme Court to uphold his right to privacy to have sex with another man in his own bedroom by declaring the anti-sodomy laws of the state of Georgia, under which he had been arrested, to be unconstitutional. The Court declined, rejecting, in more general terms, "the proposition that any kind of private sexual conduct between consenting adults is constitutionally insulated from state proscription."[28]

Although this particular ruling was later overturned, in 2003 in *Lawrence v. Texas*, when the Supreme Court pronounced a similar anti-sodomy law in Texas to be unconstitutional and upheld the right of all adults to sexual privacy, such laws used to be commonplace.[29] Legislating sexual morality was considered an essential part of good governance; it still is in many places. Sodomy has now been decriminalized across most of the globe, and many countries not only outlaw discrimination based on sexual orientation but also permit same-sex marriages.[30] But so-called alternative sexual behavior, and homosexuality in particular, is still proscribed in some sixty-nine countries (including eleven in which it is a capital offense), mostly in Africa and the Middle East.[31]

Religion and culture underpin such laws in ways that do not promise speedy reform. For example, you might expect human rights commissioners from any country to condemn discrimination on grounds of sexuality and to certainly not actively promote such discrimination. Yet that is precisely what I witnessed some years ago in a strange encounter involving members of the Iraqi Human Rights Commission, an openly gay Australian High Court judge, and a conscience-stricken interpreter. Michael Kirby, then one of Australia's most senior members of the bench, had just finished describing to the visiting Iraqi delegation the state of sexuality discrimination in Australia from both legal and personal points of view. I was chairing the meeting and had asked if our visitors had any questions. They had, and matters were proceeding normally when suddenly I noticed our interpreter—a man whom I knew to be highly competent and hitherto unflappable—becoming, well, decidedly flapped. An Iraqi delegate had just asked a question, and our interpreter was staring at the questioner, open-mouthed and seemingly unable or unwilling to translate. He recovered, stuttered a bit, and then turned to look at me (not Kirby, as would have been proper) and said something like, "Thank you for speech, it was very interesting." Now my Arabic is almost nonexistent, but even I knew that was not what had been said (whatever else it was, it was much longer and impassioned). From there things moved on to a timely and unremarkable conclusion, save a heavily sweating interpreter. It turned out that what was actually said was more along the lines of how appalled the interlocutor was to hear that Australia had openly gay judges. Our interpreter—breaching a fundamental tenet of interpreters' code of ethics, I'm sure— simply could not bring himself to convey such an insult to His Honor. A shame for many reasons, not least the fact that Kirby would almost certainly have addressed the comment with his trademark wit and trenchant rebuttal. So, alas, an opportunity went begging.

Sex Appeal

Restricting people's freedom to love as they wish by trying to police their lust has always been about control. Or *social* control, to be more precise. If not in the Orwellian sense (although that is certainly still the case for many of the above-mentioned sixty-nine countries with draconian anti-gay laws), then at least in terms of manipulating social expectations and fashioning cultural mores. Quite apart from what our legislators have to say on the matter, sex in all forms arouses intense passions far beyond its participants.

There is seemingly no end to the list of sex-related topics that agitate strong opinions, but at minimum they include abstinence, addiction, adultery, orientation, age of consent, education, masturbation, prostitution, the use of language or the use of condoms or sex toys (in Alabama it is illegal to sell sex toys of any kind unless for "medical, scientific [or] educational" purposes, while in Texas possession of more than six "obscene devices" is prohibited).[32] In some places lawmakers have been moved to legislate on permissible sexual positions or acts (oral sex is criminalized in Gambia and Indonesia and was banned in many US states until the Supreme Court decision in *Lawrence v. Texas*),[33] on tolerable public displays of affection (most Muslim countries prohibit public kissing, though holding hands is permitted provided you're married), and, as we saw earlier, what we should be allowed to do in private between consenting adults. Ahead, there are also a host of undeniably thorny questions to be added to this list regarding the impact of artificial intelligence—most especially, how should we regulate access to sexbots? Will we be able to marry robots? Is it adultery to have sex with one? What level of artificial augmentation turns our lover into a cyborg?[34]

What can be said about all this with some authority is that debate over the limits and responsibilities of our sexual freedoms is not only alive and well; it clearly has implications that reach far beyond the performance of the act itself. Like a stone thrown into a millpond, what we do in moments of passion ripples throughout our private and public worlds. The easiest way to understand how this is so is to reflect on why *others* seem to care so ardently about what happens during those moments. Why, in particular, are those who wish to police sexual activity so hell-bent on denying the pleasure it brings. Essayist and satirist H. L. Mencken's definition of puritanism, "the haunting fear that someone, somewhere, may be happy," captures the ascetic zeal that appears to drive so many social and religious conservatives. Denying, or at least controlling, sexual pleasure (your own and others) is one important way to maintain an established social order, so the reasoning goes.[35]

The argument is unashamedly moral. Planting your flag on its high ground apparently gives you the right to pronounce on many things, including, to be sure, how you and I choose to get our sexual kicks. Yet, while morality, and law, for that matter, certainly should and do have boundary-defining roles to play, both morals and laws are open questions, forever evolving, never entirely settled. Be that as it may, it can be fairly said that any quest to control love's lustful manifestations is ultimately doomed to fail precisely because of sex's innately subversive character. A vital part of its allure is its flirtation with or immersion in the forbidden. "Every model of morality or politically correct sexual behaviour *will be subverted* by nature's daemonic law,"[36] as Camille Paglia cautions all who might believe otherwise. She is surely correct.

Like flowing water negotiating any obstacle in its way, our bedroom (and elsewhere) peccadillos and perversions are too creatively agile to be effectively disciplined. And why should they be? What is so wrong, so problematic, so dangerous? Providing all the normal baseline conditions are met—between consenting adults, in private (or at least not causing public offense), and not otherwise criminal (like necrophilia or erotic asphyxiation)[37]—why concern ourselves at all with what others are doing (except, of course, for educational purposes)?

Attitudes toward sexuality have long been a litmus test of where we stand—as individuals and communities—on the question of the moral policing of sex. As indicated earlier, levels of tolerance in many countries have shifted markedly in recent years. Having watched closely the ultimately successful campaigns for same-sex marriage in surprisingly prudish Australia and in devout Ireland (both South and North, finally),[38] I, for one, found my faith in societies' capacities to overcome prejudice somewhat restored. The decisive vote in the Republic of Ireland's referendum on the matter (62 percent voted in favor) "has confirmed that our society's philosophy is one of inclusiveness," as Frances Fitzgerald, the country's minister for justice and equality, said at the time.[39]

With the dismantling of the moral and legal discriminations against those who choose to love in ways other than, or in addition to, conventional heterosexuality well under way in many places, it makes those obstacles still in place look all the more arcane and invidious. What good reasons can there have been, for instance, that twenty-eight US states until recently permitted employers to discriminate on the basis of sexuality or gender identity? In a triptych of cases brought before the Supreme Court in October 2019,[40] it was argued that such discrimination was in fact outlawed by the 1964 federal Civil Rights Act's prohibition of "discrimination because of . . . sex," which words should and could be read to encompass sexuality and gender identity.

No matter that the Court ruled in favor of this argument (and provided impetus for expanded protections of LGBTQI rights under the proposed federal Equality Act, which, as of early 2023, awaits Senate approval),[41] the fact remains that so many state legislatures believed questions about whom one has sex with or which gender one identifies with were relevant to employers when considering how well a person does their job. Workplace discrimination based on racial or religious grounds is prohibited, so why not sexuality or gender identity? What makes these grounds so different? Fear that toilets might have to be shared by members of the biologically opposite sex or that one's gender is an immutable (and binary only) gift from God just doesn't cut it.[42] And we're not talking here about some insignificant proportion of society—7.1 percent of American adults (some 18.3 million people) identify as gay, lesbian, bisexual, or transgender, or some combination.[43] The three cases referred to above attracted enormous attention—some seventy amici curiae briefs were filed with the court, representing more than one thousand individuals and organizations (corporations, trade unions, church groups, civil society, and the Department of Justice)[44]—reflecting once again the intensity of people's opinions about the proper place of sex, sexuality, and gender identity within the broader contexts of our lives.

Disputing the boundaries of sexual freedom is evidently not short of opportunities or fora in which to do so. Nor is it lacking in enthusiastic participation. In defining those boundaries, the negotiation of the responsibilities of sexual freedom, alongside love more broadly, plays a crucial part. None more so than the combustible question of whether we share our love and if so with whom.

Sharing Our Love

As a matter of fact, we are not monogamous lovers. We do spread it around. We love partners, family, friends, animals, idols, and things in different ways and often simultaneously. Mostly this is quite acceptable—to ourselves, to those we love, and to society at large. Sometimes, however, it is not, even while it happens every day and all around us. Loving more than one member of your family (hopefully all of them) equally, if differently, is quite possible and not unusual. It's the same with friends, animals, ideas, and things. But in the matter of one's chosen partner, the rules of love are entirely different. Alexandre Dumas (the younger) hit the nail on the head for more than a few of us when he wrote that "the chains of marriage are so heavy that it takes two to bear them, sometimes three," but that doesn't mean that affairs are condoned.[45] Far from it.

One Gallup poll of 1,535 American adults, for example, found that having an affair while married was considered far more morally reprehensible than abortion, teenage sex, suicide, cloning humans, or even polygamy, with 91 percent of respondents deeming it morally wrong.[46] Clearly, the breach of trust such trysts involve wounds deeply, even if their incidence is hardly uncommon. Which does rather beg the question whether we expect too much of ourselves. Celebrated relationship guru Esther Perel thinks we do. "Lovers today seek to bring under one roof desires that have forever had separate dwellings," she writes in her book *The State of Affairs*.[47]

Belgian by birth but living in the United States, Perel brings what one commentator has described as "a Continental exasperation with American mores" to her writing,[48] which might be one reason why her books are so wildly popular. She's not alone on that score, of course. Coincidentally, while writing an earlier draft of this chapter (in France, as it happens), a news story broke of a French court ruling that a company was liable to pay compensation to the family of one of its employees who had had a heart attack and died during sex with a stranger while on a business trip. The court accepted the reasoning that "Mr. X" (the employee in question) was simply engaged in a normal, everyday activity "like taking a shower or a meal," in the course of his job and so falling within the ambit of an industrial accident.[49] Readers from Anglo-Saxon jurisdictions may doubt that such an argument would ever be entertained by their courts. But despair (or rejoice) not. In reasoning almost identical to that used in the French case, an Australian court some seven years earlier had awarded workers' compensation to a federal government employee on a work trip who suffered facial and psychological injuries after a light fixture fell on her during sex with a stranger in her hotel room.[50]

Whether solemnized or not, our bonds to lovers do, or are expected to, limit our freedom. Such limitations or responsibilities are usually negotiated within the private realm. The perceived breaches of trust, however grave, are nowadays generally not the subject of legal disputes in Western countries, save as a part of divorce laws. Infidelity's threat to our emotional security, as Esther Perel puts it, is left largely to us to sort out ourselves.

The same is true in almost all instances of our nonsexual love of others, whether in platonic relations with companions or friends, or in families. The former flourish and wither according to all the usual vagaries of friendship and collegiality and, to that extent, are truly matters of our free choice. The latter, however, are in a category of their own. This is understandable given that the bonds of family are based on love born (often literally) of shared genes and that the family is, in turn, the essential building block of human society.[51] Cultures and communities across the globe and throughout history have all placed the family at the center of their social structures. The expectations made of familial bonds are therefore great: that we love our relations, no matter how varied in manner and form we express it. And, goodness me, what variety there is.

From the besotted intensity of a mother's love for her child, to the complicated but enduring feelings children have for their parents. The all-knowing, all-seeing, "you can't fool me" bonds between siblings and the "familiar alien" relationship between children and grand-parents (or parents), as well as the various permutations of attachment found throughout extended family relations however far they stretch.[52] Needless to say, little or no love (or even hate) also roam freely throughout family relationships, sometimes precipitated or accentuated by the very expectation that strong and abundant love should exist between family members. Few of us have not, at some time or other, shared George Burns's sentiment that "happiness is having a large, loving, caring, close-knit family in another city."[53]

Love's Responsibilities

There are, then, responsibilities of love that we must bear across all family relations, as well as between friends and between lovers, if love is to survive, let alone flourish. Trust, respect, compassion, care, sympathy and empathy and, perhaps above all, a sense of commitment need to be in the mix, albeit necessarily in differing proportions depending on the relationship. The obligation to love (that is, *not* to be free to choose either way) is surely strongest in the relationship parents have with their children. It is, in effect, nonnegotiable.

This means, as philosopher Matthew Liao argues, not only that children have a right to be loved but also that parents have a corresponding duty to love them.[54] What this duty entails in practice is of critical importance to both children and parents. For Liao it boils down to parents providing protection, nurture, and sacrifice in proportion to the child's needs. The more vulnerable the child, the more onerous the duty. The international human rights apparatus specializing in children's rights (headed by the UN Convention on the Rights of the Child, which promotes above all the "best interests of the child"),[55] along with rafts of domestic laws governing child protection and welfare, including authority to remove children from abusive or neglectful families, underlines the nature and extent of these obligations.[56]

The bonds of romance, as this chapter amply shows, are also tied in ways that tend very much toward obligation, at least until they are broken—a circular argument, I know, but one that seems to fairly represent how we treat such relationships. One imagines, for example, that the intentions behind each of the 700,000 or so couples who attached "love locks" to Paris's Pont des Arts before their removal in 2015, after their combined weight threatened to collapse the bridge, were indeed sincere, even if more than one or two have since gone the way feared for the bridge.[57]

Other, nonromantic loving relationships range widely, from the similarly uncompromising (devotion to deities, for example) to the more casual (as for a particular flavor of ice cream or a TV series—though I concede these can be life-or-death matters for some). In whichever form and however expressed, love is always a heartfelt impulse first and a negotiation second. When we find ourselves in its thrall, whether suddenly or by gradual realization, we may feel somewhat helpless before its onslaught: "Reason is, and ought only to be, the slave of the passions," as philosopher David Hume unsparingly warns us.[58] But love in all forms has limits and responsibilities that we are compelled to negotiate between ourselves, with others, and at times with or through the state. These are the demands that liberty makes of our love lives, yet in a matter so visceral, their fulfillment is often complicated and sometimes immensely difficult.

Communication is key. On which point I am drawn to conclude this chapter with sociologist Michelle Miller-Day's pithy representation of the many modes of communication we use as families in our efforts to "navigate cohesion and adaptability; create family images, themes, stories, rituals, rules, and roles; manage power, intimacy, and boundaries; and participate in an interactive process of meaning-making, producing mental models of family life that endure over time and across generations."[59] For as it is inside families, so it is likewise outside them, in the manner we as individuals and societies tackle the unending tasks of cultivating love's pleasures and shouldering its burdens.

10

Death
The Ultimate
Freedom?

Seeing that death, a necessary end,
Will come when it will come.
—William Shakespeare

That day in December 2010, he'd had enough. He just couldn't take it anymore. After years of almost daily harassment and extortion by the authorities of the small town of Sidi Bouzid in central Tunisia, the morning's slap in the face by a policewoman, on top of the confiscation of his weighing scales and produce for refusing to pay a bribe, sent street fruit vendor Mohamed Bouazizi over the edge. His immediate complaints to the local government officials were condescendingly dismissed. So he decided to buy a can of paint thinner, return to the local government building, pour the contents over his head and body, and set himself alight. He burned for long enough to ensure that his injuries were fatal, but not immediately. He died, in hospital, eighteen days later. He was twenty-six years old. It was a desperate act by a desperate young man.[1]

Since the age of twelve, Mohamed, the second eldest of seven children, had been his family's main breadwinner after his father had died when he was only three years old and after his elder brother moved to another town. He was an easy target for the

228

petty corruption and cruelty that so often characterizes countries
blighted by nepotistic authoritarianism, as was Tunisia at that time
under President Zine El Abidine Ben Ali.

Mohamed Bouazizi's plight was not unique. Thousands of
small traders like him were being similarly hounded everyday all
over Tunisia. He was not even the first to resort to self-immolation
in protest. But on that day on a dusty street in front of his tor-
mentors, Bouazizi's suicide struck a chord. Angry demonstrations
erupted in the town, which turned into deadly riots after Bouazizi
died. With social media recording the police firing live rounds
into the crowds, the unrest spread throughout the country with
such ferocity that just ten days later, Ben Ali was forced to flee
the country. It was the beginning of the "Arab Spring" movement,
which was to sweep across North Africa and the Middle East
throughout 2011.[2]

The Importance of Dignity

At one level you might say that Bouazizi chose to take his own
life; but equally you might argue that the choice was forced on
him. Either way, he felt compelled to act as he did. If he could
not live freely, it seems, he would end his life. At once both an
exercise of freedom and a bellow of rage and disgust. More than
poverty's daily struggle to make ends meet, what really affected
Mohamed was the humiliation, the demeaning subordination to
authority that was neither legitimate nor fair. "It got to him deep
inside, it hurt his pride,"[3] said his mother, Mannoubia, when interviewed about her posthumously famous son, adding that he
"did what he did for the sake of his dignity."[4]

In death, as in life, dignity is enormously important: whether
it is a slight to one's pride or self-esteem that prompts people to
kill others (and, my word, how history is littered with killing
to avenge bruised or battered egos) or to kill oneself, as did

Mohamed. Dignity is also a critical feature of the manner of one's demise—how you die, where, and when. Of course, these are matters we are seldom able to predict let alone dictate, but that doesn't stop us from craving their control, especially when, due to circumstances or age, mortality makes its presence more keenly felt.

It is precisely because death comes to us all, without exception, that we are lured toward wanting some degree of control over the occasion. I dare say most of us would agree with the sentiment expressed by iconic Japanese author Yukio Mishima: "If we value so highly the dignity of life, how can we not also value the dignity of death?" Even if, equally, most of us would not be keen on ritual self-disembowelment, as was Mishima's chosen means to depart this Earth in a dignified manner.[5] Less dramatical but no less telling is American medic and bioethicist Sherwin Nuland's critical examination of the common notion of "death with dignity." It is, he says, "society's expression of the universal yearning to achieve a graceful triumph over the stark and often repugnant finality of life's last sputterings." For those of us who are nodding in agreement after reading these words, however, Nuland offers a sober, scientific rebuttal. "Death is not a confrontation," he points out, but "simply an event in the sequence of nature's ongoing rhythms."[6]

Between these two representations we get glimpses of both the ethereally spiritual and the matter-of-factly physical elements of the idea of dignity surrounding death. But in the context of our quest in this book to understand living (or dying) with liberty, this takes us only so far. For so long as the freedoms and responsibilities of death are tied up with the notion of dignity, we need to know more about what both elements entail and how they relate to each other. Indeed, above all else, it is the message that human dignity transcends purely physical and factual circumstances to encompass impalpable metaphysical sentiments that makes the idea of dignity so attractive and so difficult to define.[7]

Undeniably, questions of physical comfort matter to someone entering the final chapter of life, but so—and maybe even more so—do questions of where, when, and precisely how they die, as well as with whom. For those suffering a terminal illness, for example, is it to be in hospital or at home, under palliative or resuscitative care, and alone, with loved ones, with medical staff, or with a member of the clergy? There can be few more poignant reminders of the significance of being with your loved ones (and of the significance for them too) at life's end than the many wrenching stories of self- or socially isolated people dying alone and untouched during COVID-19's global rampage.[8]

Dignity has long been associated with the soul—the essence of your being, your uniqueness, what makes you "you." And while contemplations of the soul (howsoever labeled) are important in life—as much of philosophy, religion, and the edifice of human rights all attest—it is in death that the soul takes on a special significance. The world's major religions all hold that a person's soul, in some form or other, either continues or is released by the person's physical expiration. For our souls, then, there is life after death. "We are stewards, not owners, of the life God has entrusted to us," according to the Catholic Church.[9] This sentiment is echoed in Islam through the Qur'anic pronouncement that each person's "life is God's gift," which, when ended, consigns their soul to the hereafter.[10]

Rationalist philosopher Immanuel Kant believed in the notion of stewardship of what he called our "personhood." "A man can indeed dispose over his [physical] condition," he argued, "but not over his person."[11] It is the intrinsic value carried by every human being that makes each of us an end in him- or herself, not a means to be used or abused by others. The inherent dignity of the individual is therefore preserved not only in their person when they are alive, but also after they have died. In this, Kant echoed Plato's conviction that every human has within them "a share of the divine attributes" such that their "soul exists" even after death.[12]

Killing . . .

What these prescriptions mean in terms of our freedoms and responsibilities concerning death is at its clearest when we consider the choices we make that cause or hasten our own death or the death of others. In either case, the roles we might or do play are bounded by all sorts of legal rules as well as social and ethical expectations. When the dignity of the individual is at the heart of these rules and expectations, as it so often is, the stakes are high. The array of killings relevant here is rich and varied. Murder, suicide, killing in self-defense, accidental death, capital punishment, deaths in combat, and euthanasia are some of the more obvious forms of death meticulously defined by law and hedged in social mores. But the list also extends to mercy killings, ritualistic sacrifice, killing to save others, and even the use and care of cadavers. Regarding relevant questions of dignity and liberty, however, things are not always as one might expect with some of these deadly matters.

. . . Extraordinarily

Thus, for example, exultation of respect for (and from) the victim was at the core of the Aztecs' industrial-scale programs of ritualistic sacrifice. It was an enormous honor and guaranteed passage to a blessed afterlife to be chosen to mount the altar and have your still-beating heart cut from your body and offered to the sun god Huitzilopochtli. Apparently, many did so willingly.[13] Present-day Islamist suicide bombers are also promised jihadic martyrdom (*istishhad*) to which is attached the reward of eternal bliss in the next world. Extreme though these examples are, both appeal to highly ordered sets of freedoms and responsibilities.

In which case, knowing that the majority of the Aztecs' sacrificial victims were captured enemies—indicating that they likely had little choice but to embrace the prospect of entering the sun god's kingdom—doesn't alter the fact that the manner of such deaths, no matter how brutal in our eyes, was viewed as culturally essential and religiously ordained by the Aztecs. Likewise, while many Muslims believe that only *defensive* jihad makes a martyr (offensive jihad, in contrast, is just killing and will consign the killer to the fires of Hell), many others read the Qur'an and Sunnah (social and legal custom) as endorsing the actions of suicide bombers.[14] The point is that in both of these cases the relevant communities, rightly or wrongly, are or were engaged in negotiating the boundaries between individuals' freedoms and responsibilities in death.

In a similarly bizarre vein, the responsibilities of preserving some sense of propriety or dignity are also to be found reflected in the death penalty protocols in some jurisdictions. All of the twenty-seven US states that retain capital punishment have replaced the electric chair with lethal injection as the preferred means of execution, because it is considered more humane and more effective, though still, apparently, far from painless or problem free.[15] Coincidentally, the same reasoning is used in China regarding its switch from firing squad to lethal injection as the favored means of dispatch.[16] Further, in the United States the Supreme Court has been active on this issue, ruling in 1972 that the then-prevailing laws regarding capital punishment were so arbitrary (the range of capital offenses being considered too broad and inconsistent) and discriminatory (being imposed disproportionately on Black defendants) that they transgressed the Eighth Amendment's prohibition on "cruel and unusual punishments."[17]

After these flaws were largely fixed to the satisfaction of the Supreme Court in another case four years later,[18] the Court ruled that the death penalty cannot be imposed for crimes committed by persons under the age of eighteen. Here again the Court invoked the Eighth Amendment's cruelty proscription in its reasoning, alongside what the judges referred to as "evolving standards of decency" within the United States. In addition, the Court was persuaded by the fact that internationally the death penalty of juvenile offenders has now been almost universally outlawed or disavowed, even in countries such as China and Saudi Arabia (though not yet Iran), all of which execute many more convicted criminals than does the United States.[19]

The same awkward sense of responsibility to temper suffering in death is evident in international laws covering humanitarian and criminal matters. The presumed "freedom" to kill in war and conflict may (or may not) be born of sufficiently serious grievances to justify such extreme action, but whatever the case, there are, according to international law, responsibilities that ride alongside. The freedom to kill, in other words, is not unrestricted, not even in the heat of battle and its aftermath. "*Some* humanity" must be retained, as the International Committee of the Red Cross puts it. In light of the long and dreadful history of armed conflict, this endeavor might seem forlorn, even hopeless, but it is in fact an earnest and necessary effort to reaffirm what else human civilization stands for. The 1949 Geneva Conventions and associated protocols are aimed at preserving the lives and welfare of prisoners of war, the wounded, and civilians and other noncombatants by imposing relevant duties on states themselves. States are obliged to treat everyone in the above-named categories with humanity and fairness, including prohibitions on murder and torture. States are also banned from using "weapons that cause superfluous injury or unnecessary suffering" or cause "widespread, long-term and severe damage to the natural environment."[20]

International laws covering war crimes and crimes against humanity take a different tack by focusing on making the perpetrators themselves (rather than states) responsible for their actions. While accepting that the killing of human beings can be and is legitimately pursued in war and armed conflict, these laws once again restrict what this means in practice. Beyond the many atrocities short of death prohibited by international criminal law, those specifically related to killing comprise genocide, murder (including the targeting of civilian populations during military operations), extermination (chillingly defined as including "deprivation of access to food and medicine, calculated to bring about the destruction of part of a population"), and the use of unusually cruel weapons such as poisonous gases, liquids, or other materials, or expanding, or otherwise doctored, bullets.

These are the conditions as stipulated in the 1998 Rome Statute, which established the International Criminal Court (the world's foremost international criminal law institution),[21] and while they are notable and commendable, conspicuously absent from the list of prohibitions is the use of chemical and biological weapons, nuclear weapons, land mines, and cluster munitions.[22] Restrictions on all of these were discussed during the Rome Statute's long negotiations, but none could be agreed upon, showing the still-yawning chasm that exists between hope and expectation in some areas of mass killings. Though perhaps unsurprising, the consequences of such bureaucratic impasses are nonetheless sobering. It means, for example, that as things stand, there exists not even the theoretical possibility of holding Bashar al-Assad to account before the International Criminal Court specifically for his barbarous and repeated use of chemical weapons against his own people during Syria's ongoing civil war.[23]

. . . Justifiably

In terms of the more ordinary, or at least more common, circumstances of killing, the boundaries of freedom and responsibility are often and well trammeled. In most countries, much is, in fact, already settled by laws and established social standards. Typically, therefore, criminal codes prohibit the taking of another's life under any circumstances, the only exceptions being restrictively defined and closely policed. Murder (by definition) is absolutely proscribed, while unintentional killing or killing in self-defense, though not endorsed, attracts lesser penalties or even none at all. Homicide, or the killing of another human being, is never truly freely permitted, and even where it is deemed justifiable or excusable, there are vast differences between levels of acceptable defenses.

Thus, the failure of a train driver to stop in time when someone suddenly throws themselves onto the track is of an order of responsibility completely different from the recklessness of an intoxicated driver who knocks down and kills someone on a pedestrian crossing. In both cases there is some causal connection between the driver and the deceased—both are directly responsible for the resultant death—but the culpability of the car driver is distinct and substantial, while that of the train driver is negligible if not nonexistent. Circumstances matter, as do our changing perspectives of them. So, where once a woman who killed her persistently and seriously abusive partner would be adjudged a murderer, or guilty of manslaughter at best, the evolution of the concept of "battered woman syndrome" in both legal and medical circles in recent years has led to greater consideration being given to the mitigating or even exonerating circumstances of the woman's actions.[24]

Such cases are never easily decided—having to rely on demonstrating the necessity of self-defense—and they are certainly not easy reading. But they do provide vivid illustrations of how we as individuals, and as societies more broadly, negotiate the often-complicated responsibilities that accompany actions that cause the death of another.

Take, for example, the plight of Barbara Sheehan of Queens, New York, who in February 2008 shot and killed her husband of twenty-four years in the home they shared with their two children. Mr. Sheehan was shaving at the time he was shot (his body was found on the bathroom floor with the faucet still running), so given that Mrs. Sheehan never denied shooting him, the case hinged on whether she could establish sufficient grounds to satisfy the standard for self-defense under the New York State penal code. That standard requires proof that the defendant was facing "imminent use of unlawful physical force" at the time the homicide took place.[25]

The litany of years of vicious physical abuse suffered by Barbara Sheehan tendered in court by her lawyers, including details of a ferocious argument and an assault the day before the incident, would not necessarily amount to proof of such imminent danger. What it did, however, was to provide the context in which the jury considered evidence that, following the previous day's events, Ms. Sheehan had decided to leave, retaining one of her husband's guns for protection. Upon seeing her the next day as she was preparing to leave, Mr. Sheehan picked up another gun sitting on the bathroom vanity and aimed it at her. It was then that Ms. Sheehan shot her husband. This context, including the fact that she had a gun pointed at her, convinced the jury to acquit Ms. Sheehan of the murder charges she faced. Speaking to the media after the verdict, Sheehan's lawyer was somber: "There is no joy today," he said. "The only thing that can bring joy to this family would be to bring them back 17 years before the first blow was struck."[26]

In many (though by no means all) jurisdictions today,[27] statutes and courts accommodate demonstrated histories of domestic violence in murder or manslaughter trials by way of such legal devices and provisions as self-defense (or "defensive homicide"), provocation, and diminished responsibility.[28] The arguments and debates that so often swirl around such cases reflect the dynamic processes by which the law and societal expectations are defined and redefined in this area. While the Sheehan case is an especially vivid example, it nevertheless fairly represents how the boundaries between freedom and responsibilities are negotiated in the matter of killing more broadly.

The elemental role of dignity in human rights laws also comes to the fore when considering reasons for protecting and taking lives. What, for instance, does human rights law say about legislation that permits war planes to shoot down a civilian airliner hijacked by terrorists? According to the Constitutional Court of Germany, which was faced with this very question regarding a statute enacted in the wake of the 9/11 atrocities, the law is invalid precisely because by treating human beings (the plane's passengers and crew) as expendable, it violates the notion of the inherent individual dignity that lies at the heart of the human rights protections in Germany's Constitution. The argument that "their killing [was] being used to save others" could never justify the "absolutely inconceivable" circumstance of their being "treated as objects."[29]

Similar human dignity arguments were raised against then–prime minister Boris Johnson's astonishing idea, floated during the early days of COVID-19, to let the disease spread unchecked through the United Kingdom in an effort to hasten herd immunity. The notion was soon dropped after the release of a study by scientists at Imperial College London predicting that such a strategy would likely cost 250,000 lives.[30] Whether it was the size of that number that convinced the prime minister to ditch the plan or the belated realization of the inhumanity of sacrificing any number of lives in such a manner is a moot and somewhat disturbing point.[31]

The killing of others (or the occasioning of their death) sits peculiarly in the context of this book in that liberty's baseline holds that there is no freedom to kill, just responsibilities not to and, more generally, to save life rather than take it. Negotiations over boundaries, therefore, are focused on exceptions to this general rule. However, the ground shifts somewhat when we alter our perspective to consider the libertarian connotations of killing oneself, as well as the contentious issue of enlisting the assistance of others to help one do so.

Suicide

The ground shifts because we might suppose that to kill oneself is the *ultimate* freedom. Ultimate, that is, not only in terms of the existential finality of the choice but also in terms of the presumption that if ever there was a choice for you alone to make, it is surely when and how you take your own life. Whatever the reasons and whatever the situation, it is for you, so this argument goes, to decide. It seems pretty certain that was how Mohamed Bouazizi saw it, and the choice is clearly reflected in Shakespeare's portrayal of Prince Hamlet's famous contemplation.

Facing diabolical circumstances (father murdered by tyrannical uncle; uncle now king; mother now married to said uncle; father's ghost imploring Hamlet to avenge his death), the prince of

Denmark surveys his options.[32] Top of the list is whether he should end it all: "To be or not to be, that is the question." He weighs the pros and cons of "shuffl[ing] off this mortal coil," without knowing, of course, what really lies on the other side of life ("the undiscovered country" that "puzzles the will"). It is splendidly poetic stuff, but what is of particular interest to us is Hamlet's unquestioned presumption that the decision is his to make. He mulls over the nobility of suicide and the bravery required to go through with it regardless of how desperately one might wish to end the suffering of "heartache, and the thousand natural shocks that flesh is heir to." Nary a reference is made to what might stop him, besides himself.

Yet "there's the rub" (to borrow again from Hamlet), for are we indeed free to procure our own demise? And to the extent that we are, with what attendant responsibilities? There are a number of relevant considerations here, beginning with questions of moral responsibility, moving on to calculations of the impact on others, and ending up with reflections on the legality of suicide.

With respect to morality, we have already encountered the religious perspective that we are but stewards of our souls, which belong to some higher authority and are not therefore ours to dispose of. Suicide is wrong according to the Christian Church, and in the eyes of Islam, Mohamed Bouazizi committed a sin when he burnt himself to death. Immanuel Kant added a secular but no less devout belief that we are subordinated keepers of our transcendental essence, our individual humanity, that which separates us from all other living things. There are, however, many who contest these viewpoints, including most of Kant's fellow Enlightenment thinkers. David Hume, Voltaire, and Jean-Jacques Rousseau, among others, all thought the religious (and secular) proscriptions on suicide were preposterous. In his essay *Of Suicide*, Hume, for example, debunked the idea that suicide was a transgression of our duty to God. The laws of nature, as ordained by the Deity, he argued, entrust in all humans "their own prudence and skill for their conduct in the world," which includes the free disposal of their own lives where circumstances might warrant. When they do so warrant, according to Hume, suicide ought to be understood as "our duty to ourselves" rather than a dereliction of any duty to "false religion," as he cuttingly adds.[33]

Acts of suicide, still less contemplation of it, need not be—and seldom are—as dramatic as with either Mohamed Bouazizi or Hamlet, or as profound as portrayed by priests and philosophers. But the consequences for those around suicide can be just as devastating. Accounts of the psychological impact on families and friends of those who have chosen this path are often as compellingly grave as the reasons that drove their loved one to take their own life. The toll on those left behind after a suicide can be terrible. On top of grief, many exhibit "feelings of guilt, anger, resentment, remorse, confusion over why it happened, distress over unresolved issues and in some instances, even relief."[34] When we die "the ones who love us will miss us," as actor Keanu Reeves pithily put it when tossed an unexpectedly metaphysical question during an interview on live television.[35]

The plight of these so-called suicide survivors (which, according to Harvard Medical School research, number at least six people per suicide)[36] is a critical, if often overlooked or underestimated, aspect of debates concerning the freedoms and responsibilities of suicidal death. Because so many suicides appear to be caused by severe depression or anxiety,[37] those who remain are left wondering whether they could and should have done more to help. After all, one's natural and usually overwhelming inclination is to do anything to prevent someone close to you from killing themselves. For despite the all-consuming awfulness of severe depression, which "causes one to see the entire world as pain," as clinical psychiatrist Charles Raison describes it,[38] there is always the hope, however slight it may seem at the time, that it will ease or even pass. But what are the respective rights, freedoms, and responsibilities here?

Are those around or close to suspected suicides justified in doing, or even obliged to do, whatever it takes to save them? Or might their actions be cruel, at least in some cases, by prolonging the agony of the sufferer and effectively denying them relief or escape? Dr. Raison is not alone in his profession when he confesses, "I've 'guilted' acutely suicidal patients into not killing themselves for the sake of their children and have done so with a clear conscience." We might all do the same thing if faced with such circumstances and if we have the wit and wherewithal to deploy such a technique. The patient and their children might also be inordinately grateful, and their lives might return to a more even keel. But is it—at least potentially—unfairly restricting individual freedom, selfishly imposing our will on another? It would be a brave person to argue as much, for it hinges on the near impossible calculus of weighing the present and future quality of life of *everyone* concerned. Either way, it is undeniably a factor, a relevant question to ask, even if in practice it is nearly always dismissed.

Dismissing the question is perhaps even more likely when we consider the sociological implications of suicide. From Émile Durkheim's pathbreaking account of its causes and consequences in the nineteenth century,[39] to harrowing analyses of youth suicide today (globally, fifteen to twenty-nine years old is the most susceptible age group), including outbreaks of near epidemic proportions in places as disparate as Russia, Guyana, South Africa, and Finland, there can be no doubt that the matter resonates powerfully in many societies.[40]

However one views suicide, the fact is that today the matter is much talked about. It remains a taboo in some communities and illegal in some countries, but overall the subject is now more openly discussed and better understood. The religious morality attached to its propriety has been dropped in most places (strong Muslim states excepted), and its decriminalization is now widespread.[41] The close causal connection between suicide and mental illness, especially depression, is now so universally recognized that today suicide is approached more as a medical concern than a legal one.[42] And it is within the context of mental health and all the social questions it raises that the freedoms and responsibilities surrounding people taking their own lives are now most commonly debated and expectations set.

Lending a Helping Hand

Assisting people in ending their own lives, on the other hand, is treated very differently. In view of the heavy toll suicide exacts on individuals, families, and societies, it is not surprising that assisting someone in committing the act has attracted such fierce controversy. Cases like that involving American teenager Michelle Carter, who in 2017 was convicted of involuntary manslaughter for encouraging her then-boyfriend, Conrad Roy, to commit suicide, have been lightning rods for deep concerns about permitting others to play any role in helping someone end their life.[43] Carter peppered Roy with hundreds of text messages goading him to do it right up to the point when he switched on the portable generator that pumped carbon monoxide into the pickup truck he was sitting in. There was evidence that Roy was depressed and that he had previously tried to kill himself, but the jury was nonetheless convinced that Carter's repeated and explicit interventions were critical in tipping him over the edge. It's hard not to agree given Roy's fragile state, especially when the texts included: "You need to do it Conrad. The more you push it off, the more it will eat at you." It was the apparently overwhelming effect such encouragement had on Roy's free will that has since led to the introduction of a bill into the Massachusetts legislature criminalizing coerced suicide.[44]

Such cases, however, are exceptional and by no means the whole story of "assisting" suicide or otherwise aiding another to end their life. The wider story is in part hidden behind the terminology. Euthanasia is a broader term, one that encompasses "assisted suicide" (where both choice of and action taken toward ending one's life are largely in the hands of the individual him- or herself), but it includes more besides. Given the sensitivity of the issue there are in fact a host of delicately posed terms: "cooperative euthanasia," "active" and "passive" euthanasia, and "voluntary" and "nonvoluntary" euthanasia. The core theme being that acts or omissions by one or more persons bring about the death of another in a manner desired by the latter, or that eases the latter's suffering. Actions or inactions that kill, in other words, but that do so with compassion.[45]

One can see the gray in this. It is not difficult to construe some conduct as tantamount to manslaughter or murder—a rule of thumb being that the more zealous the intervenor, the more suspect their intentions. Most jurisdictions still ban euthanasia for this very reason.[46] But, equally, there is also broad agreement on certain approaches, attitudes, and behavior that in effect condone euthanasia, whether or not it has been legalized, for the very reason that it offers relief from suffering.

It is common medical practice, for example, when attending to terminally ill patients to reach a point where the prescribed treatment, or at least a part of it, may promote their welfare *and* hasten their death at the same time. Known as the "principle of double effect,"[47] it provides an ethical framework within which it is possible to interpret treatment as promoting the patient's welfare *by* easing their passing. The most obvious and commonplace circumstances in which this occurs is in palliative care in which pain relief is a key feature of the treatment. Administering sufficient medication to alleviate the patient's pain may also (i.e., the double effect) be sufficient to end their life, painlessly. This is in fact what happens with many people under medical care in the last stages of life, whether due to age, illness, or trauma. The end is brought about by a process both unremarkable and tacitly understood by all concerned.[48]

This is a world of euphemisms laced with fine-grained medical ethics and often-hazy laws. Patients are "made comfortable," their "prolonged or unbearable suffering" is ended, and they are "allowed to slip away." It is a benevolent "culture of deception," as my Sydney Law School colleague and health law specialist Roger Magnusson calls it in his gripping book *Angels of Death: Exploring the Euthanasia Underground*, and it happens daily and everywhere. Most importantly of all, Magnusson stresses, it is the default practice of many respected, mainstream physicians, nurses, and other health care professionals, not of "isolated and wild-eyed miscreants acting from the fringes of their professions."[49]

It is partly in recognition of this routine reality that the legalization of euthanasia is now more openly debated, albeit with a focus on more active forms of assistance, particularly in situations where people are facing intolerable pain, dysfunction, or deterioration but are not yet in the terminal stages of life. In short, euthanasia debates today are about the *right* to die. International human rights laws do not expressly recognize such a right, but they do not expressly prohibit it either. Thus, for instance, euthanasia cases brought before the European Court of Human Rights in Strasbourg have invoked an array of other rights that, applicants argue, sustain an implied right to die. The rights to life, privacy, and freedom of conscience, as well as the prohibition on inhuman or degrading treatment, have all been argued to this end.

But all have been rejected.[50] This does not, however, close the door on euthanasia in Europe (Belgium, Germany, Luxembourg, the Netherlands, Spain, and Switzerland already have proactive euthanasia laws);[51] rather it forestalls any claim that the European Convention on Human Rights alone provides grounds for enactment of such laws, still less any obligation to do so.

Human rights laws, therefore, do not provide a definitive answer. Indeed, what makes euthanasia debates so difficult to settle is precisely the lack of consensus on where (or even if) a line can be drawn between acceptable and unconscionable assistance, such as rendered by Michelle Carter. It is also complicated by the above-noted, common practice of assistance provided by health practitioners to patients near death or in otherwise medically intolerable circumstances. Few jurisdictions expressly permit euthanasia (in addition to the European states listed above, the others that presently do so are Australia [mostly], Canada, Colombia, New Zealand, Japan, and a number of US states).[52] But in each case lawmakers have had to juggle often-competing freedoms and responsibilities that range across the patient's medical condition, their consent or that of their family, the role of physicians, and the nature and timing of the life-ending measures.

In euthanasia, as in so many aspects of death, considerations of individual dignity are central. The preservation of that dignity; in whose hands it lies if not the individual's; how to weigh it against the competing wishes of others and against the demands of health care? Cases like those of Vincent Lambert in France and Charlie Gard in the United Kingdom are intractable and tragic reminders of just what a legal, medical, and ethical minefield this subject can be. Both cases involved severely brain-damaged patients on life support systems whose medical teams had concluded that further treatment was pointless or possibly detrimental to the patient's welfare, and that the life support should be withdrawn and replaced by palliative care until their death. Vincent Lambert, a former psychiatric nurse, had been rendered catatonic after suffering catastrophic injuries in a road accident in 2008 when he was thirty-two years old. Charlie Gard was an infant born in August 2016 with a rare genetic disease that atrophies brain and muscle tissue so rapidly that sufferers usually die before they reach their first birthday. The parents in both cases disagreed with their medical teams and wanted life support to continue.[53]

Neither France nor the United Kingdom has legalized euthanasia, but the withdrawal of medical treatment is permissible in both countries whenever no chances of recovery are considered possible. Following separate sets of protracted, painful, and extremely public legal hearings before their respective national courts, as well as the European Court of Human Rights,[54] final authority was granted in both cases for life support to be withdrawn. Vincent Lambert died nine days later in July 2019; he had been in a vegetative state and on life support for more than a decade. Charlie Gard died the day after withdrawal in July 2017; he had been on life support for all but a few weeks of his short life of eleven months and twenty-four days.

The Point of Death

Both Vincent and Charlie had been living undeniably reduced lives, entirely dependent on the constant care of others, medical apparatus, and drugs. Their lives were very largely artificial. But were they entirely so? No matter how physically and mentally diminished, was there still subsisting a part in each representing their essence or their soul?[55] If so, to what extent might their sense of dignity be attached to it? Wider questions follow. When facing our own death or the death of others, what can, or ought, we do to preserve and respect dignity? What are our respective freedoms and responsibilities?

One's intentions regarding death and their impact on others are critical. About life or death, Charlie Gard was never able to convey his intentions, if indeed he had any. After his accident, Vincent Lambert was also unable to convey his wishes, though at least some in his family (including his wife) were certain that he did not want to live in the circumstances forced upon him. "Advance directives" setting out our health care wishes in the event of our incapacitation are certainly helpful in such situations, but even they are not definitive. One's state of mind at the time the directive was drawn up and the nature of the instructions it contains may nevertheless be questioned in the broader contexts of relevant legal prescriptions and standards of medical practice.[56] In the case of suicide—where intent seems pretty clear—there are also legal boundaries and social standards to contend with, as well as the considerations of families and friend. The killing of others against their wishes, whether intended or not, while typically prohibited, is nonetheless mitigatable, excused, or even condoned, depending on circumstances such as occur in accidents, self-defense, warfare, or the death penalty.

In contemplating the freedoms associated with death, there is light and dark—what, clearly, is possible and permitted, and what is not—but there is also much in between. The really difficult questions for liberty's assignment of freedoms and responsibilities revolve around twilight issues, such as those discussed in this chapter. As individuals, governments, and societies at large, we struggle, in our efforts to draw boundaries, with the intertwined dilemmas of respecting individual choice, preserving personal dignity, considering the impact on others, and maintaining legal, moral, and medical standards. In the matter of death, whether free or forced, prosaic or poetic, it will be ever thus.

PART III
Rehabilitating Liberty

In which I draw out lessons learnt from parts I and II by high-lighting the necessity of respect in understanding the true nature of liberty, as well as the importance of building trust if liberty is to withstand the challenges it faces today and tomorrow.

11

<hr>

Respect
Playing on a Team

No man is an island,
Entire of himself.
Each is a part of the continent,
A part of the main.

—John Donne

When I was a graduate student at university, one of my favorite places to work was in the Old Library. A set of small, musty, book-stuffed rooms with mullioned windows overlooking a manicured lawn. On the lawn stood a prancing, bronze horse,[1] which one afternoon I saw being approached by a young man with arms outstretched. He ran his hands and fingers across every inch of the sculpture until he appeared satisfied that he knew it, that he could "see" what his eyes could not. As he retrieved his white stick and walked off, it struck me how much more of the horse he now understood than I did, though I had walked past it hundreds, if not thousands, of times before. His care and attention to the detail as well as to the whole made all the difference.

The Shape of Liberty
Liberty is a bit like that. To really appreciate its contours, its strength and promise, as well as its weaker points and limitations, one must take time to study it across its whole breadth. Our journey in this book has hardly been exhaustive of such an enormous

251

subject, but from its forays into some of the chunkier questions that dominate our daily lives we have seen what those strengths and weaknesses look like. We have even caught glimpses of ways we might exploit the former and counter the latter.

As a matter of fact, the very source of liberty's greatest strength can also be the source of its greatest weakness. It is liberty's component parts of freedom and responsibility—or more especially their relationship to each other—that provides the notion with its foundational heft. From its earliest days, as the opening chapters explain, liberty has been held out as a light on the hill, both aspirational and inspirational. It has galvanized people, pooling their energies and efforts toward a common goal of a better society built on respect for, and freedom of, individuals. Implicit in the idea is an understanding of the need to assume personal and social responsibilities if the goal is to be achieved. Giving is part and parcel of receiving. As individuals we must nevertheless play as a team. Yet herein lies its potential weakness.

For a concept that advertises so appetizing a notion as individual freedom, making it conditional on you shouldering certain responsibilities sits uneasily. It seems counterintuitive, a bit of a letdown; like buying certain Swedish furniture before you realize that it comes flat packed. Liberty relies on people accepting that despite all its normal connotations, freedom is not absolute. You are not free to do whatever you want as limits of some kind are always in place. Intellectually, people may (or may not) appreciate the implications of intersecting freedoms, that some overlap or clash and that limits are therefore required if everyone is to enjoy the same access to freedom. Yet even when we understand this much in theory, taking the next steps of honoring our personal responsibilities in the ways we exercise our freedoms is much more difficult.

There are a host of reasons for this. The belligerence of freedom absolutists, for example, or overzealous policing of freedoms,

or the woolly definitions of freedoms and their attendant responsibilities and the porous boundaries between the two. The inexorable and unending debates over the edges and sometimes core
content of what being free means in social settings are also problematic. We have encountered examples of each of these issues
throughout the book, and all of them bedevil our efforts to put
the responsibilities of freedom into practice.

Second Amendment fanatics in the United States who consider
any restrictions on their right to bear and use arms as sacrilegious,
and radical anti-vaxxers whose depths of self-centeredness are
matched only by their defiance of scientific evidence. The censoring of free speech deemed offensive by means, ironically, of
speech that itself can be deemed offensive because it preferences
the rights of one speaker over another. And the extraordinary presumption of some people that others ought not to be free to love
whomever they wish should their love involve sexual relations
considered improper, despite being private and consensual and
harming no one ("harming" your religious or cultural sensibilities doesn't count—if you're offended, don't pry).

Further, defining freedom in the context of work and employment is fraught with difficulties. Not just because of the apparent
contradiction between what we normally understand by the terms
"work" and "freedom" to mean, but also because of our complicated attitudes toward what precisely constitutes work and why
we do it. What responsibilities we ought to bear—if any at all—
in our individual pursuits of happiness is a taxing question for
individuals and governments alike, especially when trying to
measure levels of responsibility that maximize collective and personal happiness. This stopped neither Jeremy Bentham, though,
nor the kingdom of Bhutan from trying to do just that.

The boundaries *between* freedoms and responsibilities can also
be opaque, the one not infrequently merging into the other.

Euthanasia debates tend to focus on the very point where the individual's freedom to choose the manner of their passing butts up against the responsibilities of others to attend to their welfare—physical, psychological, and spiritual. Freedoms to create and dispense wealth as one pleases are inextricably tied up with responsibilities to create and dispense wealth in socially acceptable ways, as backed by corporate, criminal, and taxation laws. And the freedom of people to pursue agendas of personal and collective economic development is increasingly indistinguishable from environmental sustainability responsibilities that are both global and intergenerational, no matter how poorly those responsibilities have been respected in the past (or are presently).

The Freedom Express

It is true that rather than only seeing weaknesses in the freedom-responsibility nexus, we might consider such tensions, trade-offs, and even contradictions as simply constituting the notion of liberty, as necessary and indeed desirable elements in its makeup. The very stuff of living with liberty. Certainly, arguments and debates on freedom's limits and related responsibilities are part of everyday deliberations in legislatures and courts across the globe, as much as they are discussed around dinner tables and water coolers. But as seen in chapter 1, there can be no denying the lexical preferencing of freedom above liberty in the past seventy years. The post–Second World War shift toward using "freedom" has been especially evident in the language of international human rights law, a language that has had a profound effect not only on the way we now talk about and view relations between states, but also on how we approach our individual relations with our own governments and between ourselves. Post-1945 has become the "freedom epoch."

Platitudes abound reflecting freedom's wholesale social assimilation. "It's a free country"; "land of the free"; "it's my right"; "my life, my choice"; and "I can say/do whatever I want." As platitudes go, there's not a whole lot wrong with these, and indeed in the countries in which you tend to hear them uttered, they largely reflect the daily reality for many or even most people. But, as they stand, they present only one-half of the story.

Hyperventilating one's freedoms in generally free societies with little or no accompanying recognition of their limits and responsibilities not only propagates selfishness but it is self-defeating. Manifestly, as John Donne chides us at the top of this chapter, no one lives life completely alone, "entire of him[or her]self." We are always in the company of others, however closely or remotely, and the freedoms (and responsibilities) of others must be, at base, the same as our own. As everyone cannot claim absolute freedom at the same time, so no one can. There must be debate over the need for and reasonableness of any of freedom's limits and responsibilities, but it is those very limits and responsibilities that embed freedom within society, that ensure freedom's more even distribution, and that engender respect for one another, insisting that we all shoulder burdens as well as reap rewards.

For countries in the so-called free world, this task of balancing freedoms and responsibilities is a delicate one. More art than science, and reliant on rhetoric as much as rationality, the task is nonetheless foundational to democracies, whether emerging or extant (and still working on it). Barack Obama captured the essence of the challenge when he said in his presidential nomination acceptance speech at the Democratic Party Convention in September 2012: "We, the People, recognize that we have responsibilities as well as rights; that our destinies are bound together; that a freedom which only asks what's in it for me, a freedom without a commitment to others, a freedom without love or charity or duty or patriotism, is unworthy of our founding ideals, and those who died in their defense."[2]

"Democracy is ours," he added, stressing that the work of "self-government" is hard and often frustrating. Though speaking within an American context while also, clearly, channeling some of his own first-term frustrations in trying to work with Congress and a recalcitrant Republican Party, Obama was in fact speaking for all democracies and all who believe in them. How one defines freedom really does matter, and it really matters to everyone, not just the person who is making the freedom claim. Twisting its meaning to allow you to invoke the term, to hitch the talismanic power of "freedom" to whatever wagon you want regardless of rational justification, is not just perverse; it can be very destructive.

Sarah Palin, for example, a former Republican Party vice-presidential nominee, infamously tweeted just two months before Obama's convention speech above, "Obama lies; freedom dies," in response to the Supreme Court upholding the constitutionality of the Affordable Care Act. Presumably Palin was referring to one's freedom to go without health care when sick, for there is no other explanation that makes sense of a piece of legislation that sought to extend basic health care coverage to all Americans. To be free from having to pay taxes to foot the bill of such a scheme (or any other publicly funded service from the courts to the military) may, of course, be the freedom that Palin and small-government libertarians like her had in mind. Which stance is not only as foolish as it is selfish but is also untenable. The gargantuan publicly funded health and welfare stimulus packages authorized by the US Congress throughout the early stages of the COVID-19 calamity, in an effort to avert the near-complete collapse of the nation's private sector–oriented health system, made that much abundantly clear.[3]

Flying freedom's flag for distorted, nefarious, or just plain weird reasons continues to attract subscribers. In May 2019 the US Department of Energy, evidently keen to introduce some pizzazz into its media releases, announced that it was no longer overseeing the export of humdrum liquefied natural gas, but rather was now engaged in "spreading freedom gas" around the world. We are delivering "molecules of U.S. freedom," an Energy Department official helpfully added.[4] It wasn't a joke. Nor was US senator Ted Cruz's maniacal screaming of the word "freedom" at the 2021 Conservative Political Action Conference (though many outside the conference did laugh at him).[5] Nor are the many claims to freedom made by other entities and institutions keen to cash in on the apparent unassailable righteousness of the term.[6]

The Freedom of "Others"

Not only we human beings but also many noncorporeal institutions and entities we create are keen to jump on board the freedom express. A central plank of the People's Republic of China's international relations strategy, for example, is "mutual noninterference," meaning that while it "respects" the sovereignty of other countries and leaves them alone to do whatever they wish within their own borders, China claims an equal freedom to have its sovereignty respected and be let alone to do whatever it wishes behind its borders. In consequence, China rejects out-of-hand any criticism of its domestic policies. The government's intemperate response to continuing and credible accusations of systemic human rights abuses of Muslim Uyghurs in Xinjiang province is typical in this regard, as is the heavy-handed bullying of protesters in Hong Kong and critics of its "zero-tolerance" COVID-19 policies.[7] "We will not accept the[se] politically driven accusations," as no country has the right to "dictate the definition of democracy and human rights," asserted Vice Foreign Minister Le Yucheng in response to United Nations criticism of China's human rights record, leaving no doubt that China considers itself free to do just that for itself.[8]

Yet, are not such assertive demands merely extensions of individuals' claims to absolute freedom? Are they not just as incoherent and illegitimate, but manifoldly more dangerous because they are claimed by a state? Is not the systematic operation of vast "re-education camps" for ethnic minorities and the banning of purportedly seditious books (including children's picture books)[9] precisely the sort of claimed governmental "freedoms" that the world sought to deny states after the Second World War with the establishment of the United Nations and the promulgation of universal human rights standards? In the preservation of people's liberty (that is, their freedoms and responsibilities), respect for and between individuals and communities is essential. The state plays a defining role in that quest, but not—or at least not legitimately—as a matter of self-perpetuating, dictatorial power but as one of responsive and representative authority.

Besides states and government agencies, other artificial, non-human entities, such as corporations and religious institutions, make appeals to freedom. The right to free speech, for example, is claimed by both. And so they should. But that freedom has to be conditional, and conditional, what is more, in ways that are quite different from the limits imposed on the free speech of individual human beings. No matter that corporations and religious bodies might choose at times to argue otherwise, they have no souls to damn or bodies to kick. They are legal constructs (secular or canonical), with institutional objectives and obligations. Sure, they comprise and are run by human beings, but the entities are not themselves human and are not therefore endowed with all the inherent dignity and individual agency that accompanies that singular classification.

So, while corporations engage all the time in so-called commercial speech—explaining what they do and why we simply must purchase their products—such speech is subject to stricter conditions than normal speech. Typically, it must be accurate (no "false advertising"), transparent (no covering up inconvenient truths), and fair (no gratuitous slagging off competitors). Yet companies such as Nike, Exxon, and Facebook have all sought to claim broader free speech rights when it suits them. Nike's claim to be "sweatshop-free" in its manufacturing supply chain was challenged in a court case initiated by a customer.[10] Exxon sought to resist legal demands that it release internal documents showing its prior and undisclosed knowledge of the health and environmental consequences of carbon emissions (here it was the freedom *not* to speak that Exxon sought to invoke).[11] And Facebook CEO Mark Zuckerberg's impassioned plea that technologically enhanced speech should be left free to develop as the market demands was roundly criticized as "symptomatic of our collective refusal to think of speech and the media in complicated ways."[12]

Religious organizations and their leaders have a long history of asserting the right of their organizations—that is, of the religions themselves—to be free from discrimination. This is precisely what blasphemy laws seek to protect, typically by prohibiting any adverse comment or portrayal of the institution, tenets, or teachings of the religion itself. It is to be distinguished from protecting the freedom of *people* to express themselves as their faith dictates and to be free from discrimination based on their faith. From the point of view of international law, the latter freedoms of individual persons fall squarely within the category of human rights protection, while the former freedoms are merely political claims that have no more merit or authority than the special pleadings made by any other societal group.[13]

In practice, however, this is not how many religions (and their practitioners) see it, used as they are to special treatment over hundreds of years. So, while rearguard actions are still being fought against the dismantling of blasphemy laws throughout the Western world, the fact is that the idea of "religious freedom" in these countries is now focused on protecting people from religious discrimination[14] rather than on protecting them from scrutiny, debate, insult, or even ridicule of their religion, beliefs, opinions, or ideas.[15]

Responsibility as the Mother of Freedom

This book's central argument that freedom and responsibility exist in a symbiotic relationship, such that the former is possible for any or all of us only if the latter is recognized and fulfilled, requires a degree of mutual respect between and among us as individuals. It requires a sense of community and of belonging whereby it is accepted that, at base, we all have equal claims on rights to be free and that we must therefore accept the necessity of reciprocal limitations on individual freedom to preserve it for each and all of us. This insistence on respect does not, however, command that we must all agree with one another or even disagree politely (what a soulless existence that would be), but it does require that we respect one another's inherent dignity as identifiably separate members of the same species. This rather grand, "existential" summation (as political scientist, George Kateb puts it)[16] is not quite as impenetrable and unattainable as it sounds, for it is essentially an appeal to the so-called golden rule of civility—doing unto others as you would have them do unto you.

In *Human Dignity*, Kateb goes on to characterize what this means for each of us in more prosaic and more attainable terms:

> The golden rule does not ask for heroic self-sacrifice or saintly forbearance. It asks, instead, that we be better, if only by a little, than the level we might see around us, despite all the risks of priggishness or self-righteousness, and better than we may have been

in the past. To be better is to be prepared to run some risks and make some sacrifices (none of them heroic) in order to help others, even if we cannot count on them to help us in some future need.[17]

It is at once a declaration of a necessary aspiration and an acknowledgment of human fallibility. We're all far from perfect citizens; we have our prejudices, likes and dislikes, loves and hates. It is beyond question that we *regard* people differently according to a whole host of circumstantial factors. Some we approach with open arms, utmost respect, and even reverence; others, with skepticism or outright scorn. It is, frankly, ridiculous to suppose that it could be any other way. But what we hold in our head or heart need not—and many times does not—dictate how we act in practice; how, in fact, we *treat* the people around us, near and far. For it is in the practice of engaging with others, of how we act toward them, that the matter of respect, or civility, is vital.

At base, it is to recognize others as fellow human beings, members of the same broad community, all seeking, like you, the same rights and freedoms. Qualifications to those rights or the nature of their attendant responsibilities may differ for individuals and groups according to behavior, time, and circumstances, but those are matters subject to subsequent negotiation and determination. What is critical, however, is that the initial point or baseline of mutual respect is established and upheld. This is true even of seemingly implacable foes who find they each profit by extending some form of recognition and respect for each other.

A telling illustration of this last point emanates from Johnathan Powell's reflections on his nearly three decades of experience mediating between governments and terrorist organizations from Colombia and Palestine to Sri Lanka and South Africa, as well as in his native United Kingdom.[18] He acted as the chief negotiator for the British government in the lengthy, fraught, but ultimately successful conclusion of the 1998 Good Friday Agreement between the United Kingdom, the Republic of Ireland, and the main political parties in Northern Ireland—an accord that brought relative peace to the province for the first time in thirty years. Getting the negotiating process off the ground was perhaps the single biggest challenge of all. How to get the two sides of the Northern Irish conflict to sit down together in the same room when for so long they had been at each other's throats (metaphorically and physically) meant persuading them to recognize and, at some basic level, respect each other.

Just how hard that task would be was made clear to Powell and his boss—Tony Blair, then the United Kingdom's prime minister—on a visit to the "loyalist" heartland of East Belfast in the earliest days of the negotiations. The walkabout happened immediately after a widely publicized meeting between Blair and "nationalist" hardliners Gerry Adams and Martin McGuinness. The people on the streets that day had come not to praise Blair but (in effect) to bury him . . . in latex, as it turned out! When they started throwing rubber gloves at him, Blair was confused, only to be enlightened by Powell, who explained that if he was going to make a habit of shaking hands with murderers, he needed to protect himself from the blood.[19]

Yet, despite such uncompromising opposition, hands had been shaken and more were to follow, and then there were discussions, arguments, setbacks, and, eventually, agreement. Freedoms as well as responsibilities were negotiated and settled, borne on the back of some little respect ventured by all involved in the process. Compromises, in other words, were made by everyone. Each in the end recognized that unless both shouldered some responsibility, they could hardly expect others to do so, and that if the ultimate goal is valued highly enough—be it peace, justice, or liberty—the compromise will be worth it.[20]

The Importance of Empathy

What the necessity and success of such transactional interrelations between people boil down to, according to philosopher Richard Rorty, is a sufficiency of empathy. When we empathize with others—when we try to stand in their shoes, as it were—we are better able to understand their position. We may not fully understand their circumstances, or always agree with their views or actions, but by attempting to identify with them, we build, and to some extent cross, a bridge between ourselves. Rorty refers to this process as a "sentimental education" that applies not only to those we hold near and dear but also, more especially, to strangers far and wide. It consists, he says, of "an increasing ability to see the similarities between ourselves and people very unlike us as outweighing the differences." The relevant similarities, he stresses, are not only ones that we share personally and deeply but also "such little, superficial similarities as cherishing our parents and our children."[21] Respecting and recognizing such common traits in strangers is what binds us together in a human community. It breaks down (or at least dents) the barriers created by the mentality of "us and them," which, Rorty notes, makes us less tempted to think of them as quasi-human or even subhuman.

It is indeed at the outer reaches of inhumanity that we see most clearly the need for empathy. For it is there, where empathy and compassion are obliterated by contempt and the warped rationality of "they deserve it," that atrocities occur.[22] Genocides, slavery and torture, gulags and concentration camps, alongside everyday obscenities of the systematic degradation of women, racial and ethnic groups, and LGBTQI communities. In many instances such callous disregard for others is directed at strangers precisely *because* they are different from "us." In which case, not only is no attempt made at building an empathetic bridge, but efforts are made to widen the gap and push "them" further away. The Black Lives Matter movement is a direct response to social, political, and legal systems that condone, or at least tolerate, huge disparities in treatment. When, for instance, Black and other communities of color are vastly overrepresented in national arrest and incarceration rates (as they are in the United States and Australia, for example)[23] and when, at the international level, least-developed and mostly Black countries in sub-Saharan Africa are severely disadvantaged by global tax regimes designed to protect and favor rich states at the expense of poor ones.[24]

But, in many other instances, the degradation is of those known, or even closest, to us. That sexual harassment and domestic violence, targeting especially women and children, are endemic across all cultures and societies graphically illustrates the point.[25] The "us and them" distinction is here replaced by a differential of power. The viral rise, and now global reach, of the #MeToo movement represents a widespread denunciation not only of the manipulation of such power (by men, almost exclusively) but also of its existence in the first place.[26] What could possibly justify this differential, let alone its abuse? In its place, quite simply, there ought to be a relationship of "equal respect" between genders, from which freedoms and responsibilities are more evenly divided.[27] To that end, a crucial step involves men developing a deeper empathetic understanding of women—that is, of their mothers, sisters, daughters, wives, partners, friends, and colleagues and also, thereby, of more than half of humanity. "If we as men are interested in gender equality," says William Fernando Rosero, a young worker from Ipiales in western Colombia, "everything gets better."[28]

Disrespect and Irresponsibility

It is not by chance that so many unwarranted or illegitimate claims to freedom are mounted on the pedestal of disrespecting others. For the more you denigrate those who might stand in the way of your claimed freedom—because they object to its impact on them or because they claim an opposing freedom—the more you are able to self-justify sweeping those concerns and counterclaims aside. It is, in effect, an attempt to claim a right or freedom without any attendant duty. Never mind the fact that the recognition and respect you deny others is precisely what you demand they pay you. This circularity of argument underlines the point made earlier, that responsibility is indeed the mother of freedom. Without it, when people act irresponsibly, freedom is lost; or rather, it becomes a one-way street, which, in the end, amounts to the same thing.

This is why our organs of government, community leaders, and indeed any individual or institution exercising authority needs to play such vital roles in the preservation of freedom. By formulating rules, marking out boundaries, and mediating disputes, they help set standards of respect that guide our everyday agreements and disagreements over freedoms and responsibilities. This is their supervisory role. Alongside that, however, they also have an exemplary role, whereby their own behavior sets the tone for these everyday negotiations. This is no mere trifling; what levels of respect are afforded us by our leaders affect directly our responses to authority and our relations with one another. Therefore, when those in power actively breed contempt and abnegate responsibilities, they not only fail to protect freedom but actively destroy it.

This can be seen happening all the time and everywhere, in circumstances large and small. Such challenges to people's freedoms are in fact never-ending. But it is especially concerning to see them so actively thriving in the most powerful nation on Earth and self-proclaimed leader of the free world, when it populates its highest echelons of government with officials that, by their actions, manifestly disrespect their citizens. For how else can you characterize the consigning of so many of its population to poverty, despite the country's wealth;[29] abandoning 28 million of its poorest people to life without health care coverage of any kind in the world's most expensive health care system;[30] and directing the might of the National Security Agency's electronic surveillance capabilities toward its own citizens in ways that are as opaque as they are pervasive.[31] An increasingly polarized political system so poisoned civil society with mutual disrespect that on the eve of the US midterm elections in November 2022, polls showed some 80 percent of both Republican and Democratic voters considered the political agenda of the other party "a threat that if not stopped will destroy America as we know it." And further, that roughly two-thirds of those same voters would support their party's candidate despite evidence of their "moral failure . . . not consistent with [the voter's] own values."[32] Stunningly, America's political culture has become so debased, it can now accommodate, even encourage, a pretender potentate of starkly limited abilities beyond boundless selfishness, first to preside over the country for four years and thereafter to continue to wield a malign influence over politics and society at large. It is a polity in the grip of "megalomaniacal authoritarianism," as Robert Reich labels it.[33]

On this last point, two coinciding viewpoints from either side of the Atlantic bear out the dire consequences for people's freedoms, not just in the United States but for all who are affected by its providence (which means most of us). First, from American political scientist Jonathan Kirshner, who bemoans "Trump's long shadow and the end of American credibility" by pointing out the uncomfortable truth that even after it ended, "the world cannot unsee the Trump presidency." He continues: "Trump is the United States—or at least a very large part of it. Many Americans will choke on that sentiment, but other countries don't have the luxury of clinging to some idealized version of the United States' national character."[34] Second, from Fintan O'Toole, Ireland's foremost political commentator, who travels down the same cataclysmic path as Kirshner in despairing of Trump's legacy. "He has successfully led a vast number of voters along the path from hatred of government to contempt for rational deliberation to the inevitable endpoint: disdain for the electoral process itself. . . . Trump has unfinished business. A republic he wants to destroy still stands. It is, for him, not goodbye but hasta la vista. Instead of waving him off, those who want to rebuild American democracy will have to put a stake through his heart."[35] Perhaps most damning of all, O'Toole's earlier reflections on the United States when Trump was still in office boiled down to "The world has loved, hated and envied the US. Now, for the first time, we pity it."[36]

In America, then, as elsewhere, to greater and lesser extents, liberty, and the claims to freedoms and bearing of responsibilities that it entails, is endangered when leaders and followers lose respect for each other, when political hypocrisy carries no shame,[37] and when society veers toward what Hobbes described as a "war of all against all."[38] Our institutions of government as well as the inherent civility within our communities and ourselves—as shown often enough throughout the pages of this book—can help save us, and it is on them that we must rely for reform and renewal.

Toward Reform and Renewal

In Svetlana Alexievich's remarkable collection of verbatim accounts of life during and after the Soviet Union, she writes that when she asks young Russians today (that is, those born in or after 1990) what "freedom" means, they say, "It's when you can live without having to think about freedom. Freedom is normal."[39] As appealing a notion as that might sound, freedom is in fact a perpetual "work in progress"; we all have to tend to it often and carefully.

Invocations of freedom, the attributions ascribed to it, whether and how it is defined, by whom and under what circumstances are all important matters. They are important because they bear directly on how we understand the broader concept of liberty and how we go about the never-ending process of its revision and re-invigoration. There will always be debate and discussion over the extent of freedoms and their attendant responsibilities in all facets of our daily lives. Whether such exchanges are ephemeral—over the scope of your choice in food, music, clothes or hobby—or foundational—your freedom to choose whom to love, what religion to practice, or how and when to die. What, however, is critical to shaping the outcome of each deliberation is the manner in which the exchange is conducted. Under what rules, presumptions and expectations, in other words, do the negotiations take place?

These deliberative processes or systems are vital in their own right. The more they are regarded as "fair"—inclusive, respectful, rational, and efficient—the more faith people have in the results they yield, whether they like or agree with them or not. When these characteristics are diluted or missing altogether—when the process is "mostly people yelling at each other and living in bubbles of one sort or another," as former CIA-analyst-cum-author Martin Gurri puts it—[40]division and disrespect run deeper and freedoms shrink. The integrity of the system itself, therefore, really matters. Our preparedness to live with limits on our freedoms—to bear liberty's responsibilities—depends directly on our perceptions of the system's integrity. If it is seen as reasoned and fair as well as efficient and timely, if its institutions of political, legal, and social intermediation are considered to be open and responsive, then people will more likely engage with the system, understand and support it. They will, in other words, trust it. So it is to consideration of the critical importance of trust—its presence and absence—in the fortunes of liberty that we now turn, in the book's concluding chapter.

12

Trust
Liberty's Keystone

Because you believed I was capable of behaving decently, I did.
—Paolo Coelho

One's life has value so long as one attributes value
to the life of others, by means of love, friendship,
indignation and compassion.
—Simone de Beauvoir

"Look After Her"

Although you are unknown to me, I imagine you as a man and a woman who will, as a father and mother, care for my only child. She has been taken from me by circumstance. May you, with the best will and wisdom, look after her.

With these words Lien de Jong's mother passed her daughter into the hands of strangers, neither knowing that they would never see each other again. It was August 1942, in German-occupied Holland. Lien was eight years old and Jewish. Her mother's words were written on a letter folded into a pocket of Lien's coat and addressed to "Most honored Sir and Madam," beseeching them to "imagine for yourself the parting between us." Lien became a "hidden child," one of the thousands of Jewish children taken in by non-Jewish families across Europe before and during the Second World War. Recognizing, if not

269

fully comprehending, the horror of the pogroms, especially after *Kristallnacht* on November 9, 1938, Jewish parents were faced with an agonizing choice: surrender their children to the relative safety of sympathetic strangers who would become in loco parentis, or keep the family together and risk their children's lives as well as their own.[1]

In choosing the former, Lien's parents were evidently torn: "When will we ever see her again?" her mother asked rhetorically. But in end they had decided to venture all in their trust of Lien's new guardians. That much is clear in what must have been the hardest words of all to write: "I want to say to you that it is my wish that she will think only of you as her mother and father."

Lien's parents died in Auschwitz, together with almost all her extended family. Lien survived the war, though with such a profound sense of loss that "nothing anyone said seemed important."[2] Today she is a mother and grandmother and still lives in the Netherlands.

Ernest Hemingway was undoubtedly correct when he pronounced, with characteristic swagger, that "the way to make people trust-worthy is to trust them."[3] But the investment takes faith and often courage from all parties and such outlays are not always repaid in the ways we hope for or expect.

In "Trust" We Must Trust

Trust really is liberty's sine qua non: the essential ingredient in liberty's freedom-responsibility calculus, no matter where or when liberty is sought, the gravity of the circumstances, or the mix of deliberative processes in play. Thus, for example, while there are some "hard laws" restricting our freedom to dress as we wish (the public nuisance offense of nudity is designed to curb notions you might have in that direction), ultimately it is a combination of prevailing social mores, comfort, and the opinions of friends (be they candid or diplomatic) that likely has greater influence on our sartorial preferences. Whereas, in contrast, the extent of our freedom to practice any or no religion is more likely to rely on explicit legal provisions for protection than it is on social mores or peer pressure.

Whether concerning apparel or prayer (or anything else), the drawing of lines of freedom and responsibility is workable only if people trust in the line-drawing process, be that the frankness of friends or the strictness of laws. Such levels of trust, it must be said, are hard won and easily lost. In the winning and losing, much hangs on how disagreements over freedom's limits are handled and disputes resolved.

This book offers numerous examples of contentious issues in which this negotiation has been done relatively well (vaccine programs and euthanasia practices) and done badly (gun ownership and tax equity). Certain issues—like countries' handling of the coronavirus pandemic—have yielded examples across the spectrum. South Korea's preparedness and speed and efficiency in screening, testing, tracking, quarantining, hospitalizing, and funding, especially in the contagion's early stages, managed to contain its spread far more successfully than almost any other country. Its citizens bought into the draconian demands made of them—including the public sharing of the detailed movements of infected persons—quickly and often with little dissent, largely because they trusted their government. There certainly were privacy and human rights concerns, but research showed that in these straitened circumstances, "most preferred the public good to individual rights."[4]

In the United States, by contrast, the inept and negligent responses by relevant health care agencies at federal and state levels during the first year of the crisis, coupled with presidential self-aggrandizement and willful ignorance so profound it didn't even qualify as sciolism, engendered neither confidence nor trust in public authorities. The US response to COVID-19 was then dominated—and still is—more by party politics than science. As a result, not only did the United States quickly become the disease's global epicenter, but freedoms, livelihoods, and lives of Americans were lost that could and should have been saved.[5] Actively encouraging people to demand purported freedoms to socialize as you please and to refuse to wear a mask or be vaccinated no matter the protection these afford yourself and others is not only hubris but manipulative and ultimately self-defeating. "There is no subjection so complete as that which preserves the forms of freedom; it is thus that the will itself is taken captive," as Jean-Jacques Rousseau daringly warned in *Émile* 260 years ago, when talking of the malignancy of educating children by appearing to give them the freedom to learn but all the while retaining mastery over their instruction.[6] The subterfuge in that message was well heeded on a wider social plane by America's Founding Fathers a decade or so later when they began their efforts to enshrine freedom in a new constitution, the integrity of which is today being sorely tested.

Whether contemplating freedom and responsibility in times of pestilence and upheaval or peace and calm, trust-building techniques of negotiation exist in various forms. They can be legal and formalized; for example, the "margin of appreciation" device used by the European Court of Human Rights to extend to states some elbow room in their interpretation and enforcement of such rights as free speech, freedom of movement, and privacy in the interests of preserving public order or protecting public health.[7] Or they can be informal social practices—such as how we accommodate shifting attitudes toward what constitutes work, or satisfactory levels of personal happiness (self-help books notwithstanding), or community perspectives on wealth inequality (how much is too much?).

Building Trust

Trust is the glue that binds us to one another. It is the foundation of friendships, families, and love affairs, as well as communities, constitutions, and churches. That we "believe" in one another in the manner as expressed by Paolo Coelho at the head of this chapter and do so by the means listed by Simone de Beauvoir in the quote following Coelho's helps ensure, quite simply, the things that make life worth living. It is unsurprising, therefore, to see trust so intimately connected to notions of personal and political liberty. In political philosophy, it is regarded as a cardinal principle of democracy that people trust one another and that together they entrust their collective will to representatives who govern in their name. Likewise, the worlds of law and commerce revolve around the ancient moral code of your word as your bond. The responsibilities of our freedoms, whether individual or communal, are built on trust.

Rousseau's idea of a "social contract" is a signature expression of the multilayered relationships of trust that must exist between people and their governments if together they are to construct a workable notion of liberty. It presumes a lot, not least that in the formation of a society of free and equal persons we all agree (by way of the social contract) that our individual wills yield, to some extent, to the collective will.[8] But it also presumes broad consensus on moral notions of right and wrong, support for utilitarian considerations of fairness and equity, and faith in rational argument as the means of debate and dispute settlement. Each and all of these features are necessary for a well-ordered society built on trust and sustained by liberty.[9]

What makes trust such an intriguing and important part of our personal and political relations is that it is, at base, a source of power. When we trust someone we invest in them a degree of authority over some aspect of our lives while believing that they will not abuse that authority. From babysitters and weather forecasters, lovers and police officers, to priests, teammates, and online content moderators, we live our lives through a web of relationships of personal and social trust.

Politicians, more than most, understand very well the relationship between power and trust. It is perhaps no surprise, therefore, that Benjamin Disraeli, a consummate nineteenth-century politician, believed "that all power is a trust; that we [elected representatives] are accountable for its exercise; that from the people and for the people all springs, and all must exist."[10] You might say, of course, that while politicians may well claim to appreciate the importance of trust, such claims are no guarantee that they will not abuse or betray it. But our political leaders are hardly alone in that regard. We all know the weight of responsibility we bear when people trust and rely on us, and the bitterness we feel when our own trust in others is betrayed. For not only is trust extremely useful—by depending on others we can leverage opportunities and expand freedoms—but it can also be extremely dangerous. That same dependency can lead to exploitation and enslavement. This highly charged dichotomy is one of the reasons we have such carefully worded constitutions. It is also a major reason that relationship counselors and divorce lawyers are never short of business.

Sticking to constitutions for the time being, they are crucial not just because they carve out the legal boundaries of political trust but also because they are also societies' mission statements, as it were—reflections of how they see themselves, or how they wish to appear to others. To be sure, they dryly describe the organs of government, detail their functions, and delimit their powers. And, yes, they parse out details of how political disputes are to be settled and what rights and freedoms of the people they must protect and promote. But, in so doing, a constitution also tells us much about the country's values, the principles it holds dear, and its goals and aspirations.[11]

In this way, the *sovereignty* of the people is retained: the vesting of all powers in the organs of government is by way of delegation, not surrender; adherence to the rule of law applies to those same organs as it does to the people themselves; and above all, the purpose of government, the authority on which it rests, is to serve the people—all of them—to protect their rights and freedoms, and to promote their welfare and safety. While this necessarily entails setting limits on certain freedoms and imposing some responsibilities on all of us, the expectation is that, in so doing, governments act fairly, openly, and rationally.[12]

For a handy summation of how constitutions deal with the balancing of freedoms by limiting them, we need go no further than the following from the US Supreme Court in 1890: "Even liberty itself, the greatest of all rights, is not unrestricted license to act according to one's own will. It is only freedom from restraint under conditions essential to the equal enjoyment of the same right by others. It is then liberty regulated by law."[13] A clear enough statement of principle, and yet in its application in practice the history and facts of the case illustrate how dependent we are on trust between citizens and their governments on getting the balance right. The Supreme Court was here condoning the prohibition of the sale of alcohol in California as constitutionally permissible. The case was a forerunner, as it turned out, to the eventual adoption of the Eighteenth Amendment to the US Constitution in 1919, prohibiting the sale of "intoxicating liquors" across the country. Although it was a long-sought victory for the Temperance Movement, which railed against the evils of alcohol, it was short-lived: the Eighteenth Amendment was repealed in 1933. Trust in the organs of government getting it right in their reading of the collective wishes of the citizenry on matters of liberty at any one time can never be assured, especially when certain sections of the community make loud and special pleadings.

Constitutions are imperfect documents, sometimes by accident, sometimes by design. While the Second and Eighteenth Amendments to the US Constitution might fall into the latter category, even more peculiar provisions can be found elsewhere.

During one of my trips to Myanmar, this one in 2012, I met with Aung San Suu Kyi in her new home in the newly established capital of Naypyidaw. It was a year or so after she had been officially released from long-term house arrest, and she was in a relaxed mood. We sat at her kitchen table, and as she poured tea, I ventured some small talk. Nodding to the puppy who had so enthusiastically greeted us at the door, I asked whether she was having fun with him. "Oh yes," she replied, "and he chews my copy of the new Constitution, you know, so he's clearly very intelligent!" Section 59(f) of the Constitution of Myanmar (2008) effectively bars Suu Kyi from ever being elected president of Myanmar. Inserted with her specifically in mind, the provision stipulates that no person married to a foreign national or having children who hold another nationality (she fell into both categories),[14] is eligible for election to the presidency. That said—and reflecting the flexibility of constitutions in matters of liberty when there is sufficient public trust and political will (and a prescient pooch)—Aung San Suu Kyi was for some time president in all but name, being both foreign minister and minister of the president's office, until the military coup in February 2021, whereupon she found herself once again incarcerated by Myanmar's generals.

Some constitutional provisions are so closely tied to the notion of liberty and the freedoms and responsibilities it comprises that their interpretation has implications far beyond the material facts of any specific case or cases before a court. The Fourteenth

Amendment to the US Constitution is one such provision. In its protection of people's privileges and immunities, and of their rights to life, liberty and property, all in accordance with due process and under the equal protection of the laws, this amendment is doing a lot.

The body of jurisprudence it has generated is understandably large, but in terms both of defining liberty and in forging an interpretation of the Fourteenth Amendment that accords with, and builds on, the trust people have invested in their organs of government, the case law that established the right to abortion in the United States was compelling. In *Planned Parenthood of Southeastern Pennsylvania v. Casey* (1992), for example, a case that upheld and clarified the right to abortion as formulated in *Roe v. Wade* (1973), the Supreme Court declared: "These matters, involving the most intimate and personal choices a person may make in a lifetime, choices central to personal dignity and autonomy, are central to the liberty protected by the Fourteenth Amendment. At the heart of liberty is the right to define one's own concept of existence, of meaning, of the universe, and of the mystery of human life." As a definition of what, fundamentally, the notion of personal liberty entails, this could hardly be bettered, accepting, as it does, that while the state has no authority to "define the attributes of personhood," individuals nevertheless have responsibilities to bear in the life choices they do make. A woman who opts for abortion "must live with the implications of her decision" however she makes it, as the Court added.[15]

More's the pity, therefore, that this monument to trust in citizens to make such existential choices as they see fit should have been recently brutalized by the current US Supreme Court. First, by its endorsement of a Texas statute that doesn't just disenfranchise women of that choice but outsources that choice to others—indeed anyone—to make for them. Astonishingly, the act actively encourages citizens to file civil lawsuits against any person who has "aided and abetted" an abortion, for which suit, if successful, they will be rewarded with a $10,000 bounty.[16] Although this law is medieval (or Wild West) in form, and despite excoriating dissents from the minority judges, the majority of the Court nevertheless declined to strike down the act in an eleventh-hour case brought by a group of Texan abortion providers seeking to prevent it coming into force.[17] And second, by the Court's wholesale removal of the constitutional protection of a woman's choice in *Dobbs* (2022), despite, once again, vehement dissent.[18]

What, above all, our constitutions and laws should be are reflections of society's prevailing opinions, respecting thereby the trust society as a whole has placed in the lawmakers themselves. The same goes for the judiciary entrusted with interpreting and applying the law. In terms of the scope of freedom and weight of responsibility, not everyone, of course, will be content with laws as they stand, or with how they are interpreted and applied. But that is inevitable and is in any case the basis on which continuing (and unending) arguments and negotiations over liberty are made. That said, both civil and common law systems are replete with what we might call "negotiating techniques," interpretive devices that allow government officials, judges, and others some flexibility in how to apply laws across different circumstances.

We have encountered some of these techniques already. The European Court of Human Rights' use of "margin of appreciation," noted earlier,[19] is perhaps the most elastic (and therefore controversial) of these techniques.[20] Other examples commonly employed by many courts include "proportionality" (the idea that legal sanctions fit the nature of the harm they seek to address), "foreseeability" (of the consequences of one's actions), and "reasonableness," perhaps the broadest of all, which seeks to keep the law connected to the ordinary person. The United Kingdom's Bribery Act of 2010 provides a good example of the use of reasonableness in its description of what test is to apply when deciding whether a public official has been induced (bribed) to act improperly, namely, "what a reasonable person in the United Kingdom would expect."[21]

The point is that all such devices and techniques are legal expressions of democracy in action. They are in fact necessities given the inherent indeterminacy of language, regardless of the statutory drafters' best efforts to make it otherwise. But they also permit the law to respond to shifts in public opinion in ways that are not dissimilar to how we ourselves negotiate difficult questions of freedom and responsibility. For example, how often do we find ourselves setting boundaries and expectations with such intonations as "Be reasonable," "What did you expect would happen?" and "That's way over the top"? The social contact of trust, between ourselves and with our governments, is genuinely populist in nature. But populist in the sense of building consensus, not breaking it.

Breaking Trust

There is a scene in *The Simpsons* where Homer opens the dishwasher to deposit his single dirty plate only to be confronted by racks full of clean dishes. He hesitates and then moves to the fridge, gathers whatever he can find and returns to the dishwasher. Contentedly humming to himself, he grates cheese, chops carrots, grinds pepper, and squirts ketchup over the clean crockery before finishing the job by spitting on them. He inserts his own dirty plate and restarts the dishwasher. It's trademark Homer—lazy, selfish, and fake. When Marg walks in and thanks him for doing the dishes, he replies, "No problem; you can unload."

When people breach the trust of others, whether over household chores or constitutional propriety, freedoms are twisted and responsibilities skewed. The ever-delicate balance that the practice of liberty strives to maintain is compromised or even broken. Winners become more entitled and selfish, and losers more embittered. If the upset is fueled by careless or deliberate disregard for the truth or rational argument, the divide grows ever wider, and distrust ever more damaging.[22] Even commandeering the label of populism to describe this calumny is disingenuous. It feigns a bond with democracy, whereas it is, in fact, a perversion of democracy. Populism focuses on the accrual of power by certain individuals or groups to promote their specific interests, rather than exercising power in ways that promote the welfare of society as a whole. It is a toxic and dangerous mix, but it works for some, at least in the short term.

"If citizens doubt everything, they cannot see alternative models beyond [their] borders, cannot carry out sensible discussions about reform, and cannot trust one another enough to organize for political change. A plausible future requires a factual present." This is what historian Timothy Snyder argues in *The Road to Unfreedom*.[23] Was he talking about Trump's America, or Johnson's United Kingdom during the latter's throes of exiting the European Union? No. He's referring to Putin's Russia and what he calls Putin's mission to destroy the very ideas of fact and truth, whether by lying to the world about the downing of the passenger plane MH17, lying to his people over the extent of COVID-19's penetration in the country, or the reasons for Russia's invasion of Ukraine.[24] The Russian leader, Snyder says, is intent on creating "a bond of willing ignorance with Russians, who were meant to understand that Putin was lying but to believe him anyway." Yet Snyder might just as well be talking about polities in the present-day United States and United Kingdom, or many other countries for that matter (Brazil, Belarus, Poland, Hungary, Syria, China, and Venezuela leap to mind).

In China, for example, the government's future plans for an already formidably weaponized internet are truly dystopian. Its 2017 white paper titled "A Next Generation Artificial Intelligence Development Plan" is eye-popping in its frankness. "AI technologies," the white paper says, will "grasp group cognition and psychological changes in a timely manner; and take the initiative in decision-making and reactions—which will significantly elevate the capability and level of social governance, playing an irreplaceable role in effectively maintaining social stability."[25] Subsequent governmental blueprints and guidance on the development and control of AI bear out the earnest intent to deliver on these words, which, as John Lanchester notes, amount to "as pure a dream of a totalitarian state as there has ever been—a future in which the state knows everything and anticipates everything, acting on citizens' needs before the citizen is aware of having them."[26]

The Chinese authorities are already using the predictive and anticipatory dimensions of AI in their ongoing social control of the Uyghur Muslim minority groups in Xinjiang province. Algorithm-based models of preemptive crime control are identifying when, where, and by whom laws might be broken and are initiating arrest and detention orders accordingly. As a result, it is believed, among the up to one million Chinese citizens detained in Xinjiang's "reeducation camps" are many whose only "crime" was a robocop flagging that they might be about to commit one.[27] At one level, this is all so extraordinary that, paradoxically, it is easy to deny as outrageously false, which is precisely what the Chinese government continues vociferously to do regarding the camps in Xinjiang.[28] But at another level, and one occupied by many Chinese, it seems an appropriate response.

On my last (pre-COVID) visit to China, a colleague there told me of an inquiry he had received from a local journalist who wanted to discuss Western attitudes towards "reeducation." She was genuinely surprised, my colleague told me, that Westerners saw it as a problem at all. "This is a classic case of Chinese mind-set," he explained, alluding to the Confucian principle of respect for authority, "where people are trouble-makers, they need to be reset, to be re-educated." In other words, the Chinese government has so successfully exploited the paramountcy of social stability in the minds of the Chinese citizenry that many now regard any disruptive exercise of free thought, voice, or action challenging political authority as necessarily illegitimate.

When, on December 30, 2019, Li Wenliang, a physician at Wuhan Central Hospital, used a chat group to warn colleagues of a possible outbreak of a new SARS-like virus, he could not have imagined that five weeks later that virus would claim his life or that the full weight of China's Cybersecurity Defense Bureau would be brought to bear on silencing his voice for "making false claims" and disrupting public order. The fact that Li was right about this novel coronavirus (and the COVID-19 disease it caused), together with an unusually vocal public outcry following his death, led the authorities to partially absolve him posthumously after an official investigation. But in declaring merely that Li was incorrectly charged, the official report maintained that he had failed to follow correct procedures in relaying his concerns and criticized his subsequent activities in talking openly about his censorship experiences.[29] Li's proclamation that "I think a healthy society should not have just one voice"—which of course the report did not care to repeat—was clearly the object of this official rebuke.[30]

Such authoritarianism, plus widespread "big baby" subservience in China,[31] reflects a break in trust between citizens and their rulers in ways that the former scarcely realize, let alone effectively object to, beyond exceptional cases such as that of Dr Li.[32] This is hardly a phenomenon alien to Western democracies. Indeed, some Western leaders in recent years have shown themselves adept at bolstering their own positions by belittling public opposition, no matter the latter's relative merits.

Dumbing down politics and political messages is nothing new, of course. But simpering references to "quiet Australians," for example, as that country's former prime minister Scott Morrison called those whom he believed must support all he stood for on account of their silence, borders on asinine.[33] Especially, that is, when he invoked this bizarre logic in efforts to silence those who protested against his government's endemic climate change denialism. Such "progressive" thinking, as he disparagingly (but confusingly) called it, is a "worrying development" that seeks to "deny the liberties of Australians." By that he meant, presumably, the freedom of Australians to retain their position as the world's second most profligate per capita carbon emitter without being too worried about it. During the same debate Morrison's then deputy, Michael McCormack, dismissed those who suggested that climate change might have contributed to the devastating bushfires Australia suffered during the 2019–20 summer as "raving inner-city lefties."[34] Such commentary from the leadership of an open democracy like Australia amply illustrates how to erode trust between citizens and their government by promoting willful ignorance and fomenting division.[35]

No stranger to division and ignorance, Donald Trump's presidency was not so much a textbook example of how to destroy trust in a democracy as the predictably disastrous consequences of "electing the most politically inexperienced candidate ever to the highest elected office in the world," as journalist and presidential historian Nancy Gibbs noted. The president's witlessness coupled with his "distant acquaintance with actual truth," Gibbs wrote, amounted to "the most frightening characteristic of this presidency."[36]

It was frightening for many reasons, but chief among them is the ongoing corrosive effect his infantilism has had on the long-term credibility of institutions of government in the United States. That is, the institution of the American people *as a whole* believing in the authority of a system of government founded on serious debate, evidence-based argument, and respect for the truth rather than vaudevillian gibberish. For if trust in *that* institution is damaged or forfeited, fair and effective negotiations over freedom and responsibility (and much else besides) become difficult if not impossible. The costs can be enormous, as illustrated by the unfathomable spectacle of a political system crippled by the obdurate refusal of a president to concede electoral defeat and his subsequent incitement of a mob attack on the US Capitol, alongside his holding to ransom an entire political party despite facing an array of recent, existing, and pending lawsuits that beggars belief, including but not limited to allegations of insurrection, espionage, incitement to assault, theft, criminal obstruction, sexual assault, defamation, wire, tax, and insurance fraud, embezzlement, electoral fraud, perjury, and contempt of court.[37] In light of this litany of political and legal degeneracy it is no wonder that the United States currently faces such eviscerating losses of people's faith in their system of government, mainstream media, and even one another.[38]

Thus, as political partisanship has deepened, trust has plummeted. Typically, in recent years, according to the Pew Research Center, when a Democrat is in the White House the percentage of Republican supporters who trust the federal government to do what's right (as Pew puts it) is in the low teens or even single digits, and the figures are the same when the roles are reversed. Worryingly, even when the presidential incumbent is from their preferred party, few Americans (28–36 percent) trust in the integrity of the government.[39] The politicization of everything, from race, religion, COVID-19, and climate change, to inauguration crowd sizes, high school history curricula, fast-food favorites, and pillow brands,[40] has jaundiced the polity such that, two years after Donald Trump lost the 2020 election, 35 percent of all Americans (including an astonishing 68 percent of Republicans) still believe that he is the real president,[41] and just over one-third (36 percent) of all Americans trust mass media organizations.[42] The "soul of the nation" really is at stake, as President Joe Biden put it when he warned that "democracy cannot survive when one side believes there are only two outcomes to an election: either they win or they were cheated. . . . You can't love your country only when you win."[43] Compassion and decency have also become so debased that in the fall of 2021 a largely maskless crowd at a public school board meeting in Tennessee felt no shame in laughing, jeering, and yelling "shut up" at a masked high school student who was explaining how his grandmother's recent death from COVID-19 was the reason why he supported a school mask mandate.[44] On both sides of the political divide, it seems, people don't just disagree; they now abhor each other.[45]

A big part of the reason for this political paralysis concerns the absence or abuse of "information." "Whenever the people are well informed, they can be trusted with their own government," wrote Thomas Jefferson in a letter to Richard Price in January 1789. Price, an English theologian and philosopher, shared with Jefferson a belief in republican virtues, most especially the responsibilities of citizens to make their governments accountable. Jefferson was the United States' minister to France at the time, and his words were inspired as much by his witnessing the building of revolutionary fervor in France as by his reflections on the new republic he had helped establish back home. But, whatever the inspiration, when he added, "that whenever things get so far wrong as to attract their notice, they [the people] may be relied on to set them to rights," it is unlikely he would have imagined what was to come to pass in his homeland exactly 240 years later.

A time when the forty-fifth president of the United States, on the eve of his first impeachment trial, tweeted, "I am coming to the conclusion that what is taking place is not an impeachment, it is a COUP, intended to take away the Power of the People, their VOTE, their Freedoms, their Second Amendment, Religion, Military, Border Wall, and their God-given rights as a Citizen of the United States of America!"[46] Or, for that matter, when the same president declared a little later, "I don't take responsibility at all," in response to a question about the acute shortage of coronavirus testing kits over which his administration had authority, when the need was so desperate in the early days of the crisis.[47]

You have to worry about the state of mind both of a president and of all those inside and outside Congress who supported him then and now when you read such smorgasbord drivel or reflect on such reprehensible shirking of duty. Negotiating liberty and holding a government to account in a political arena based on such divided and perverted trust were and are perilous endeavors that test Jeffersonian principles of governance in ways that Mr. Jefferson himself would have had trouble imagining.

Technology to the Rescue?

If our trust in human institutions is wavering, might machines help shore up our faith? Film script dialogue from *Hobbs and Shaw* might not be your first choice of where to look for an answer, and yet the cyborg in pursuit of our eponymous heroes turns out to be something of a closet philosopher. "The more machine I am; the more humane I become," it snarls at one point while surrounded by such carnage and destruction of its own doing that you wonder if it might also be a closet wit.

As a matter of fact, this is pretty much what artificial intelligence guru Stuart Russell (who is both philosopher and wit) argues in his book *Human Compatible*. If anything, Russell tells us, we are more likely to produce robots that are *overly* altruistic than not enough. He calls this the "Somalia Problem," whereby in our enthusiasm to program robots with suitably high-minded and egalitarian algorithms, we create domestic help bots compelled to race off to assist vulnerable humans in Somalia rather than prepare their owner's dinner or clean their home. While Russell believes that such inadvertent impracticality could be programmed out, he is nonetheless optimistic about the benign effect such relentless altruism might have on us mortals. Daily exposure to singularly empathetic machines, he suggests, just might help us all be less driven by envy and pride.[48]

Well, maybe. But if better programming is the answer to perfecting AI, it remains shackled to the problem of human fallibility. For, no matter how technically proficient the machines we build are, so long as human play a part in their construction or maintenance, errors are possible and will occur. *We* become the weakest link. Racial and gender prejudices, for example, find their way into facial recognition technology, with tests repeatedly showing identification error rates significantly higher for women and darker-skinned people.[49] In one test of Amazon's "Rekognition" system conducted by the American Civil Liberties Union (ACLU), comparing the scanned faces of 535 members of the US Congress with 25,000 police mugshots, the system generated 28 false matches. While startling enough, what is especially shocking about this error rate is that it was so racially biased: 11 of the 28 false matches were of people of color (almost 40 percent of the error sample size), whereas only 20 percent of the members of Congress at that time were people of color.[50]

Such skewed results arise directly from the "dirty data" sets on which the system is built: the more data supplied on Caucasian and other lighter-skinned people, the more accurate the system for those groupings. The fact that more data from these groupings are used may stem from the conscious or unconscious prejudices of the programmer—a profession typically dominated by white men.[51] It's one example of the "discrimination feedback loops" that exist in many aspects of our lives, from job applications and search engine predictions to assumptions about someone's need for financial and medical services.[52]

Other human frailties such as carelessness and greed can also undermine our trust in machines. It was this combination that undid Boeing's new 737 MAX8 airplanes. In a five-month period between late 2018 and early 2019 two of these planes were forced to crash by a faulty computer override system installed, ironically, to prevent the engines on planes from stalling and causing the planes to fall out of the sky. Everyone on both planes died—348 people in total. Boeing's "Maneuvering Characteristics Augmentation System" (MCAS) was designed to bypass the pilot when it detected certain unsafe combinations of speed and angle. So efficient is MCAS that once it has been triggered—even when based on false data (neither plane was in danger of stalling)—nothing the pilot can do will prevent the system repeatedly forcing the plane's nose downward. Black-box data from the Lion Air jet involved in the first of the crashes shows a heartbreaking tussle between pilot and autopilot occurring twenty-one times in the seven minutes the plane was in the air before it plummeted into the sea at more than 500 miles per hour.[53]

None of this would have happened if the "System Safety Analysis" of MCAS that Boeing filed with the US Federal Aviation Administration had not contained a number of crucial flaws. Such safety analyses are explicitly intended to guard against catastrophic design and technical failures. Yet it seems clear from documents leaked to the press that due to a lack of funding of the Federal Aviation Administration (FAA), coupled with Boeing's haste to have the 737 MAX approved as soon as possible so as to compete with the rival Airbus 320neo (already nine months ahead in its development), the safety screening was fatally compromised.[54] Here again, human frailty undoes technical competence, and once more commercial imperatives are at the heart of the matter.

To be sure, the free market and technology have together proven to be a potent mix. It has led to the private sector development and commercialization of many features of modern existence that we consider essential to exercising our freedom today. How we travel, communicate, learn, earn, play, treat illness, stay safe, and try to live more sustainably are all actions underpinned by the commercial exploitation of technology. But it has also created new and serious problems for the state of liberty. Error-prone facial recognition and autopilot apparatus aside, technology has enormously enhanced our capacities to harm the environment and thereby curtail the freedoms and pile on the responsibilities of future generations. It has created such enormous rivers of communication and reservoirs of information that we are ever more reliant on the companies that control the technology to sort and filter what we see, hear, and say. Perhaps most significant of all, we have opened wide the door on our privacy through our wholesale addiction (or surrender) to the indispensable role technology plays in our everyday lives.

As the end of chapter 2 (on responsibility) and chapter 7 (on security) show, the extent of digital surveillance we are all subject to today is astonishing and, for some, like journalists, activists, and critics operating in nondemocracies, even life threatening.[55] Nearly all of this surveillance happens without our consent or even knowledge, and much of it is made possible by private sector innovation and the pursuit of profit. What makes this situation so troubling in terms of our liberty is that it serves the interests of both control-driven governments and profit-driven corporations to ensure the surveillance sector is subject to as little supervision and public scrutiny as possible. The result, as David Kaye, the former UN special rapporteur on the right to free speech, noted in his damning 2019 report on surveillance and human rights, is that "private industry has stepped in, unsupervised and with something close to impunity."[56]

Trust in our institutions of government and our technology service providers under such accommodating conditions is limited if not impossible. And we know it. "Techlash," such as was directed at Cambridge Analytica's brazen attempts to influence the US presidential election and UK Brexit referendum in 2016 by manipulating personal data harvested from some 50 million Facebook accounts,[57] is now a real and growing phenomenon. The *Oxford English Dictionary* (*OED*) recognized the term as runner-up for its "Word of the Year" in 2019, defining it as a "strong and widespread negative reaction to the growing power and influence of large technology companies." The Edelman Trust Barometer, in a nod to the *OED*, noted in its 2019 report that for the first time "significant cracks" are appearing in our trust in tech.[58] Edelman pursued the point in its "2021 Trust Barometer" by headlining what it called a state of global "information bankruptcy" caused by the toxic mix of institutional tendencies not to "provide truth, unbiased and reliable information" and the enormous electronic capacity to spread such calumny.[59]

One might suppose that tighter and more thorough regulation would help. It almost certainly would with technologies that we already know reasonably well. But regulation is far less likely to be the answer with frontier AI technologies, precisely because we don't yet know all the questions we need to ask.[60] Driverless cars, surveillance drones, digital data mining, and predictive medical treatment, as well as text generator chatbots, domestic-help robots, facial recognition, and autopilot systems, are all throwing up learn-as-we-go problems. Putting our faith in technology to safeguard our freedom of movement, information exchange, personal safety, and privacy will always be restricted by the unavoidable compromises that make up any form of regulation. Speed and convenience versus security and confidentiality, as well as competing questions of ownership, control, and cost, yield myriad tensions that must be reconciled through some form of negotiated settlement. Calls for "ethical tech"[61] and "trustworthiness" in the governance of technology[62] are all welcome (and I certainly am glad to hear them), but they leave unanswered the difficult questions of detail.[63]

In the end, neither technology nor its oversight can be foolproof. Faults and abuses will occur in both. We may seek to minimize their instance and impact, of course, but we will never remove them altogether. No geek, no matter how starry-eyed, can rightly tell you otherwise. The possibility of error in technology is always present, even if we continually strive to reduce the probability of it happening. Perhaps the most important lesson we should draw from our reliance on technology is to manage our expectations of it. To be wary of its fallibility. To recognize that even if technology is more reliable than a human being, it can nonetheless fail, not least because of human intervention in its design or operation. Even at its most optimistic, Amazon promises only 95 percent accuracy from its facial recognition system, and the FAA's categorizations of risk for aircraft manufacturers are designed to minimize rather than eliminate certain outcome probabilities (such as "catastrophic" and "hazardous").[64] The mantle of responsibility to handle the part technology plays in promoting or retarding our freedoms ultimately rests on our shoulders.

All of us. Individually and collectively, it will be up to us to decide how far technology helps or hinders how we live with liberty.

Sharing the Sunlight

In one of the most famous tales of antiquity, Alexander III visits the celebrated philosopher, eccentric, and vagabond Diogenes. At the time, Alexander was setting out on his extraordinary empire-building journey that would earn him the sobriquet "The Great," while Diogenes was simply enjoying a lie-down in the sun. Upon seeing the approaching entourage, Diogenes raised himself up on one elbow, wondering who had come to disturb his peace. Alexander introduced himself and asked Diogenes if there was anything he could do for him. "Yes," replied Diogenes, "stand a little less between me and the sun."[65]

As with the sunshine, so with liberty. We all deserve to feel its warmth on our skin, but for each of us to enjoy it, we must accept that there will be times when others stand in front of us, with still others standing beside and behind us. We may bask in the light a lot or a little, but however much, there are always others around us to consider. Sometimes it is those who govern us that stand in the way; at other times it is our family, friends, neighbors, strangers, or enemies who cast shadows. Whichever, each will likely plead necessity or fairness (though some will try to steal it or take it by force). But it is inevitable that each of us spends time in the shade. How much time and how much shade are matters for us—alone and together—to determine as best we can. These are the responsibilities that come with freedom. Sometimes onerous, often negotiable, and always present, these are responsibilities shared by all, so all can enjoy the freedoms they uphold. This is living with the paradox of liberty.

Acknowledgments

I began writing this book in the pre-COVID freedom of Paris, mostly at a table in the enchantingly elegant Bibliothèque Richelieu. I finished it in post-lockdown Sydney amid the shambolic clutter of my study. As contemporary symbols of the roller-coaster ride that is any enterprise seeking to pin down the essence of liberty, these do very nicely. Along the way I have incurred many debts to those who kept the project, and me, from going off the rails. They read, listened, challenged, suggested, corrected, and encouraged, some from the very beginning to the very end, others without even knowing.

To all the following I offer my thanks and appreciation: Nicole Abadee, Dennis Altman, Daniel Augenstein, Steven Baker, Ann Barger Hannum, Simon Bronitt, Micah Burch, Larry Catá Backer, Josh Dowse, Catherine Drayton, Lydie Duverne-Polilat, Valerie Duverne-Polilat, Nick Fowler, Catherine Giraud-Kinley, Nikki Goldstein, Hurst Hannum, James B. Hill, Aimilia Ioannidou, Helen Irving, Rowan Jacob, Judith Kinley, Martin Krygier, Juliana McCarthy, Stephen McGlinchey, Neil Murphy, Lucy Nason, Justine Nolan, Pip O'Keefe, Geeta Pathak Sangroula, Philip Pettit, Fergus Pickles, Anne Pierce, Pete Pierce, Wojciech Sadurski, Yubaraj Sangroula, Ben Saul, Patti Sellers, Kym Sheehan, Chris Sidoti, Shiyan Sun, Charlie Taylor, Kevin Walton, and Leif Wenar. I'm also indebted to my students over many years and in many places for all that I've learned from them while debating the boundaries of freedom.

Finally, I am especially grateful to my former agent Jim Hornfischer, who died tragically in June 2021; to my current agents, Chris Newson and Nick Wallwork; and to Robin Coleman, my editor at Johns Hopkins University Press, each of whom has shown faith in me and in the book beyond deserving.

293

Notes

Prologue

1. It is sobering to recall that the disease was not even formally named as COVID-19 (or SARS-CoV-2, as it is officially known) by the World Health Organization (WHO) until February 11, 2020, before being declared a pandemic barely four weeks later, on March 11 (again by the WHO).
2. A label favored by right-wing populists whose uncompromising demands for freedom make frequent appearances throughout the book and that are addressed accordingly.
3. I must confess, for example, to wondering long and hard whether such notable concerns as privacy and fairness deserved dedicated chapters, but in the end I saw their particular importance lying in their ubiquity rather than specificity, being elemental features of many, if not all, of the other domains.

Introduction. Tea with a Dictator

1. But as one of my colleagues on these trips, Chris Sidoti, reminds me, General Khin Nyunt, then chief of intelligence and de facto prime minister, as well as Tin Hlaing's superior, was ultimately responsible for the program's approval.
2. See UN Commission on Human Rights, Commission on Human Rights Resolution 2000/23: Situation of Human Rights in Myanmar, April 18, 2000, E/CN.4/RES/2000/23.
3. One which led me to a somewhat soul-searching article written with Trevor Wilson (then Australia's ambassador to Myanmar and a crucial supporter of the program) on why and how we as human rights practitioners and advocates engaged with the military dictatorship. See David Kinley and Trevor Wilson, "Engaging a Pariah: Human Rights Training in Burma/Myanmar," *Human Rights Quarterly* 29, no. 3 (2007): 368–402.
4. "No more than a show of objectivity separating self-consciousness from possession," as philosopher G. W. F Hegel dismissively put it, in *Phenomenology of Spirit* (1807), para. 583.
5. Thus, for example, whereas the English Bill of Rights in 1690, together with, a century later, the American Declaration of Independence and the US Constitution, referred to both "freedom" and "liberty" sparingly but in roughly equal measure, the UN Universal Declaration of Human Rights in 1948 refers to "freedom" or "free" thirty times and "liberty" just once. Thereafter, the preference for freedom over liberty in landmark rights documents and in political speech more generally has, if anything, gained

further traction. The implications of this lexical shift are discussed in chapter 1.

6. See chapter 6, on work, under the heading "A Working Future."

Chapter 1. From "Liberty Dogs" to "Freedom Fries"

1. Plato, *The Republic* (circa 380 BCE), trans. Benjamin Jowett (1998), VIII and IV.6, respectively, Project Gutenberg, https://www.gutenberg.org/files/1497/1497-h/1497-h.htm.

2. Thomas Hobbes, *Leviathan* (1651), ed. Edward White and David Widger (2002), chapter XIV, Project Gutenberg, https://www.gutenberg.org/files/3207/3207-h/3207-h.htm.

3. John Locke, *Second Treatise of Government* (1690), ed. Chuck Greif (2017), chapter VI, sec. 57, Project Gutenberg, https://www.gutenberg.org/files/7370/7370-h/7370-h.htm.

4. Immanuel Kant, "What Is Enlightenment?" (1784), at 8.36.

5. Immanuel Kant, *Critique of Practical Reason* (1788), 5:19–30.

6. We return to the remarkable story of Paine's devotion to liberty, as well as what it cost him, in the opening pages of chapter 8 on voice.

7. Mary Wollstonecraft, *A Vindication of the Rights of Women* (London: J. Johnson, 1792), chapter 2.

8. Bearing testimony to Lincoln's words, the very first iteration of the Pledge of Allegiance of the United States, formulated some thirty years later, declared "liberty and justice for all," which phrase remains to this day despite several amendments to the Pledge.

9. Bentham, *Principles of the Civil Code* (1843), part 1, chapter 1.

10. Most famously in *A Room of One's Own* (London: Hogarth Press, 1929); on which see the further discussion in the opening pages of chapter 5.

11. For a pair of excellent surveys of divergent views on freedom in contemporary philosophical thought, see Leif Wenar, "The Meanings of Freedom," in Laurence Thomas (ed.), *Contemporary Debates in Social Philosophy* (New York: Wiley-Blackwell, 2007), 43–53, and Katrin Flikschuh, *Freedom* (Cambridge: Polity Press, 2007).

12. Which boundaries, he argued, "should absolutely govern how society deals with its individual members in matters involving compulsion and control, whether through physical force in the form of legal penalties or through the moral coercion of public opinion." John Stuart Mill, *On Liberty* (London: John W. Parker, 1859), chapter 1.

13. Isaiah Berlin, *Two Concepts of Liberty* (Oxford: Clarendon Press, 1958).

14. In *Just Freedom: A Moral Compass for a Complex World* (New York: W. W. Norton, 2014), Pettit employs the notion of liberty as a moral compass by which we measure and hold accountable our organs of government as they go about the business of negotiating freedom's limits.

15. Edmund Fawcett, *Liberalism* (Princeton, NJ: Princeton University Press, 2014), 1–4.

16. Hanna Fenichel Pitkin, "Are Freedom and Liberty Twins?" *Political Theory* 16 (1998): 523–52, at 543.

17. Friedrich A. von Hayek, *The Constitution of Liberty* (Chicago: University of Chicago Press, 1960), 15.

18. Adolf Hitler's May 1, 1939, address to German youth, in Max Domarus (ed.), *Hitler: Speeches and Proclamations, 1932–1945: The Chronicle of a Dictatorship*, vol. 3 (Wauconda, IL: Bolchazy-Carducci, 1997), 1603.

19. J. V. Stalin, *Works* (London: Red Star Press, 1978), vol. 14, Marxist Internet Archive, https://www.marxists.org/reference/archive/stalin/works/1936/03/01.htm. Echoes of the same blithe disingenuity are found in Vladimir Putin's reasoning for invading Ukraine in February 2022: "Freedom guides our policy, the freedom to choose independently our future and the future of our children," he said. "We believe that all the peoples living in today's Ukraine . . . must be able to enjoy this right to make a free choice." "Transcript: Vladimir Putin's Televised Address on Ukraine," *Bloomberg News*, February 24, 2022.

20. For an excoriating critique of both these twisted views of liberty, it's hard to go past Aldous Huxley: "We are asked by the supporters of Stalin's government to believe that the best and shortest road to liberty is through military servitude; that the most suitable preparation for responsible self-government is a tyranny employing police espionage, delation, legalized terrorism and press censorship; that the proper education for future freemen and peace-lovers is that which was and is still being used by Prussian militarists." Aldous Huxley, *Ends and Means* (New York: Harper, 1937).

21. Google Books Ngram Viewer charts the steady decline of the use of "liberty" in published works from 1800 (when its incidence was approximately 2.5 times that of "freedom") to 2019 when "freedom" appeared some 3.5 times more often than "liberty." Interestingly, the crossover point was in 1914. See https://books.google.com/ngrams/ (search: liberty, freedom).

22. Altogether, the words "free" and "freedom" appear nine times in the UN charter. "Liberty" is not mentioned at all in the charter and just once in the UDHR—in Article 3: "Everyone has the right to life, liberty and security of person."

23. See, for example, the "Travaux Préparatoires" for the International Covenant on Civil and Political Rights (ICCPR), archived in "UN Human Rights Treaties," University of Virginia School of Law, accessed January 28, 2023, http://hr-travaux.law.virginia.edu/document/iccpr/.

24. The European Convention on Human Rights (1950), for example, which focuses on civil and political rights, refers to freedom no less than fifty times, whereas liberty is mentioned on only six occasions and exclusively in respect to the right against arbitrary detention and free movement.

25. Bruce Sterling, "Charter 08: The Most Politically Explosive Tract Ever Published on the Internet," *Wired*, October 13, 2010.

26. It is a little shocking to note that Mandela was in fact ten years older than King. Mandela's death at age ninety-five in 2013 underlined not only how much and for how long he had fought for freedom, but also what we all lost when King's life was cut short by an assassin in 1968 at the age of thirty-nine.

27. Treaty of Rome (1957), titles I and III.

28. In another sign of the times, and possibly outdoing the freedom fries saga, was the Trump administration's preposterous dubbing of liquefied natural gas in 2019 as "freedom gas" when announcing an increase in overseas exports of the commodity. Department of Energy, media release, May 29, 2019; for further discussion, see chapter 11, on respect, under the heading "The Freedom Express."

29. "The Nation: Freedom vs. Liberty; More Than Just Another Word for Nothing Left to Lose," *New York Times*, March 23, 2003.

30. In respect of which and the subsequent case of *Bruen*, decided by the Supreme Court in 2022, see the further discussion in chapter 7, on security, under the heading "Bearing Arms."

31. As explored more fully throughout chapter 8, on voice.

32. The fact that homosexuality remains a criminal offence in sixty-nine countries testifies to the residual power of religion of all stripes over institutions of government. See "Map of Countries That Criminalise LGBT People," Human Dignity Trust, accessed January 28, 2023, https://www.humandignitytrust.org /lgbt-the-law/map-of-criminalisation. I return to this topic in chapter 9, on love, under the heading "What's Sex Got to Do with It?"

33. See John Schoen, "States with Strict Gun Laws Have Fewer Firearms Deaths; Here's How Your State Stacks Up, *CNBC*, February 27, 2018, https://www .cnbc.com/2018/02/27/states-with-strict-gun-laws-have-fewer-firearms-deaths -heres-how-your-state-stacks-up.html. The freedom consequences of gun control, or its lack, are discussed further in chapter 7, on security, under the heading "Bearing Arms."

34. That is, according to the *Oxford English Dictionary*: "The state of being able to act without hindrance or restraint."

35. As part of its Freedom 2014 initiative, the BBC asked the public to submit their images of what freedom meant to them. Although there were, of course, a huge variety (including, delightfully, a broken egg shell with the number of incubating days scored on the inside), the most common theme was open space. See "Freedom2014: What Freedom Looks Like to You," *BBC News*, April 1, 2014, https://www.bbc.com/news/magazine-26614481.

36. Berlin, *Two Concepts of Liberty*, 54.

37. Karl Popper, *The Open Society and Its Enemies* (London: Routledge, 1945), chapter 7.

38. See chapter 12 of this volume, on trust.

39. In fact, regarding the scope of free speech the Chinese Constitution goes further than nearly all others by adding (in Article 41) that "citizens of the People's Republic of China have the right to criticize and make suggestions regarding any State organ or functionary."

40. See, for example, Kai Strittmatter, *We Have Been Harmonised: Life in China's Surveillance State* (Exeter, UK: Old Street Publishing, 2019). The frankly terrifying extent to which the Chinese Communist Party has weaponized the internet to regulate and silence the voices of its own citizens is explored in chapter 8, on voice, and chapter 12, on trust.

41. For discussion on the bendability these qualifications lend to the interpretation of human rights laws, see chapter 2 under the heading "The Bendability of Human Rights."

42. *On Liberty*, chapter 4.

43. Jean-Jacques Rousseau, *On the Social Contract* (1762), book 1.6 ("The Social Compact").

Chapter 2. There Are No Robinson Crusoes

1. See Grimshaw's autobiography, *A Grain of Sand: The Story of One Man and an Island* (Nairobi: Camerapix International Publishers, 1996), and his feature documentary of the same name on YouTube, accessed November 7, 2022, https://www.youtube.com/watch?v=GjRke2b36tM.

2. *The Second Treatise of Government* (1690), chapter II.

3. In light of the following catalog of tyrannical infamy it is sobering to note that leaders who claim to have "the right to do whatever I want" can also be found in modern democracies. Former president Donald Trump uttered these very words in 2019, albeit based on a fundamentally erroneous reading of Article II of the US Constitution. See Michael Brice-Saddler, "While Bemoaning Mueller Probe, Trump Falsely Says the Constitution Gives Him 'the Right to Do Whatever I Want,'" *Washington Post*, July 24, 2019.

4. Suetonius, *Lives of the Caesars*, vol. 1, trans. J. C. Rolfe, Loeb Classical Library (Cambridge, MA: Harvard University Press, 1914).

5. "Autocracy crept in, like the coward it is," as Nadya Tolokonnikova writes about Putin's Russia, but also in warning against complacency in democracies. "I'm an Activist in Russia: I Can't Believe What My Life Has Become," *New York Times*, August 26, 2020.

6. See Shirer's entry for June 22, 1940, in *Berlin Diary: The Journal of a Foreign Correspondent, 1934–1941* (New York: Alfred A. Knopf, 1941).

7. Li Zhi-Sui, *The Private Life of Chairman Mao* (New York: Random House, 1994), x.

8. *The Republic*, Book IX. Demonstrating the acuity and timelessness of his observations on human nature, Plato says of tyrants-in-the-making: "When such men are only private individuals and before they get power, this is their character; they associate entirely with their own flatterers or ready tools; or if they want anything from anybody, they in their turn are equally ready to bow down before them: they profess every sort of affection for them; but when they have gained their point they know them no more." Of the many modern politicians who might fit this description, I ask you who jumps to mind as the best fit of all?

9. I'm drawing on Plato's *Gorgias*, in which he depicts Socrates in dialogue with Polus on this question, at 466a4–468e5. See also James Doyle's interpretation of this interaction in "Do Tyrants Do What They Want?" Academia, accessed November 5, 2022, https://www.academia.edu/11974538/Do_Tyrants_Do_What_They_Want_Gorgias_466a4-468e5.

10. On the many and varied legal implications of the free will question, see Allan McCay and Michael Sevel (eds.), *Free Will and the Law* (Abingdon, UK: Routledge, 2019).

11. Or, as Hegel presents it, a tad more dramatically, the consequence of a "pure *being-for-self* which has thrown off all community with others . . . is that the individual has simply perished, and the absolute unyieldingness of individual existence is pulverized on the equally unrelenting but continuous world of actuality." *Phenomenology of Spirit* (1807), para. 364.

12. Hannah Arendt, "Freedom and Politics: A Lecture," *Chicago Review* 14, no. 1 (Spring 1960): 28–46.

13. As of 2019, however, trucks have now been banned from the city between 7 a.m. and 7 p.m., which has helped.

14. See World Health Organization, *Global Status Report on Road Safety 2018*, table A2, at 302.

15. Reflecting, in part, John Locke's grandiose proclamation that "where there is no law, there is no freedom"—or, rather, "no *liberty*," as I see the respective meanings of the two terms. See Locke, *Second Treatise of Government*, chapter VI.

16. George Bernard Shaw, *Maxims for Revolutionists* (Cambridge: Cambridge University Press, 1903).

17. In *Civilization and Its Discontents* (London: Hogarth Press, 1930), 25, 33, Sigmund Freud professes to be astonished "that so many people have come to take up this strange attitude of hostility to civilization," as reflected in their "urge for freedom" from the "demands" it makes of them.

18. There are today, writes Fintan O'Toole, "very powerful interests who demand 'freedom' in order to do as they like with the environment, society, and the economy. They have infused a very large part of American culture with the belief that 'freedom' is literally more important than life. My 'freedom' to own assault weapons trumps your right not to get shot at school." See his article, "Donald Trump Has Destroyed the Country He Promised to Make Great Again," *Irish Times*, April 25, 2020.

19. David Boaz, *The Libertarian Mind: A Manifest of Freedom* (New York: Simon & Schuster, 2015), 1.

20. This simple, incontrovertible truth seems so often to escape the minds of many rabid American libertarians that one cannot but salute the depth of their commitment to incoherence. Thus, for example, former US senator and Republican presidential candidate Ron Paul, in his feted manifesto *Liberty Defined* (New York: Grand Central, 2011), holds (at xi) that to believe in liberty is to "trust in the spontaneous order that emerges when the state does not intervene in human volition and human cooperation." Yet, barely a page later, he laments that "powerful special interests rule, and there seems to be no way to fight against them." Well, yes, indeed and it is precisely those "private interests" of all kinds that would devour one another (in a "war of all against all," as Thomas Hobbes warned some 370 years ago) if let loose in the sort of ultraminimalist state envisioned by Mr. Paul. He might presume, of course, that he and his kin would triumph in such confrontations and devour more than most, but that is a testimony to selfishness, not liberty.

21. On which points of distinction, see Herbert McClosky and Dennis Chong, "Similarities and Differences between Left-Wing and Right-Wing Radicals," *British Journal of Political Science* 15, no. 3 (1985): 329–63.

22. What Williams wanted, it transpires, was to take her "sweet time" eating a "delicious" meal at "a crowded Red Robin." See Tina Nguyen, "A New MAGA Movement Debate: Is Trump Overdoing It?" *Politico*, March 22, 2020.

23. "Florida Gov. DeSantis to School Officials: Enforce Mask Mandate, Get Your Salaries Withheld," *USA Today*, August 9, 2021. An injunction against the relevant provision in DeSantis's executive order (dubbed the "Parents' Bill of Rights") was subsequently granted by a Florida state circuit court judge who,

after taking care to recognize the importance of parents' right to choose, added that such a right can nonetheless be restricted if "exercising that right is harmful to other people." See Ana Ceballos and Jeffrey Solochek, "Florida Judge Rules That DeSantis Overreached on School Mask Debate," *Miami Herald*, August 27, 2021.

24. For my take on the wider political and policy implications of this bendability, see David Kinley, "Bendable Rules: The Development Implications of Human Rights Pluralism," in Brian Z. Tamanaha, Caroline Mary Sage, and Michael J. V. Woolcock (eds.), *Legal Pluralism and Development: Scholars and Practitioners in Dialogue* (Cambridge: Cambridge University Press, 2012), 50–65.

25. See, for example, Articles 2, 17, 18, 19, 21, and 22 of the UN International Covenant on Civil and Political Rights. No such qualifications apply to one's freedom from torture, slavery, nondiscrimination, or arbitrary detention as protected in the same treaty.

26. See, for example, Articles 7, 8, 9, 11, 12, and 13 of the UN International Covenant on Economic, Social, and Cultural Rights.

27. See Mary Ann Glendon, *A World Made New: Eleanor Roosevelt and the Universal Declaration of Human Rights* (New York: Random House, 2002), 42.

28. Chris Welch, "Google Just Gave a Stunning Demo of Assistant Making an Actual Phone Call," *The Verge*, May 8, 2018.

29. Natasha Lomas, "Duplex Shows Google Failing at Both Ethical and Creative AI Design," *TechCrunch*, May 11, 2018.

30. Josh Gillin, "The More Outrageous, the Better: How Clickbait Ads Make Money for Fake News Sites," *Politifact*, October 4, 2017.

31. Educators have been especially animated in these debates, and for good reason. See, for example, Chris Gilliard and Pete Rorabaugh, "You're Not Going to Like How Colleges Respond to ChatGPT", *Slate*, February 3, 2023.

32. The Center for Humane Technology's mission is neatly captured by the pronouncement in its newsletter, *Catalyst* (March 31, 2022), that AI "neutrality is a myth . . . we shape technology and technology shapes us." And in response to the ethical challenges posed by the rise of generative AI, such as ChatGPT, Tristan Harris is no less forthright: "We are the ones who decide what it will mean to be human going forward and what it means to be a machine." Center for Humane Technology, "Synthetic Humanity and AI: What's at Stake," February 16, 2023, podcast transcript, 1, https://www.humanetech.com /podcast/synthetic-humanity-ai-whats-at-stake.

33. To which end, see the excellent *State of AI Ethics* reports published regularly by the Montreal AI Ethics Institute, accessed November 5, 2022, https:// montrealethics.ai/state/.

34. Which debate bodies like the UK government's Centre for Data Ethics and Innovation are expressly tasked to facilitate; see https://www.gov.uk /government/organisations/centre-for-data-ethics-and-innovation (accessed November 5, 2022).

35. The Australian government's algorithmically automated welfare debt recovery process (dubbed "Robodebt") is but one catastrophic example. Erroneously and illegally targeting some 400,000 welfare recipients, the scheme was labeled a

"massive failure of public administration" in a 2021 court-ordered settlement worth AUD1.8 billion and is now subject to an ongoing royal commission. See "A Robodebt Royal Commission Has Been Announced: Here's How We Got to This Point," *ABC News*, August 26, 2022.

36. See "You Won't Believe What Obama Says in This Video," YouTube, accessed February 2, 2023, https://www.youtube.com/watch?v=cQ54GDm1eL0; and a whole series of clips on the *deeptomcruise* TikTok account, at https://www.tiktok.com/@deeptomcruise (accessed November 5, 2022).

37. Schick, interviewed on "American Deepfake," *Foreign Correspondent*, ABC, June 25, 2021. See also her book *Deep Fakes and the Infocalypse* (London: Monoray, 2020).

38. Shoshana Zuboff, *The Age of Surveillance Capitalism* (London: Profile Books, 2019), 11.

39. Zuboff defines surveillance capitalism, succinctly and stylishly, as "the ubiquitous computational, sensate, actuating architectures of Big Other" (496).

Chapter 3. Health

1. Published as a white paper and titled *Social Insurance and Allied Services* (Cmd. 6404; 1942) (hereafter cited as Beveridge Report).

2. Roderick Floud, *Height, Health, and History: Nutritional Status in the United Kingdom, 1750–1980* (Cambridge: Cambridge University Press, 1990).

3. In particular, Beveridge highlighted the fact that compared to other industrialized nations, the provision of publicly funded medical services in Britain "fall[s] seriously short of what has been accomplished elsewhere." Beveridge Report, para. 3.

4. See *OECD Health Statistics 2021*. In the United States, however, national health expenditure accounts for a staggering 17.7 percent (or $3.8 trillion) of GDP (2019 data). See also "NHE Fact Sheet," US Centers for Medicare and Medicaid Services, December 16, 2020, https://www.cms.gov/Research-Statistics-Data-and-Systems/Statistics-Trends-and-Reports/NationalHealth ExpendData/NHE-Fact-Sheet.

5. See Ben Saul, David Kinley, and Jacqueline Mowbray, "The Right to Health," chapter 14 in *International Covenant on Economic, Social, and Cultural Rights: Commentary, Cases, and Materials* (Oxford: Oxford University Press, 2014).

6. Soobramoney v. Minister of Health KwaZulu Natal, November 27, 1997, 1998 (1) SA 765 (CC).

7. See Magdalena Sepúlveda, "Colombia: The Constitutional Court's Role in Addressing Social Justice," in Malcolm Langford (ed.), *Social Rights Jurisprudence: Emerging Trends in International and Comparative* Law (Cambridge: Cambridge University Press, 2008), 152–53.

8. Amy Davidson-Sorkin, "Trump's Reckless Rush to Reopen," *New Yorker*, March 24, 2020.

9. For an early harbinger of how countries might measure up against these standards, see "The Politics of Pandemics," *The Economist*, March 12, 2020. For real-time data on how countries are performing in terms of managing infections, hospitalizations (US only), and deaths, see the John Hopkins Coronavirus Resource Center, accessed November 5, 2022, https://coronavirus

.jhu.edu/map.html; and for vaccine rollouts worldwide, see "Coronavirus (COVID-19) Vaccinations," Our World in Data, accessed November 5, 2022, https://ourworldindata.org/covid-vaccinations, which highlights the huge and unconscionable disparities in vaccination rates and totals between high- and low-income countries.

10. An overabundance of which, according to philosopher John Rawls in his iconic *Theory of Justice* (Cambridge, MA: Harvard University Press, 1971), "is more likely to be a positive hindrance, a meaningless distraction at best if not a temptation to indulgence and emptiness" (§44, pp. 257–58).

11. See, for example, Steve Salerno, *Sham: How the Self-Help Movement Made America Helpless* (New York: Crown, 2006).

12. Sugar taxes have focused on sweetened beverages; some fifty countries have now adopted such a tax; see the "Countries That Have Taxes on Sugar-Sweetened Beverages (SSBs)," Obesity Evidence Hub, August 2021, https:// www.obesityevidencehub.org.au/collections/prevention/countries-that-have -implemented-taxes-on-sugar-sweetened-beverages-ssbs.

13. Currently twenty-four countries prohibit abortion under any circumstances (consisting mostly of states heavily dominated by Christian or Muslim mores), to which one must now add a quickly growing number of states within the United States, following the *Dobbs* decision in 2022 (see further below). For a running tally of those US states, see "After *Roe* Fell: Abortion Laws by State," Center for Reproductive Rights, accessed February 3, 2023, https:// reproductiverights.org/maps/abortion-laws-by-state/.

14. According to the global market research and consulting firm Ipsos ("Global Views on Abortion in 2021"), the global country average of support for abortion rights stands at 71 percent.

15. In *Dobbs v. Jackson Women's Health Organization* (597 U.S. __ [2022]), the Supreme Court overturned (6–3) the abortion rights established in *Roe v. Wade* (410 U.S. 113 [1973]), and *Planned Parenthood of Southeastern Pennsylvania v. Casey* (505 U.S. 833 [1992]). A CNN-SSRS opinion poll taken one month after the *Dobbs* decision recorded 63 percent of Americans disapproving the overturning of *Roe v. Wade* and only 37 percent approving the decision. See the SSRS survey results, July 28, 2022, reported at https://s3 .documentcloud.org/documents/22122830/abortion.pdf.

16. In a telling deconstruction of this incongruous position, ethicists Tina Rulli and Stephen Campbell conclude that in fact "anti-vaxxers who are ultimately concerned about vaccine mandates' restriction on their bodily autonomy should be pro-choice." See "Can 'My Body, My Choice' Anti-vaxxers Be Pro-life?" *Bioethics* 36, no. 6 (2022): 708, 714.

17. This is the case even in the United States where federal, state, and local government spending combined accounts for 45.1 percent of total health care expenditure. Private health care insurance amounts to 31 per cent of that total, while the balance comprises household out-of-pocket expenses, philanthropic health care spending, and worksite- or school-sponsored health care programs. See "NHE Fact Sheet"; and Congressional Research Service, "U.S. Health Care Coverage and Spending," *In Focus*, April 1, 2022.

18. World Health Organization, *World Health Statistics 2022*.

19. "Health" (continually updated), World Bank, accessed November 5, 2022, https://data.worldbank.org/topic/health.

20. On pneumonia, see David McAllister et al., "Global, Regional, and National Estimates of Pneumonia Morbidity and Mortality in Children Younger than 5 Years between 2000 and 2015: A Systemic Analysis," *Lancet Global Health* 7, no. 1 (2019): PE47–PE57. On diarrhea, see Report of the Global Burden of Diseases, Injuries, and Risk Factors Study 2016: "Estimates of the Global, Regional, and National Morbidity, Mortality, and Aetiologies of Diarrhoea in 195 Countries," *Lancet Infectious Diseases* 18, no. 11 (2018): P1211–P1228.

21. Save the Children UK, reports that globally the disease kills "close to 1 million" children under the age of five each year: "Pneumonia: The Silent Killer," Save the Children, April 12, 2017, https://www.savethechildren.org.uk /blogs/2017/pneumonia-silent-killer.

22. At 5.4 deaths per 1,000 live births (0.54 per cent), compared to the best performers—Estonia, Norway, Finland, and Japan, all of which are at less than 2.0 deaths per 1,000 live births (0.2 per cent). See "Infant Mortality Rates" (2021 data), OECD Data, accessed November 5, 2022, https://data.oecd.org /healthstat/infant-mortality-rates.htm.

23. OECD, *Health at a Glance 2021: OECD Indicators—Life Expectancy by Sex and Education Level.*

24. See "Nombre de centenaires: évolution et projection," Institut national d'études démographiques, March 2021, https://www.ined.fr/fr/tout-savoir -population/chiffres/france/structure-population/centenaires/.

25. The British medical journal *The Lancet* proclaimed this to be so in its *Global Burden of Disease 2010 Report* 380, no. 9859 (December 15, 2012): 2053–260; since then, obesity rates have continued to increase.

26. According to the World Health Organization, "Non-communicable diseases (NCDs) kill 41 million people each year, equivalent to 71 per cent of all deaths globally." See WHO, *Factsheet: Non-communicable Diseases* (April 13, 2021).

27. See WHO, *Global Antimicrobial Resistance and use Surveillance System (GLASS) Report 2021* (June 9, 2021).

28. The percentage can be lower and still be effective; for polio, for instance, the figure is around 80 percent. The figures are rubbery—there "isn't a 'magic threshold'" percentage, as epidemiologists Gypsyamber D'Souza and David Dowdy point out—because they depend on a host of factors including community make-up and behavior and the nature of the disease. See "What Is Herd Immunity and How Can We Achieve It with COVID-19?" Johns Hopkins Bloomberg School of Public Health, April 6, 2021. See also Christine Aschwanden, "Five Reasons Why COVID Herd Immunity Is Probably Impossible," *Nature*, March 18, 2021.

29. The herd immunity threshold for MMR is believed to be between 93 and 95 percent. See Lavanya Vasudevan and Gavin Yamey, "The Myth about Herd Immunity," *Global Health Now*, December 11, 2019, which also discusses the declining rates of measles vaccinations.

30. WHO, *Ten Threats to Global Health 2019.*

31. "Attitudes to Vaccines," chapter 5 in *Wellcome Global Monitor 2018* (London: Wellcome Trust, June 18, 2019), https://wellcome.org/reports/wellcome-global -monitor/2018.

32. Julio S. Solís Arce et al., "COVID-19 Vaccine Acceptance and Hesitancy in Low- and Middle-Income Countries," *Nature Medicine* 27 (2021): 1385–94.

33. This level of skepticism appears to have been translated into practice, with just 67 percent of the population being fully vaccinated for COVID-19 by late August 2022 (albeit 79 percent have had a least one dose); see "COVID-19 Vaccinations in the United States," in "COVID Data Tracker," Centers for Disease Control and Prevention, accessed November 6, 2022, https://covid.cdc.gov/covid-data-tracker/#vaccinations_vacc-people-additional-dose-totalpop.

34. See Danielle McLaughlin, Jack Mewhirter, and Rebecca Sanders "The Belief That Politics Drive Scientific Research and Its Impact on COVID-19 Risk Assessment," *PLOS One* 16, no. 4 (2021). The consequences of this rift in public trust are further considered in chapter 12.

35. "Western Europeans Have Least Trust in Vaccines Worldwide: Report," *Al Jazeera*, June 19, 2019.

36. Data drawn from WHO, "Tuberculosis Profile: Bangladesh," in *Global Tuberculosis Report 2021*.

37. Lena Sun and Amy Brittain, "Meet the New York Couple Donating Millions to the Anti-vax Movement," *Washington Post*, June 19, 2019, https://www.washingtonpost.com/national/health-science/meet-the-new-york-couple-donating-millions-to-the-anti-vax-movement/2019/06/18/9d791bcc-8e28-11e9-b08e-cfd89bd36d4e_story.html.

38. "Hanging Out with Anti-vaxxers," *The Economist*, March 29, 2019. And while the number of anti-vaxxers peddling such deranged nonsense may be few in number, the damage they do is immense. See Shannon Bond, "Just 12 People Are Behind Most Vaccine Hoaxes on Social Media, Research Shows," *NPR*, May 14, 2021.

39. Jacobson v. Massachusetts, 197 U.S. 11 (1905), at 26. In terms of its uncompromising validation of the program, the court was echoing a long history of community support for smallpox inoculation in America dating back at least to the time of the American Revolution when, as Andrew Wehrman puts it in his *The Contagion of Liberty* (Baltimore: Johns Hopkins University Press, 2022), there was a "violent insistence for freedom from disease" among colonists.

40. *Jacobson*, at 11–12.

41. Vavřička and Others v. the Czech Republic (ECHR, Application nos. 47621/13 and five others), April 8, 2021, at para. 284. In reaching its decision, the Court's Grand Chamber considered that in respect of questions as to how states might choose to go about administering their child vaccination programs the "margin of appreciation" (that is, permitted differences between states) "should be a wide one" (at para. 280).

42. Laura Eggertson, "*Lancet* Retracts 12-Year-Old Article Linking Autism to MMR Vaccines," *Canadian Medical Association Journal* 182, no. 4 (2010): E199–E200.

43. "Rubella in the U.S.," CDC, 2020, https://www.cdc.gov/rubella/about/in-the-us.html.

44. According to the WHO, there were 7 million such cases in 2016. See WHO's *Measles Fact Sheet*, December 6, 2019.

45. The WHO estimates that global rates of severe reactions to vaccines for measles to be 1 in 1 million doses; for the oral polio vaccine, 1 in 2 to 3

million doses; and for the DTP vaccine (diphtheria, pertussis [whooping cough], and tetanus), 1 in 750,000. For the BCG (tuberculosis) vaccine, out of 117 million doses administered in the United Kingdom between 1997 and 2003, there were only 130 reported cases of severe (anaphylactic) allergic reaction (roughly 1 in 900,000). See "Vaccine Knowledge Project: BCG Vaccine," University of Oxford, accessed November 6, 2022, https://vk.ovg.ox .ac.uk/vk/bcg-vaccine. For COVID-19 vaccinations in the United States, anaphylaxis occurs in approximately 5 people per 1 million vaccinated. See *Selected Adverse Events Reported after COVID-19 Vaccination* (continually updated), CDC, accessed November 6, 2022, https://www.cdc.gov/coronavirus /2019-ncov/vaccines/safety/adverse-events.html.

46. See at note 54 in this chapter and accompanying text.
47. See "Measles Cases and Outbreaks" (continually updated), CDC, accessed November 6, 2022, https://www.cdc.gov/measles/cases-outbreaks.html.
48. See "Study Finds Vaccine-Hesitant Public in France and U.S.," Kantar, February 4, 2021, https://www.kantar.com/inspiration/society/study-finds -vaccine-hesitant-public-in-france-and-us; and "Global Vaccine Tracking" (continually updated), Morning Consult, accessed November 6, 2022, https://morningconsult.com/global-vaccine-tracking/. On some of the more outrageous anti-vaxxer theories, see Tim Dickinson, "How the Anti-vaxxers Got Red-Pilled," *Rolling Stone*, February 10, 2021.
49. See "Health Care Utilisation: Immunisation," OECD Health Statistics 2022; and *OECD Family Database: Childhood Vaccination*, OECD, accessed November 6, 2022, https://stats.oecd.org/.
50. "The Message of Measles," *New Yorker*, August 26, 2019.
51. One could see signs of this phenomenon happening throughout 2021 when, for example, in France (one of the world's most vaccine-skeptical nations) COVID-19 vaccine rates had reached beyond 90 percent of the adult population by early September 2021 (see "COVID-19 Vaccine Tracker" (continually updated), European Centre for Disease Prevention and Control, accessed November 6, 2022, https://vaccinetracker.ecdc.europa.eu/public/extensions /COVID-19/vaccine-tracker.html#uptake-tab, despite one survey conducted just six months earlier showing that 37 percent of people in France were either definitely or probably not going to get the vaccine (see "Study Finds Vaccine-Hesitant Public in France and U.S.").
52. "Country Level Data: France," in "Attitudes to Vaccines."
53. See Solís Arce et al., "COVID-19 Vaccine Acceptance and Hesitancy in Low- and Middle-Income Countries," "Table 2: Vaccination Beliefs and Coverage for the Countries Studied."
54. See "Factbox: Countries Making COVID-19 Vaccines Mandatory," *Reuters*, October 8, 2021.
55. See "The Message of Measles." Mulligan is a professor of medicine and director of New York University's Langone Vaccine Center.
56. "Hey, Anti-vaxxers, Are You Ready to Get Your Shots Yet?" (editorial), *Los Angeles Times*, March 18, 2020.
57. "America's Vaccination Crisis Is a Symptom of Our Broken Society," *The Guardian*, April 2, 2019.

58. Albeit in many different forms. See Douglas Vakoch (ed.), *Altruism in Cross-Cultural Perspective* (New York: Springer, 2013).

59. UN Convention Relating to the Status of Refugees (hereafter cited as Refugee Convention), 1951, Art. 1(A)(2). For estimates of the number of all forcibly displaced persons, see UN Office of the High Commissioner for Refugees, *Global Trends Report 2021* (June 2022).

60. Offenses, 8 U.S.C. § 1324(A) (1907).

61. See Office of the Attorney General, "Memorandum: Renewed Commitment to Criminal Immigration Enforcement" US Department of Justice, April 11, 2017, at https://www.justice.gov/opa/press-release/file/956841/download.

62. Lorne Matalon, "Extending 'Zero Tolerance' to People Who Help Migrants along the Border," *All Things Considered*, NPR, May 28, 2019.

63. Ryan Devereaux, "Criminalizing Compassion," *The Intercept*, August 10, 2019, and "Humanitarian volunteer Scott Warren reflects on the borderlands and two years of government persecution," *The Intercept*, November 23, 2019.

64. For further discussion, see Hannah Hamley, "The Weaponization of the 'Alien Harboring' Statute in a New Era of Racial Animus towards Immigrants," *Seattle University Law Review* 44 (2020): 171.

65. Devereaux, "Criminalizing Compassion."

66. I return to the question of how we treat others when I consider the importance of respect in liberty's makeup in chapter 11.

Chapter 4. Happiness

1. "Anne, 104, 'Arrested' for Being an Upstanding Citizen," *BBC News*, March 20, 2019.

2. See Chanuki Illushka Seresinhe, Tobias Preis, George MacKerron, and Helen Susannah Moat, "Happiness Is Greater in More Scenic Locations," *Scientific Reports* 9 (2019): 4498. Results were drawn from data collected via a "Mappiness" app.

3. Alex Bryson and George MacKerron, "Are You Happy While You Work?" *Economic Journal* 127, no. 599 (2015): 106–225.

4. See J. H. Burns, "Happiness and Utility: Jeremy Bentham's Equation," *Utilitas* 17, no. 1 (2005): 46–61.

5. Jeremy Bentham, *An Introduction to the Principles of Morals and Legislation* (1781), chapter IV.

6. Adam Phillips, *Missing Out: In Praise of the Unlived Life* (London: Penguin, 2013), 1–33. On the nature of frustration and our lifelong awareness of the exquisiteness of longing, he writes, "We quickly notice as children—it is, perhaps, the first thing we do notice—that our needs, like our wishes, are always potentially unmet" (xi).

7. *A Point of View: Clams Are Happy* (podcast), BBC Radio 4, 2007, republished in Listener's Guide, November 29, 2019, http://www.listenersguide.org.uk/bbc/podcast/episode/?p=p02plkmf&e=m000cqf3.

8. See "The Science of Happiness Course," offered by Berkeley's Greater Good Science Center, accessed February 22, 2023, https://ggsc.berkeley.edu/what_we_do/online_courses_tools/the_science_of_happiness.

9. See *World Happiness Report 2022*, accessed November 16, 2022, https://worldhappiness.report/ed/2022/.

10. Katia Hetter, "This Is the World's Happiest Country in 2019," *CNN*, March 26, 2019.

11. For an intriguing analysis of the correlation between a country's levels of taxation and happiness, see Alan Kohler, "The Secret to Happiness Is More Taxation," *New Daily*, April 7, 2022. Notable too is the fact that common to all the top-ranking happy countries are people's strong perceptions of both "freedom to make life choices" and "social support," which factors are correspondingly meager or absent in the lowest-ranking states (see *World Happiness Report 2022*).

12. This is known as the "Easterlin Paradox," after economist Richard Easterlin, whose work showed that increasing levels of per capita income do not necessarily translate to rising averages of people's happiness. See his "Explaining Happiness," *Proceedings of the National Academy of Sciences* 100, no. 19 (2003): 11176–83.

13. The *Journal of Happiness Studies* is a flagship scholastic enterprise for this discipline.

14. The so-called U-shaped happiness curve—where after the first flush of childhood, one's level of contentment tracks south, plateauing in one's forties, before steadily rising from roughly fifty onward—though especially persistent, turns out to be something of a myth. Or at least applicable only to those comfortable enough to indulge in the luxury of a midlife slump in satisfaction, as Susan Krause Whitbourne demonstrates in her article "That Midlife Happiness Curve? It's More like a Line," *Psychology Today*, September 15, 2018.

15. Yielding, thereby, to the "inner curmudgeon in us all," as Andrew John and Stephen Blake put it in their wry take on the appeal, history, and science of grumpiness, *Are You a Miserable Old Bastard?* (Guilford, CT: Lyons Press, 2010).

16. See Philip Brickman, Dan Coates, and Ronnie Janoff-Bulman, "Lottery Winners and Accident Victims: Is Happiness Relative?" *Journal of Personality and Social Psychology* 36 (1978): 917–27. The difficulties inherent in the subjectivity of one's self-declared happiness set point are matters of endless study. See, for example, Frank Fujita and Ed Diener, "Life Satisfaction Set-Point: Stability and Change," *Journal of Personality and Social Psychology* 88 (2005): 158–64.

17. Even during a pandemic, the UN's *World Happiness Report 2021* noted that in 2020 "global life evaluations [on a scale of 1 to 10] have shown remarkable resilience in the face of COVID-19," being on par with the averages across the three years prior. In addition, the same study found that for 2020 "positive emotions [whether we "smiled or laughed a lot" yesterday] were almost three times more frequent (global average of 0.71) than negative emotions [whether we were "sad, worried or angry" yesterday] (global average of 0.27)"; chapter 2, "Happiness, Trust and Deaths under COVID-19."

18. Vaillant, *Aging Well: Surprising Guideposts to a Happier Life from the Landmark Study of Adult Development* (Boston: Little, Brown Spark, 2002), quoted in Joshua Wolf Shenk, "What Makes Us Happy?" *The Atlantic*, June 1, 2009.

Vaillant was the longtime director of the Harvard Study of Adult Behavior, a more than eighty-year study of the lives of 268 "Harvard men" who entered college in the late 1930s.

19. Which is the subtitle of her book *Happiness around the World* (New York: Oxford University Press, 2009).

20. About which skill Arthur C. Brooks, "happiness columnist" for *The Atlantic*, suggests that immigrants—who by definition are living "start-up lives"—are often especially good at assessing risk, putting their faith in the future, and duly reaping happiness rewards. See his "What Immigrants Know about Happiness," *The Atlantic*, July 29, 2021.

21. John Ingraham, "There Are Now More Guns than People in the United States According to a New Study of Global Firearm Ownership," *Washington Post*, June 19, 2018. Pro-gun advocates see this extraordinary circumstance as cause for celebration rather than alarm. The National Rifle Association's Institute of Legislative Action, for example, boasted that 2020 was "the year of the gun" and quoted data showing that by 2021 there were more than 21 million active "concealed carry" permits in the United States, "a 48% increase since 2016." See "The Year of the Gun—Record Number of Carry Permits in 2020," NRA-ILA, October 18, 2021, https://www.nraila.org/articles/20211018/the -year-of-the-gun-record-number-of-carry-permits-in-2020.

22. "Gun Deaths by Country 2022," *World Population Review*, accessed November 6, 2022, https://worldpopulationreview.com/country-rankings/gun-deaths -by-country.

23. Sixty-seven percent, to be precise. See John Gramlich, "7 Facts about Guns in the U.S.," *Pew Research Center*, December 27, 2017.

24. Megan Brenan, "Americans Remain Largely Dissatisfied with U.S. Gun Laws," *Gallup*, February 19, 2021.

25. "Muslim Women Defy Ban to Swim in Burkinis at French Pool," *BBC News*, June 24, 2019. The same ban in the same pool is still being resolutely defied two years later. See "Women in France Fined for Wearing 'Burkini' Swimsuits at Pool," *Euronews*, July 22, 2021.

26. The Conseil d'État (France's highest administrative court) had previously ruled against the imposition of burkini bans on public beaches: Décision No. 402702, 402777 (August 26, 2016). For further discussion, see Mariëtta D. C. Van der Tol, "Intolerance Unveiled? Burkini Bans across France," *Revue du Droit des Religions* 6 (2018): 139–49.

27. Carol Graham, *Happiness around the World* (New York: Oxford University Press, 2009), 216.

28. See, for example, Carl Anderson, "Locus of Control, Coping Behaviors, and Performance in a Stress Setting: A Longitudinal Study," *Journal of Applied Psychology* 62, no. 4 (1977): 446–51.

29. See Frederick Rauscher, "Kant's Social and Political Philosophy," in Edward N. Zalta (ed.), *The Stanford Encyclopedia of Philosophy* (revised, 2022), accessed November 2, 2022, https://plato.stanford.edu/entries/kant -social-political/.

30. Anthony Kenny and Charles Kenny, *Life, Liberty, and the Pursuit of Utility* (Exeter, UK: Imprint Academic, 2006).

31. See Julie McCarthy, "The Birthplace of 'Gross National Happiness' Is Growing a Bit Cynical," *NPR*, February 12, 2018.

32. UN General Assembly Resolution 65/309, "Happiness: Towards a Holistic Approach to Development," A/RES/63/309 (July 19, 2011).

33. In large part this low ranking is due to discrepancies in the methodologies employed by the World Happiness Report teams as compared to that used in Bhutan's own Gross National Happiness index; see "Known as The Kingdom of Happiness, Why Is Bhutan Ranked 95th in the World Happiness Report 2019?" *Daily Bhutan*, April 3, 2019.

34. The UK Office of National Statistics continues to track Britons' levels of "personal wellbeing." See "Personal Well-Being in the UK: April 2020 to March 2021," Office of National Statistics, October 15, 2021, https://www.ons .gov.uk/peoplepopulationandcommunity/wellbeing/bulletins /measuringnationalwellbeing/april2020tomarch2021.

35. For a somewhat damning review of how the policy is faring, see Tess McClure, "New Zealand's "Wellbeing Budget" Made Headlines, but What Really Changed?" *The Guardian*, April 10, 2021.

36. See Alfred Webb, *A Compendium of Irish Biography* (Dublin: M. H. Gill & Son, 1878), 219–22.

37. On which, see also Leong Ching, "The Paradox of Social Resilience: Explaining Delays in Water Infrastructure Provision in Kathmandu," *Water Alternatives* 11 (2018): 61–85.

38. On which, see Thomas Piketty, *Capital in the Twenty-First Century* (Cambridge, MA: Harvard University Press, 2014), discussed in chapter 5 of this book, before the callout for note 45.

39. See chapter 5, at note 35 and accompanying text.

40. As if to foreshadow her own fate, Article 10 of her *Déclaration* reads: "No one should be disturbed for their fundamental opinions; woman has the right to mount the scaffold, so she should have the right equally to mount the rostrum."

41. Jill Filipovic, *The H-Spot: The Feminist Pursuit of Happiness* (New York: Nation Books, 2017); the quotes that follow have been taken from chapter 1, pp. 11–31.

42. Which reiterates a point made at the end of chapter 6, on work, at note 46.

43. See, for example, Cordelia Fine, "Agenda Bender," *The Monthly* (Australia), August 2022.

44. "This is a relatively under-researched field and . . . there is no clear-cut solution" is the frank assessment of Allie Reynolds and Alireza Hamidian Jahromi, in "Transgender Athletes in Sports Competitions: How Policy Measures Can Be More Inclusive and Fairer to All," *Frontiers in Sports and Active Living*, no. 3 (2021), article 704178.

45. For academic studies of the freedoms and responsibilities associated with both of these activities, see Jarrett Rudy, *The Freedom to Smoke: Tobacco Consumption and Identity* (Montreal: McGill-Queen's University Press, 2005); and Bouke de Vries, "The Right to Be Publicly Naked: A Defence of Nudism," *Res Publica* 25 (2019): 407–24.

Chapter 5. Wealth

1. Virginia Woolf, *A Room of One's Own*, new ed. (London: Hogarth Press, 1935), 163.

2. It was in search of all that is trampled, and what might be done to find other ways to make money and do good at the same time, that I wrote *Necessary Evil: How to Fix Finance by Saving Human Rights* (New York: Oxford University Press, 2018).

3. A view advocated most notably by Milton Friedman in *Capitalism and Freedom* (Chicago: University of Chicago Press, 1962). Friedman's distinctive contribution to the relationship was to argue that it works best when capitalist enterprise is as free as possible from governmental interference, though such free enterprise must itself be secured by way of governmental regulation.

4. As elegantly explained by Peter Dougherty, in *Who's Afraid of Adam Smith?* (Hoboken, NJ: Wiley, 2002), and upon which theme and its human rights implications I expatiate in *Civilising Globalisation* (Cambridge: Cambridge University Press, 2009).

5. Society's "disposition to admire, and almost to worship, the rich and the powerful, and to despise, or, at least, to neglect persons of poor and mean condition," he wrote, is "the great and most universal cause of the corruption of our moral sentiments." *The Theory of Moral Sentiments* (1759), Part I, Section III, Chapter III, Para. 1.

6. *An Inquiry into the Nature and Causes of the Wealth of Nations* (1776), Book I, Chapter VIII, Para. 36.

7. *Theory of Moral Sentiments*, Book IV, Chapter 1, Para. 10.

8. *Wealth of Nations*, Book IV, Chapter II, Para. 9.

9. For further discussion, see Joseph Stiglitz, "Are Markets Efficient or Do They Tend toward Monopoly? The Verdict Is In," *World Economic Forum*, May 18, 2016.

10. For a survey of the variety of such necessary interventions, see Johan Graafland and Harmen Verbruggen, "Free-Market, Perfect Market, and Welfare State Perspectives on 'Good' Markets: An Empirical Test," *Applied Research in Quality of Life* 17 (2022): 1113–36.

11. See "GDP, PPP (constant 2017 international $)," World Bank, accessed November 6, 2022, https://data.worldbank.org/indicator/NY.GDP.MKTP.PP .KD?end=2020&start=1990; and "World GDP over the Last Two Millennia" (figures are inflation adjusted and expressed in 2011 dollars), Our World in Data, accessed November 6, 2022, https://ourworldindata.org/grapher/world -gdp-over-the-last-two-millennia. Total global household wealth is even more spectacular (albeit extremely unevenly distributed), measuring $463 trillion in 2021, according to Credit Suisse's *Global Wealth Report 2022*.

12. Max Roser, "The Short History of Global Living Conditions and Why It Matters That We Know It," *Our World in Data*, updated 2020, accessed November 6, 2022, at https://ourworldindata.org/a-history-of-global-living -conditions-in-5-charts.

13. "GDP, PPP (constant 2017 international $)."

14. See McKinsey Global Institute Discussion Paper, *Inequality: A Persisting Challenge and Its Implications* (June 2019).

15. Based on analyses of electoral processes, political participation, freedom of expression and belief, the rule of law, and associational and group rights, as well personal autonomy and individual rights. Information is gathered from local consultations, news stories, governmental and NGO sources, expert advisers, and regional specialists. See "Freedom in the World 2022," Freedom House, February 2022, https://freedomhouse.org/report-types/freedom-world.

16. "Freedom in the World" (historical data), Freedom House, accessed November 6, 2022, https://freedomhouse.org/report-types/freedom-world.

17. See section headed "Freedom" in Roser, "The Short History of Global Living Conditions."

18. Laurie Macfarlane, "A Spectre Is Haunting the West—The Spectre of Authoritarian Capitalism," *openDemocracy*, April 16, 2020, https://www.opendemocracy.net/en/oureconomy/a-spectre-is-haunting-the-west-the-spectre-of-authoritarian-capitalism/.

19. See Roberto Stefan Foa and Yascha Mounk, "When Democracy Is Longer the Only Path to Prosperity," *Wall Street Journal*, March 1, 2019.

20. Or, as Robert Cooper wryly puts it, "Marx was wrong according to John Kampfner. It is not religion that is the opium of the people but capitalism. Give them good shopping opportunities and they will forget about liberty, equality and fraternity, and cease to care about who governs them and how." See Cooper's review of Kampfner's book *Freedom for Sale* (London: Simon & Schuster, 2009), in *Sunday Times* (London), September 6, 2009.

21. For one of his more recent contributions on the topic, see Emmie Martin, "Warren Buffett and Bill Gates Agree That the Rich Should Pay Higher Taxes—Here's What They Suggest," CNBC, February 26, 2019.

22. See Credit Suisse, *Global Wealth Report 2021*, Figures 1 and 4, pp.17–22. Among this number there are 295,450 so-called ultra-high net worth individuals (each with net worth in excess of USD$30m), whose combined wealth in 2020 was a staggering $35.5 trillion; see X-Wealth, *World Ultra Wealth Report 2021*.

23. See Rachelle Alterman and Cygal Pellach, "Beach Access, Property Rights, and Social-Distributive Questions: A Cross-National Legal Perspective of Fifteen Countries," *Sustainability*, no. 14 (2022): 4237.

24. See Trump Golf Count, accessed November 6, 2022, https://trumpgolfcount.com/. This figure amounts to nearly three times the number of golf club visits made by fellow golf-loving president Barack Obama during his first term in office.

25. "Court Circular," *Private Eye*, no. 1500 (July 12–15, 2019). Members of the royal family receive what are in effect stipends paid out of the Sovereign Grant, which for 2021–22 totalled £86.3 million. *The Royal Family Financial Reports 2021–22*.

26. Geoffrey Ward and Ken Burns, *The Roosevelts: An Intimate History* (New York: Alfred A. Knopf, 2014), 135.

27. The 2020 US federal elections cost $14.4 billion, which is two and half times more than the next most costly, being those of 2016 at a total of $5.9 billion; see "Cost of Election," *OpenSecrets*, accessed November 6, 2022, https://www.opensecrets.org/elections-overview/cost-of-election.

28. On the corrupt and broken nature of campaign financing regulation in the United States, see David Frum, "The Good That Ted Cruz's Win Can Do," *The Atlantic*, May 18, 2022.

29. Noah Smith, "It's Gotten Too Hard to Strike It Rich in America," *Bloomberg Opinion*, August 14, 2019, quoting research undertaken by the Federal Reserve Bank of Minneapolis.

30. The marginal income tax rate for the highest earners in the United States has dropped from 70 percent in the early 1970s to 37 percent today, and long-term capital gains taxes rates have dropped from 40 percent to 20 percent over the same period. As Robert Bellafiore points out, however, the rate at which the rich actually pay tax (their "effective tax rate") is consistently well below these levels. See Bellafiore, "The Top 1 Per Cent's Tax Rates over Time," *Tax Foundation*, March 5, 2019.

31. Catarina Saraiva, "How a 'K-Shaped' Recovery Is Widening U.S. Inequality," *Bloomberg*, December 10, 2020.

32. Davide Scigliuzzo, "The Rich Are Minting Money in the Pandemic Like Never Before," *Bloomberg Wealth*, January 17, 2021.

33. Former President Trump's characterization of his 2019 proposal to buy Greenland from Denmark (presumably on behalf of the United States rather than for himself, though that was not made immediately clear at the time) as "essentially a large real estate deal" exquisitely portrays the perversity of a "money talks" perspective on life and its infinite complexities. The proposal was rebuffed by the Danish prime minister, Mette Frederiksen, who described it as "absurd." See "Trump Cancels Denmark Visit amid Spat over Sale of Greenland," BBC, August 21, 2019.

34. Amartya Sen, *Development as Freedom* (Oxford: Oxford University Press, 2002), 3, 5.

35. See World Bank, *Poverty and Shared Prosperity 2020: Reversals of Fortune* (2021), 1–5; and Yonzan et al., "The Impact of COVID-19 on Global Poverty and Inequality," *World Bank Data Blog* (January 18, 2022). Both of these works stress how the COVID-19 pandemic has halted or reversed the steady decline in global poverty rates in recent decades. The World Bank classified extreme poverty as living on less than $1.90 per day until September 2022, when it "updated" its base global poverty line to $2.15 per day (at 2017 prices). See "Factsheet: An Adjustment to Global Poverty Lines," World Bank, updated September 14, 2022, https://www.worldbank.org/en/news/factsheet/2022/05 /02/fact-sheet-an-adjustment-to-global-poverty-lines.

36. See "Distribution of Poverty between Different Poverty Thresholds, World, 1820–2018," Our World in Data, accessed November 6, 2022, https:// ourworldindata.org/grapher/distribution-of-population-between-different -poverty-thresholds-historical?country=~OWID_WRL. Drawing on the work of economic historian Michail Moatsos and using figures historically adjusted for inflation, the graph's authors calculated that in 1820, 79.36 percent of people were living on under $1.90 per day (at 2011 prices) and a further 16.92 percent were living on between $1.90 and $5 per day.

37. World Bank, *Poverty and Equity Brief—India* (April 2021). The range reflects discrepancies in data collection in India in recent years.

38. See Wealth-X, *Billionaire Census 2021.*

39. See US Census Bureau, *Income and Poverty in the United States 2021* (2022).

40. See Stone Shi, "The Great Divide between China's Rich and Poor," Zhongguo Institute, November 21, 2018; and Branko Milanovic, "China's Inequality Will Lead It to a Stark Choice," *Foreign Affairs*, February 11, 2021.

41. Eurostat, "Living conditions in Europe - material deprivation and economic strain" (February 2022).

42. "Poverty and Equity Data Portal—South Africa," World Bank, accessed November 6, 2022, https://povertydata.worldbank.org/poverty/home/.

43. Marigold Warner, "South Africa's Born Free Generation," *British Journal of Photography*, May 8, 2019.

44. "To 11 Million Brazilians, the Earth Is Flat," *France24*, February 28, 2020. Olavo de Carvalho's wide appeal stems not just from his warped sense of astronomy (he also believes the sun revolves around the Earth) but especially his readiness to blame almost everything he dislikes on Marxism—from climate change and COVID-19 (both hoaxes) to R-rated movies, women using Gothic makeup, and the threat posed by a dynastic consortium "of large-scale capitalists and international bankers committed to establishing a worldwide socialist dictatorship." See Mitchell Abidor, "The Gramsci of the Brazilian Right," *Dissent* (Summer 2020).

45. What he refers to as a "potentially explosive process." Piketty, *Capital in the Twenty-First Century* (Cambridge, MA: Harvard University Press, 2014), 444.

46. Literally: "It's yellow, it's ugly, it goes with nothing, but it can save your life."

47. "How Life Became an Endless, Terrible Competition," *The Atlantic*, September 15, 2019. Markovits is himself a law professor at Yale.

48. Mandela, quoted in Amy McKenna, "15 Nelson Mandela Quotes," *Britannica*, accessed November 6, 2022, at https://www.britannica.com/list/nelson-mandela-quotes.

49. Friedman, *Capitalism and Freedom*, 15.

50. Nelson Mandela, *The Long Walk to Freedom* (London: Little, Brown, 1994), 138.

51. Friedman, *Capitalism and Freedom*, 133.

Chapter 6. Work

1. Gloria Steinem, *Outrageous Acts and Everyday Rebellions* (New York: Holt, Rinehart & Winston, 1983), 155.

2. See Richard Donkin, *The History of Work* (New York: Palgrave Macmillan, 2010), 3–4.

3. The citation of the 65 percent figure in the World Economic Forum's report *The Future of Jobs* (2016) was perhaps its loudest broadcast, but the source cited in the report and other related sources have since proved to be nonexistent or baseless. See the perceptive blog: "The Undead Factoid: Who Decided 65% of the Jobs of the Near Future Don't Exist Today?" *Edtech Curmudgeon*, July 6, 2017, http://edtechcurmudgeon.blogspot.com/2017/07/the-undead-factoid-who-decided-65-of.html.

4. See "Have 65% of Jobs Not Yet Been Invented?" *More or Less*, BBC World Service, May 26, 2017, at https://www.bbc.co.uk/sounds/play/p053ln9f. In a

recent survey of 32,517 workers across nineteen countries worldwide, PricewaterhouseCoopers (PwC) found an astonishing 39 percent of respondents believed that their job would be obsolete within five years: "Hopes and Fears 2021," PwC, accessed November 6, 2022, https://www.pwc.com/gx/en/issues/upskilling/hopes-and-fears.html.

5. See "Time Tracking Statistics," Clockify.me, accessed November 6, 2022, https://clockify.me/time-tracking-statistics. See also the World Health Organization, *Global Strategy on Occupational Health for All: The Way to Health at Work* (1995).

6. On the study, undertaken by KPMG, see Simon Jessup, "UK Financial Services? It's a Family Affair: Report," *Reuters*, April 21, 2019.

7. See Mercer, *Global Talent Trends 2019*. Another global survey, conducted by Imperial, also a careers and recruitment firm, this time of 26,000 LinkedIn members, reflected similar results. See Lauren Vesty, "Millennials Want Purpose over Pay Checks; So Why Can't We Find It at Work?" *The Guardian*, September 14, 2016.

8. Namely: Baby boomers (born 1944–64); Generation X (born 1965–79); and Generation Y (born 1980–94). Members of Generation Z (born 1995–2010), were apparently not surveyed.

9. PricewaterhouseCoopers' "Hopes and Fears 2021" survey, mentioned above, underlines this point, showing that 54 percent of those aged 55-plus preferred "doing a job that makes a difference" over "maximising my income," while for 18-to-34-year-olds the same preference was made by only 43 percent. A 2022 survey by Glassdoor, however, suggests some blurring of the divide in its recording of Generation Zers being "most satisfied in roles that provide them with the opportunity to shape company culture and have social impact." See Richard Johnson, "A Change of Pace for Gen Z Employees Entering the Workforce," *Glassdoor Economic Research*, August 16,2022.

10. Joseph Conrad, *Heart of Darkness* (1902; reprinted, Auckland: Floating Press, 2008), 56.

11. Derek Thompson, "Workism Is Making Americans Miserable," *The Atlantic*, February 24, 2019.

12. As outlined in *Bullshit Jobs: A Theory* (London: Allen Lane, 2018), chapter 2.

13. Regarding universities, see, for example, Richard Vedder, "Who Is Ruining Our Universities? Administrators!" *Forbes*, August 3, 2020; and Gwilym Croucher and Peter Woelert, "Administrative Transformation and Managerial Growth: A Longitudinal Analysis of Changes in Non-academic Workforce at Australian Universities," *Higher Education* 84 (2022): 159–75.

14. Graeber, *Bullshit Jobs*, 37, 67.

15. For an excellent overview of the industry in the region, see International Labour Organization (ILO), *Brick by Brick: Environment, Human Labour, and Animal Welfare* (2017).

16. In Nepal, one remarkable organization that tries to alleviate some of these problems is Better Brick Nepal (accessed November 6, 2022, https://goodweave.org/bricks/), not least by providing free day care at some kiln sites for the youngest children of the workers. For further discussion, see Shilpa Shrestha and Steven M. Thygerson, "Brick Kilns of Nepal: A Non-governmental

Organization Perspective," *Open Journal of Safety Science and Technology* 9 (2019): 1–6.

17. With staff of such NGOs as the Child Development Society (accessed February, 23 2023, https://www.cds.org.np/) and the above-mentioned Better Brick Nepal, I have visited many brick kilns in the Kathmandu Valley over the years, and it is from my notes of these visits and other sources cited that I draw in making these observations. For descriptions of the very similar conditions in Indian brick kilns, see J. John, "Brick Kilns and Slave Labour: Observation from Punjab," *Labour File* 9, nos. 1–2 (2014): 15–26.

18. ILO, *Brick by Brick*, 30.

19. F. A. Hayek, *The Constitution of Liberty* (London: Routledge, 1960), 70–71.

20. On which topic, let me recommend Richard Beasley's *Hell Has Harbour Views* (Sydney: Macmillan, 2001) as an entertaining but cautionary tale for anyone considering a career in high-end corporate law.

21. So named, as it happens, in honor of two of Watterson's philosopher heroes: John Calvin and Thomas Hobbes.

22. Kenyon College Commencement Speech, May 20, 1990.

23. The history and details of the universal basic income are explained by Matthew Thompson in "Money for Everything? Universal Basic Income in a Crisis" *Economy and Society* 51, no. 3 (2022): 353–74. Thompson notes the "astonishing levels" of public support for the idea, reaching 71 percent in one Europe-wide survey published in 2020. See also Rutger Bregman, "Why We Should Give Everyone a Basic Income," *TEDx Talks*, October 21, 2014.

24. Daniel Markovits, *The Meritocracy Trap* (New York: Penguin, 2019).

25. On which see further details in the previous chapter on wealth, at note 47 and accompanying text, drawing on statistics cited by Markovits.

26. In Volume 1 of *Capital* Marx devised a complex series of formulae to explain what he meant by the exploitative nature of profit. See Jon Elster, *An Introduction to Karl Marx* (Cambridge: Cambridge University Press, 1986), chapter 4, for an explanation of Marx's explanation.

27. See "Decent Work," International Labour Organization, accessed November 6, 2022, https://www.ilo.org/global/topics/decent-work/lang--en/index.htm. This definition is itself drawn from the prescriptions of the ILO's many conventions on labor rights and standards, including, in particular, its eight so-called Fundamental Conventions.

28. See "85% of American Workers Are Happy with Their Jobs, National Survey Shows," *CNBC*, April 2, 2019; the other job satisfaction factors surveyed were pay, opportunity, contribution, and autonomy.

29. Graeber, *Bullshit Jobs*, xxi–xxii. The sample size for the UK figure was 849 working adults; see "YouGov Survey Results," YouGov, August 10–11, 2015, https://d25d2506sfb94s.cloudfront.net/cumulus_uploads/document/g0h77ytkkm/Opi_InternalResults_150811_Work_W.pdf.

30. To which mix one might add the intriguing insight from the PwC survey mentioned above, "Hopes and Fears 2021," that while globally some 75 percent of us want work that "makes a positive contribution to society," that sentiment is strongest in the major emerging economies of China (87 percent), India, and South Africa (both 90 percent).

31. On the origins and operation of these "Factory Acts" in Britain, as they were originally known, see Elizabeth Leigh Hutchins and Amy Harrison Spencer, *A History of Factory Legislation* (Westminster, UK: P. S. King & Son, 1903; 3rd edition, London: Routledge, 2013).

32. See Max Beer's classic text, *General History of Socialism and Social Struggles* (New York: Russell & Russell, 1957).

33. On which point, conservative critic Tom Nichols laments: "The Republican Party has, for years, ignored the ideas and principles it once espoused, to the point where the 2020 GOP convention simply dispensed with the fiction of a platform and instead declared the party to be whatever . . . Donald Trump said it was." Tom Nichols, "The Republican Party Is Now in Its End Stages," *The Atlantic*, February 26, 2021.

34. Vannak Anan Prum, *The Dead Eye and the Deep Blue Sea* (New York: Seven Stories Press, 2018).

35. See Walk Free Foundation, ILO, and UN International Organization of Migration, *Global Estimates of Modern Slavery: Forced Labour and Forced Marriage* (September 2022).

36. According to the Walk Free Foundation, Africa, Europe and Central Asia, and the Americas have comparable numbers of people in modern slavery: 7 million, 6.4 million, and 5.1 million, respectively. Asia and the Pacific states are host to by far the largest number: 29.3 million. Notably, while the Arab states register the lowest numbers of modern slaves in any region (1.7 million), in terms of prevalence (that is, taking into consideration the population sizes of each region), they record the highest levels: 5.3 per thousand persons in forced labor and 4.8 per thousand persons in forced marriages. Walk Free Foundation, ILO, and UN International Organization of Migration, *Global Estimates of Modern Slavery*, 18.

37. Walk Free Foundation, ILO, and UN International Organization of Migration, 17.

38. For a fine global overview of the topic, see Justine Nolan and Martijn Boersma, *Addressing Modern Slavery* (Sydney: University of New South Wales Press, 2019).

39. The Cambodian League for the Promotion and Defense of Human Rights. After Prum jumped overboard to escape the fishing boat, his Malaysian rescuers sold him to the owner of a palm oil plantation where he was forced to work for another four months. It was from there that he was eventually rescued by LICADHO. Such local advocacy and action groups fighting modern slavery are truly heroic organizations, achieving remarkable results on shoestring budgets. I well know three such organizations: Shakti Samuha in Nepal (accessed November 6, 2022, http://shaktisamuha.org.np/) rescues and rehabilitates sex-trafficked women and girls. Cisarua Learning Center in Indonesia (accessed November 6, 2022, https://cisarualearning.com/) facilitates education of the children of stranded Afghan refugees by the refugees themselves. And the Institute for Ecosoc Rights, also in Indonesia (accessed November 6, 2022, http://ecosocrights.blogspot.com/), champions reforms for workers on palm oil plantations.

40. Carl Benedikt Frey and Michael Osborne, "The Future of Employment: How Susceptible Are Jobs to Computerisation?" working paper, Oxford Martin School, Oxford University, September 17, 2013.

41. Jeremy Bowles, "Chart of the Week: 54% of EU Jobs at Risk of Computerisation," *Brugel Blog*, July 24, 2014, https://www.bruegel.org/blog-post/chart-week-54-eu-jobs-risk-computerisation.

42. See World Economic Forum, *The Future of Jobs 2019*, 10–12. Regarding "augmentation" and "productivity," see, for example, James Manyika et al., *A Future That Works: Automation, Employment, and Productivity* (Washington, DC: McKinsey & Company, 2017).

43. Certainly safer than the wildly optimistic views of some futurists. See, for example, Elisa Camorani, "Will Artificial Intelligence Provide Us with More Freedom?" *Medium*, March 11, 2019.

44. See Marshall Sahlins, "Notes on the Original Affluent Society," in R. Lee and I. DeVore (eds.), *Man the Hunter* (New York: Routledge, 1968), 85–9.

45. See his essay *In Praise of Idleness* (1935). In truth this was a curious topic to be so devoutly defended by Russell when you consider how prolific, hardworking, and long was his working life. His published writings span seventy-five years and comprises some seventy books, more than two thousand articles, and thousands of other commentaries, pamphlets, and reviews, including one lengthy and animated statement on the Arab-Israeli conflict two days before his death on February 2, 1970.

46. Or both, if that's possible, on which point, see Anne-Marie Slaughter, "Why Women Still Can't Have It All," *The Atlantic*, July–August 2012.

47. Emily Maitlis, "COVID-19 Is Not a 'Great Leveller,' as Some Say; It's Much Harder If You're Poor," BBC *Newsnight*, April 9, 2020, posted to YouTube, accessed November 6, 2022, https://www.youtube.com/watch?v=L6wIcpdJyCI.

Chapter 7. Security

1. See Stephanie Boltje, "Former Navy Diver Paul De Gelder Reveals the Three Things He Learned from Being Attacked by a Shark," ABC, January 19, 2019. Because it occurred during a training exercise conducted by the navy, the incident was filmed. It makes for an uncomfortable few seconds of viewing, not least because the grainy quality of the images leaves much to the imagination. *Channel 10 News*, posted on YouTube, accessed November 6, 2022, https://www.youtube.com/watch?v=y7uSvQUJTZE.

2. Robert Burns, "Man Was Made to Mourn: A Dirge" (1784).

3. For a classic account of the origins and importance of the notion of *mens rea*, see Francis Bowes Sayre, "*Mens Rea*," *Harvard Law Review* 45, no. 6 (1932): 974–1026.

4. According to Equality Now, spousal or de facto rape is still legally permissible in Ghana, India, Indonesia, Jordan, Lesotho, Nigeria, Oman, Singapore, Sri Lanka, and Tanzania. See Equality Now, *The World's Shame: The Global Rape Epidemic* (2019).

5. On the complicated issues of negligence and foreseeability in criminal law, see Alexander Greenberg, "Why Criminal Responsibility for Negligence Cannot Be Indirect," *Cambridge Law Journal* 80 (2021): 1–26. And on the equally complex place of *mens rea* in tort (negligence) law, see Peter Cane, "*Mens Rea* in Tort Law," *Oxford Journal of Legal Studies* 20, no. 4 (2000): 533–56.

6. But, as with many things "put simply," the reality in legal practice is often a good deal more complicated. See David Crump, "What Does Intent Mean?" *Hofstra Law Review* 38 (2010): 1059–82.

7. See Eduardo Levy Yeyati and Federico Filippini, "Social and Economic Impact of COVID-19," *Brookings*, June 2, 2021.

8. According to the IMF, lost economic output worldwide for 2020 amounted to almost $3 trillion (or 3.2 percent of global GDP); see IMF, *World Economic Outlook 2021* (July Update). The IMF's *Fiscal Monitor* (April 2021), for an overview of countries' fiscal responses to COVID-19. The IMF also credits "the lingering . . . pandemic" as a key factor in the marked slowdown of global economic growth across 2022 and as projected for 2023; see IMF, *World Economic Outlook 2022* (October).

9. According to a global survey conducted by McKinsey in July 2021, "The Coronavirus Effect on Global Economic Sentiment," McKinsey & Company, accessed November 6, 2022, https://www.mckinsey.com/business-functions /strategy-and-corporate-finance/our-insights/the-coronavirus-effect-on-global -economic-sentiment.

10. See Fabian Mendez Ramos and Jaime Lara, "COVID-19 and Poverty Vulnerability," *Brookings*, May 18, 2022.

11. On which point compare the optimism of Steven Lee Myers et al., in "Power, Patriotism, and 1.4 Billion People: How China Beat the Virus and Roared Back," *New York Times*, February 2, 2021, with the later and more damning view of Xianbin Yao, in "Why Does China Persist with Its 'Zero-COVID' Strategy?" *Brink News*, September 13, 2022. China's strict anti-COVID-19 restrictions were eventually rolled back in early December 2022.

12. "Rethinking the Coronavirus Shutdown" (editorial), *Wall Street Journal*, March 19, 2020.

13. And in terms of the relationship between the economy and human rights, not a dichotomy but rather a relationship of mutual reliance, argues Juan Pablo Bohoslavsky, in "COVID-19 Economy versus Human Rights: A Misleading Dichotomy," *Health and Human Rights Journal* (April 20, 2020).

14. On March 24, 2020, when President Trump declared that he intended to lift movement and social-distancing restrictions by Easter Sunday (enabling churches to be "packed" that day, as he put it), the United States' COVID-19 total infections stood at approximately 53,700, and deaths at 704. By Easter Sunday, three weeks later (April 12), these figures were 555,313 and 22,020, respectively. By Election Day, November 3, 2020, some 9.2 million Americans had been infected by COVID-19 and 231,599 had died. Finally, as of late October 2022, the figures were some 98 million infections and nearly 1.1 million deaths in the United States. John Hopkins Coronavirus Resource Center, accessed November 1, 2022, https://coronavirus.jhu.edu/map.html.

15. Of the many publications on this era in Northern Ireland, David McKittrick and David McVea's *Making Sense of The Troubles*, revised ed. (London: Viking, 2012) is a standout.

16. On the continuing opacity of the term, see Alan Greene, "Defining Terrorism: One Size Fits All?" *International and Comparative Law Quarterly* 66, no. 2 (2017): 411–40.

17. See Boaz Ganor, "Defining Terrorism: Is One Man's Terrorist Another Man's Freedom Fighter? *Police Practice and Research* 3, no. 4 (2002): 287–304, https://doi.org/10.1080/1561426022000032060.

18. Despite several attempts, and the existence of its own Office of Counter-Terrorism, even the United Nations has been unable to conclude any international agreement on a universal legal definition of the term. See UN Global Counter-Terrorism Strategy, General Assembly Resolution, A/RES/60/288 (September 20, 2006).

19. J. Cofer Black, Unclassified Testimony before the Senate Intelligence Committee, 107th Congress, 2nd sess., September 26, 2002, https://fas.org/irp/congress/2002_hr/092602black.html.

20. Reed Brody et al., "Getting Away with Torture? Command Responsibility for the U.S. Abuse of Detainees," *Human Rights Watch* 17, no. 1(G) (April 2005), https://www.hrw.org/reports/2005/us0405/us0405.pdf.

21. See "A Guide to the Memos on Torture," *New York Times* (2005), accessed November 6, 2022, https://archive.nytimes.com/www.nytimes.com/ref/international/24MEMO-GUIDE.html.

22. Reproduced in "Letter: Retired Military Leaders to Presidential Candidates," Human Rights First, February 16, 2016, https://humanrightsfirst.org/library/letter-retired-military-leaders-to-presidential-candidates/.

23. A and others v. Secretary of State for the Home Department (the "Belmarsh Detainees" case) [2004] UKHL 56, at para. 97. The statute in question was the Anti-terrorism, Crime and Security Act 2001 (per sec. 23, defining the government's power to detain suspected international terrorists).

24. Patrick Toomey, "The NSA Continues to Violate Americans' Internet Privacy Rights," American Civil Liberties Union, August 22, 2018.

25. Jianan Qian, "Feeling Safe in the Surveillance State," *New York Times*, April 10, 2019. The consequences of this level of surveillance on freedom of expression in China are discussed in the following chapter, on voice, under the heading "Voice Control."

26. This is what Zuboff refers to as the revenue value of "behavioural surplus." See *The Age of Surveillance Capitalism* (London: Profile Books, 2019), 82–85.

27. Ilija Trojanow, "Security versus Freedom: A Misleading Trade-off," *Eurozine*, May 15, 2015.

28. Which is how Edward Snowden describes himself in his autobiography, *Permanent Record* (New York: Metropolitan Books, 2019). Many others see him either as a patriot or a traitor.

29. To which topic I return and in greater depth in chapter 12, on trust.

30. Weber, *Politics as a Vocation* (1919). On this matter, the philosopher giants' shoulders upon which Weber stood included, in particular, Jean Bodin, in *Les Six livres de la République* (1576), and Thomas Hobbes, in *Leviathan* (1651).

31. See Lydia Saad, "What percentage of Americans own guns?" *Gallup*, November 13, 2020.

32. See Jonathan Masters, "U.S. Gun Policy: Global Comparisons," *Council for Foreign Relations*, Backgrounder, June 10, 2022. What is more, the pace of guns sales has been increasing in recent years, with 2020 and 2021 marking the highest annual sales of firearms in US history; see "U.S. firearms sales

December 2021: Slight fall from December 2020. Year closes out with nearly 20 million firearms sold," *Small Arms Analytics*, January 5, 2022.

33. "Canada: Gun Facts and Stats," *TheGunBlog.ca*, News Update, September 2, 2021, https://thegunblog.ca/facts-stats/.

34. See "Gun Ownership by Country 2022," *World Population Review*, accessed November 6, 2022, https://worldpopulationreview.com/country-rankings/gun -ownership-by-country. The figures quoted for the United Kingdom are based on 2021 data, and the figure for gun ownership in Australia is drawn from "Australia—Gun Facts, Figures, and the Law," GunPolicy.org, accessed November 6, 2022, https://www.gunpolicy.org/firearms/region/australia.

35. Gun death rate is measured by "violent deaths by firearm" per 100,000 of population in 2020. For the United States that year, there were a total of 23,224 gun homicides, at a rate of 7.0 deaths per 100,000 of population (rising sharply from 2019 when there were 17,270 gun homicides, at a rate of 5.2 per 100,000 people). For all the figures quoted here, see "Global Violent Deaths (GVD)" database, compiled by Small Arms Survey, accessed November 6, 2022, https://www.smallarmssurvey.org/database/global -violent-deaths-gvd. The 2020 data for the United States published by the US Centers for Disease Control and Prevention (CDC) differ: 19,384 firearm homicides, at a rate of 5.9 deaths per 100,000 of population, which was also a marked increase of 35 percent over the CDC's 2019 data; see "Assault or Homicide (U.S.)," CDC, accessed November 6, 2022, https://www.cdc.gov /nchs/fastats/homicide.htm.

36. Chelsea Bailey, in "More Americans Killed by Guns since 1968 than in All U.S. Wars—Combined," *NBC News*, October 5, 2017, draws on data from the CDC and the Department of Veterans Affairs.

37. When you add accidental and suicide gun deaths to the numbers of gun homicides, the statistics are even more alarming, totaling 45,222 gun-related deaths in 2020 in the United States, at a rate of 124 deaths per day. See John Gramlich, "What the Data Says about Gun Deaths in the U.S.," *Pew Research Center*, February 3, 2022. The annual numbers of mass shootings (defined as four or more people injured or killed, excluding shooter[s]) have also risen markedly in the United States in recent years, from 349 and 336 in 2017 and 2018, respectively, to 690 and 647 in 2021 and 2022. See "Past Summary Ledgers," Gun Violence Archive, accessed February 25, 2023, https://www .gunviolencearchive.org/past-tolls.

38. For a wry take on the absurdity of this type of argument, see Sarah Hutto, "Guns Don't Kill People; People Kill People: It's Time We Get Rid of People," *McSweeney's Internet Tendency*, October 1, 2019.

39. The Center for Homeland Defense and Security's K–12 School Shooting Database (accessed February 15, 2023, https://k12ssdb.org/all-shootings) recorded 303 school shootings for 2022, reflecting a dramatic increase over the previous five years (there were 58 such incidents in 2017). "Since Sandy Hook," writes David Frum, "this country has plunged backward and downward toward barbarism." See his "America's Hands Are Full of Blood," *The Atlantic*, May 25, 2022.

40. District of Columbia v. Heller, 554 U.S. 570 (2008).

41. New York State Rifle & Pistol Association v. Bruen, 597 U.S. __ (2022), at 62–63. The ramifications of the case are profound as it effectively renders unconstitutional similar "proper cause" statutes in other states. See Lisa Vicens and Samuel Levander, "The *Bruen* Majority Ignores Decision's Empirical Effects," *SCOTUSblog*, July 8, 2022, https://www.scotusblog.com/2022/07/the -bruen-majority-ignores-decisions-empirical-effects/.

42. See Giffords Law Center's "Annual Gun Law Scorecard," in "National Release: Despite Disruptions of State Legislatures in 2020, New Annual Gun Law Scorecard Reveals Progress, Opportunities for Biden Administration to Save Lives from Gun Violence" (press release), Giffords, accessed November 8, 2022, https://giffords.org/press-release/2021/02/national-release-new-annual -gun-law-scorecard-reveals-progress/.

43. See, for example, "America's Gun Culture in Charts," *BBC News*, April 8, 2021.

44. It is estimated that Earth has existed for 3.6 billion years. For an informative and entertaining representation of the estimates used in this paragraph (and many more besides), see Tim Urban, "Putting Time in Perspective—Updated," Wait But Why, August 22, 2013, at https://waitbutwhy.com/2013/08/putting -time-in-perspective.html.

45. As Rebecca Dean puts it, the "study of anthropogenic environments is primarily concerned with the coevolution of human communities and their landscapes, the dialectic between ecology and society." See Dean, "Anthropogenic Environments, Archaeology of," in Claire Smith (ed.), *Encyclopedia of Global Archaeology* (New York: Springer, 2014).

46. As documented in various reports of Working Group II of the United Nations' Intergovernmental Panel on Climate Change, which is mandated to "assesses the impact, adaptation and vulnerabilities related to climate change."

47. Calibrated as carefully as scientific methodology permits by the Intergovernmental Panel on Climate Change. See, for example, the report of its Working Group I, *Climate Change 2021* (August 2021), covering current and projected changes in greenhouse gas emissions, global warming, glacial retreat, rising sea levels, and extreme weather events.

48. See Yadvinder Mahli, "The Concept of the Anthropocene," *Annual Review of Environment and Resources* 42, no. 1 (2017): 77–104.

49. Steven Vogel, *Thinking like a Mall: Environmental Philosophy after the End of Nature* (Cambridge, MA: MIT Press, 2016).

50. Vogel, 199.

51. Ambelin Kwaymullina, "Seeing the Light: Aboriginal Law, Learning, and Sustainable Living in Country," *Indigenous Law Bulletin* 6, no. 11 (2005): 12.

52. More than focusing primarily on the mitigation of climate change, we should perhaps be concerned with the "potential impacts of climate change on social behaviour and psychosocial wellbeing." See Kim-Pong Tam, Angela Leung, and Susan Clayton, "Research on Climate Change in Social Psychology Publications: A Systematic Review," *Asian Journal of Social Psychology* 24, no. 2 (2021): 117–43.

53. On which, see chapter 11, on respect.

54. See Stephen Porges, "Vagal Pathways: Portals to Compassion," in Emma M. Seppälä et al. (eds.), *The Oxford Handbook of Compassion Science* (Oxford: Oxford University Press, 2017), 189–202.

Chapter 8. Voice

1. Thomas Paine, "In a French Prison, 1794," in E. C. Stedman and E. M. Hutchinson (eds.), *A Library of American Literature*, vol. 3 (New York: Charles L. Webster & Company, 1891), reproduced on Bartleby.com, accessed November 15, 2022, https://www.bartleby.com/400/prose/453.html.

2. Paine's appointment with the guillotine had been scheduled for July 24, 1794; Robespierre was arrested on July 27 and guillotined the following day. Paine was eventually released from prison, on November 4, 1794.

3. John Keane, *Tom Paine: A Political Life* (London: Bloomsbury, 1995), chapter 12.

4. Robert Ingersoll, "Thomas Paine," *North American Review*, August 1892.

5. For a fascinating and authoritative survey of the scope of the First Amendment, see Mark Tushnet, Alan Chen, and Joseph Blocher, *Speech beyond Words: The Surprising Reach of the First Amendment* (New York: New York University Press, 2017).

6. Such "shield laws" are permissible but not required under the First Amendment; thus, while they currently exist in thirty-nine US states (as well as the District of Columbia), the remaining eleven states do not have them, nor does the federal government. See Hank Nuwer, "Understanding Shield Law," *Quill*, April 8, 2021.

7. 319 U.S. 624 (1943).

8. Christopher Hitchens, "Why Even Hate Speech Needs to Be Protected," *Reader's Digest*, December 2011.

9. Benjamin Franklin, "On Freedom of Speech and the Press," *Pennsylvania Gazette*, November 17, 1737.

10. Stanley Fish, *Why There's No Such Thing as Free Speech . . . and It's a Good Thing Too* (New York: Oxford University Press, 1994), 102–4.

11. It is with a sense of pained resignation as I write these words in late 2022 that while SLORC may have gone, the authoritarian impulses of the country's military have not.

12. See the further discussion of this topic later in this chapter under the heading "Voice Control," and in chapter 12, on trust, under "Breaking Trust."

13. See Sarah Repucci, "Freedom and the Media 2019: A Downward Spiral," Freedom House, accessed February 17, 2023, https://freedomhouse.org/sites/default/files/FINAL07162019_Freedom_And_The_Media_2019_Report.pdf.

14. "2021 World Press Freedom Index: Journalism, the Vaccine against Disinformation, Blocked in More than 130 Countries," RSF: Reporters without Borders, accessed February 16, 2023, https://rsf.org/en/2021-world-press-freedom-index-journalism-vaccine-against-disinformation-blocked-more-130-countries.

15. Verisk Maplecroft, *Human Rights Outlook 2019*, accessed November 13, 2022, https://www.maplecroft.com/insights/analysis/human-rights-outlook-2019/.

16. Generally for this paragraph, see "The New Censors: The Global Gag on Free Speech Is Tightening," *The Economist*, August 17, 2019.

17. The International Federation of Journalists (IFJ) recorded 94 murders of journalists worldwide in 2018, up from 82 the year before. See "2018 Reverses Downward Trend in Killings of Journalists and Media Staff with 94 Victims

of Violence" (press release), International Federation of Journalists, December 31, 2018. Although in 2021 the IFJ recorded a reduction in killings (47), it also noted a "significant increase" in intimidation and detention, with 365 journalists behind bars. See "The IFJ Killed List 2021," International Federation of Journalists, February 8, 2022, https://www.ifj.org/media-centre/news/detail/category/health-and-safety/article/ifj-killed-list-report-2021.html.

18. "Internet Shutdowns in 2021: The Return of Digital Authoritarianism," Access Now, April 22, 2022.

19. See Julia Bergin, Louisa Lim, Nyein Nyein, and Andrew Nachemson, "Flicking the Kill Switch: Governments Embrace Internet Shutdowns as a Form of Control," *The Guardian*, August 29, 2022.

20. See Sophia Nazalay, "'Strongmen' Regimes Lead Charge against Freedom of Speech and Privacy," in Verisk Maplecroft, *Human Rights Outlook 2019*.

21. On Egypt and Saudi Arabia, see Wafa Ben Hassine, "The Crime of Speech: How Arab Governments Use the Law to Silence Expression Online," accessed February 17, 2023, Electronic Frontier Foundation, https://www.eff.org/pages/crime-speech-how-arab-governments-use-law-silence-expression-online.

22. The Murdoch News Corporation media empire, for example, stretches across Australia, the United Kingdom, and the United States and is a powerful and influential political player in each. Just how powerful and influential it is in the United States is damningly exposed by Sarah Ferguson in "Fox and the Big Lie (Parts 1 & 2)," *ABC Four Corners*, August 23, 2021, https://www.abc.net.au/news/2021-08-23/fox-and-the-big-lie:-how-the-network-promoted/13510238.

23. For a global overview, see "How Public Service Broadcasting Shapes Up Worldwide," *The Guardian*, July 20, 2015.

24. A phenomenon that Sean Illing refers to as "free speech devouring itself," in "What the 2020 Debate over Free Speech Missed," *Vox*, December 22, 2020.

25. E. S. v. Austria, ECtHR, App. no. 38450/12 (October 25, 2018). Coincidentally, the very next day a referendum in Ireland returned a vote to remove the offense of blasphemy from the country's constitution.

26. "The absence of a uniform European conception of the requirements of the protection of the rights of others in relation to attacks on their religious convictions broadens the Contracting States' margin of appreciation when regulating freedom of expression in relation to matters liable to offend personal convictions within the sphere of morals or religion," as the Court put it in *E. S. v. Austria*. "Just because you are offended doesn't mean you're right," as writer and comedian Ricky Gervais puts it; this might be considered another way of expressing the same sentiment. See Christopher Hooton, "Ricky Gervais on Outrage Culture: 'Offence Is the Collateral Damage of Freedom of Speech,'" *The Independent*, April 13, 2016.

27. International Covenant on Civil and Political Rights, Articles 19(2) and 20, respectively.

28. That is, especially, the UN Human Rights Committee, which oversees the implementation of the ICCPR, General Comment 34 (2011) on Article 19: Freedom of Opinion and Expression, as well as the committee's jurisprudence of individual complaint cases relating to Articles 19 and 20, searchable via this database: United Nations Human Rights, Office of the High Commissioner,

accessed November 15, 2022, https://juris.ohchr.org/BasicSearch. There is also the UN Special Rapporteur on the Promotion and Protection of Freedom of Opinion and Expression, the mandate of which has been in continuous existence since 1993.

29. On the inscrutability of drafting hate speech laws, see Nadine Strossen, *Hate: Why We Should Resist It with Free Speech, Not Censorship* (New York: Oxford University Press, 2018), chapters 4 and 5.

30. See the report published by the NGO Article 19 entitled *Responding to "Hate Speech": Comparative Overview of Six EU Countries* (2018), https://www .article19.org/wp-content/uploads/2018/03/ECA-hate-speech-compilation -report_March-2018.pdf.

31. "Germany Is Silencing 'Hate Speech' but Cannot Define It," *The Economist*, January 13, 2018.

32. "Former French Star Bardot Fined over Racist Remarks," *France24*, June 3, 2008.

33. Alexander Stille, "Why French Law Treats Dieudonné and Charlie Hebdo Differently," *The New Yorker*, January 15, 2015. The various dimensions of burkini bans in France are discussed in chapter 4, on happiness, in the section headed "In Pursuit of Happiness."

34. Sarah Souli, "The Netherlands' Burgeoning Free Speech Problem," *New Republic*, March 14, 2019.

35. Irving v. Penguin Books Ltd & Deborah Lipstadt (2000) EWHC QB 115.

36. See "Holocaust Denier Irving Is Jailed," *BBC News*, February 20, 2006.

37. For example, see Christopher Hitchens, "Hitler's Ghost," *Vanity Fair*, June 1996.

38. See, for example, *Dennis v. United States* (341 U.S. 494 [1951]), restricting the speech of the Communist Party USA.

39. 343 U.S. 250 (1952), in which Justice Felix Frankfurter wrote for the Court.

40. Garrett Felber, "Integration or Separation? Malcolm X's College Debates, Free Speech, and the Challenge to Racial Liberalism on Campus," *Journal of Social History* 53, no. 4 (2020): 1033–59.

41. Brandenburg v. Ohio, 395 U.S. 444 (1969). It is precisely this immanency of lawlessness that some lawyers argue would deny former President Trump the protection of First Amendment free speech should he be prosecuted for inciting the storming of Capitol Hill on January 6, 2021 immediately following his speech at a rally earlier that day during which he exhorted his supporters to "fight like hell." See Bent Kendall, "Incitement Case against Trump for Capitol Riot Would Present Challenges," *Wall Street Journal*, February 21, 2021.

42. Garrett Epps, "Free Speech Isn't Free," *The Atlantic*, February 7, 2014.

43. Jones faced three separate defamation trials brought by families of the victims in 2022 and 2023, after the conclusion of two of which he incurred damages awards totaling more than $1 billion. See Aaron Katersky and Meredith Deliso, "Alex Jones Ordered to Pay $965 Million in Sandy Hook Defamation Trial," *ABC News*, October 13, 2022.

44. Which was the sentiment behind the "Letter on Justice and Open Debate," signed by 150 American academics, writers, and activists denouncing "forces of

illiberalism" that attempt to confront "bad ideas . . . by trying to silence them or wish them away," rather than "by exposure, argument, and persuasion," published in *Harper's Magazine*, July 7, 2020.

45. Such intensity (and controversy) is, however, now also a feature of free speech debates in many universities elsewhere, including the United Kingdom (see Matthew Goodwin, "How Universities Were Corrupted," *UnHerd*, June 24, 2022) and Australia (see *NTEIU v. University of Sydney* [(2021) FCAFC 159], in which the Federal Court ruled against Sydney University's dismissal of a lecturer who, among many such intemperate communications, displayed in class a swastika superimposed on an Israeli flag, on the grounds that his right of intellectual freedom to such "speech" was protected under the conditions of his employment with the university).

46. Zack Beauchamp, "The Myth of a Campus Free Speech Crisis," *Vox*, August 31, 2018 ("several dozen incidents"). See also Beauchamp, "The 'Free Speech Debate' Isn't Really about Free Speech," *Vox*, July 22, 2020. Survey data covering Americans generally show a steady increase over the past fifty years in people's willingness to allow platforms for speakers identified as communists, militarists, homosexuals, and antitheists. "Racists" was the group people favored least allowing to speak, and that view remained steady over the same period. See Matthew Yglesias, "Everything We Think about the Political Correctness Debate Is Wrong," *Vox*, May 12, 2018.

47. See Erwin Chemerinsky and Howard Gillman, "What's at Stake?" chapter 6 in *Free Speech on Campus* (New Haven, CT: Yale University Press, 2017).

48. On the commanding role played by social media in mainstreaming the absurd, see Kamile Grusauskaite, Jaron Harambam, and Stef Aupers, "Picturing Opaque Power: How Conspiracy Theorists Construct Oppositional Videos on YouTube," *Social Media + Society* 8, no. 2 (2022), https://doi.org/10.1177/20563051221089568.

49. See "Donald Trump," *Politifact*, accessed February 18, 2023, https://www.politifact.com/personalities/donald-trump/.

50. Glenn Kessler, Salvador Rizzo, and Meg Kelly, "Trump's False or Misleading Claims Total 30,573 over 4 Years," *Washington Post*, January 24, 2021, citing data drawn from the *Washington Post*'s Fact Checker database.

51. Bella DePaulo, "I Study Liars; I've Never Seen One like Donald Trump," *Chicago Tribune*, December 8, 2017. DePaulo is a psychologist and author specializing in "deceiving and detecting deceit."

52. Not counting, of course, the biggest lie of all, which came thereafter—that he won the 2020 presidential election. Patent though that lie is, a staggering 56 percent of Republican voters say they believe it. See Neil Barron, "The Founders Anticipated—and Feared—Trump's 'Big Lie,'" *The Hill*, June 30, 2021. As of August 2022, that figure still stood at 51 percent. See "Traits of the Parties: Trump and the GOP," Pew Research Center, August 9, 2022, https://www.pewresearch.org/politics/2022/08/09/2-traits-of-the-parties-trump-and-the-gop/.

53. For example, Karen Greenberg, "There's Philosophy behind Trump's Lies," *The Nation*, November 25, 2019.

54. In her essay "Lying in Politics," in *Crises of the Republic* (New York: Harcourt, 1972), 45.

55. Susan Glasser, "The Awful Truth about Impeachment," *The New Yorker*, November 22, 2019.
56. See FiveThirtyEight's rolling tallies of leading polls, "Latest Polls," updated October 28, 2021, 9:01 p.m., https://projects.fivethirtyeight.com/polls/trump -approval/.
57. The president's campaign of misinformation on the COVID-19 crisis is "gonna cost lives," as MSNBC journalist Rachel Maddow put its. Marty Johnson, "Maddow Hits Trump's 'Happy Talk' on Virus: 'I Would Stop Putting Those Briefings on Live TV,'" *The Hill*, March 21, 2020. See also Jeff Tollefson, "How Trump Damaged Science—And Why It Could Take Decades to Recover," *Nature*, October 5, 2020. Reflecting on Trump's gross mishandling of the pandemic as revealed in the numerous interviews Bob Woodward recorded with the president between late 2019 and August 2021,Woodward called Trump's actions "a moral crime," adding, "I've never heard about or read anywhere in my own reporting or in history where a president was so negligent." Woodward, quoted in David Smith, "'It's on the Tape': Bob Woodward on Donald Trump's 'Criminal Behavior,'" *The Guardian*, November 20, 2022.
58. As one former senior party official put it, in the lead-up to the 2020 presidential election, "To pledge allegiance to a political party, void of principle or honor, is an empty oath that will not serve country or conscience. Where once we stood together to advocate for responsible governance, individual liberty, equal justice and opportunity for all, today's GOP platform is nothing more than a vow to support, protect, defend and defer to Donald Trump." Jennifer Horn, "Former New Hampshire GOP Chair: My Fellow Republicans, Trump Does Not Deserve Your Loyalty," *USA Today*, October 16, 2020.
59. A dangerously unfunny "Tower of Babel," as Johnathan Haidt writes in his damning article "Why the Past 10 Years of American Life Have Been So Uniquely Stupid," *The Atlantic*, April 11, 2022. See also Wojciech Sadurski, "The War on Institutions," chapter 2 in *A Pandemic of Populists* (Cambridge: Cambridge University Press, 2022).
60. Simona Kralova and Sandro Vetsko, "Ukraine: Watching the War on Russian TV—A Whole Different Story," *BBC News*, March 2, 2022; Joscha Weber, "Fact Check: Russia's False Case for a Dirty Bomb in Ukraine," *Deutsche Welle*, October 29, 2022.
61. George Orwell, "Looking Back on the Spanish Civil War" (August 1942), in *George Orwell: Essays* (London: Penguin with Secker & Warburg, 2000). See also Mark Satta, "Putin's Brazen Manipulation of Language Is a Perfect Example of Orwellian Doublespeak," *The Conversation*, March 15, 2022.
62. The government's standover tactics regarding Sadurski somewhat prove his point. See John Morijin and Barbara Grabowska-Moroz, "Supporting Wojciech Sadurski in a Warsaw Courtroom," *Verfassungsblog*, November 28, 2019; and, more generally, Dariusz Kalan, "Poland's State of the Media," *Foreign Policy*, November 25, 2019. Sadurski has since been acquitted of the criminal charge. Max Shanahan, "USyd Professor Sadurski Acquitted of Criminal Defamation," *Honi Soit*, September 26, 2021.
63. Ed Bracho-Polanco, "How Jair Bolsonaro Used 'Fake News' to Win Power," *The Conversation*, January 9, 2019.

64. Joshua Zitser, "Brazil's Jair Bolsonaro Bizarrely Suggests That COVID-19 Vaccines Could Turn People into Crocodiles or Bearded Ladies," *Business Insider*, December 20, 2020. Brazilian Federal Police have since sought to prosecute Bolsonaro for spreading misinformation about the pandemic that killed 680,000 Brazilians. Tom Philips, "Police Call for Bolsonaro to Be Charged for Spreading Covid Misinformation," *The Guardian*, August 19, 2022.

65. Nir Eisikovits and Dan Feldman, "AI Is Killing Choice and Chance: Which Means It Is Changing What It Means to Be Human," *The Conversation*, February 25, 2021.

66. John Lanchester, "Document Number Nine," *London Review of Books*, October 10, 2019.

67. For an extensive list of censored words and terms born of breathtaking paranoia, see "Little Red Book Censorship Encyclopedia: Leaked Documents Reveal China's Sophisticated Censorship Machine," *China Digital Times*, July 14, 2022. For an overview of the various techniques used by the Chinese government to restrict online freedom of expression, see Harriet Moynihan and Champa Patel, *Restrictions on Online Freedom of Expression in China: The Domestic, Regional, and International Implications of China's Policies and Practices*, Chatham House Research Paper, International Law Programme, Asia-Pacific Programme, March 2021, 1–7.

68. Such fake posts number in the hundreds of millions each year. See Gary King, Jennifer Pan, and Margaret Roberts, "How the Chinese Government Fabricates Social Media Posts for Strategic Distraction, Not Engaged Argument," *American Political Science Review* 111, no. 3 (2017): 484–501. On the regime's extensive use of social media influencers to skew public debate about its treatment of Uyghurs in Xinjiang province, see Fergus Ryan, Daria Impiombato, and Hsi-Ting Pai, *Frontier Influencers: The New Face of China's Propaganda*, Policy Brief Report 65 (Canberra: Australian Strategic Policy Institute/2022). For discussion of China's monumentally dystopian plans for future state surveillance, see chapter 12 of this book, on trust, under the heading "Breaking Trust."

69. "WHO Chief's Remarks on China's COVID Policy Blocked on Country's Social Media," *Reuters*, May 11, 2022.

70. John Milton, *Areopagitica* (1644).

71. Including the notorious "Good Samaritan" protection against civil suits provided to social media companies when censoring certain content, under section 230(C) of the United States' Communications Decency Act of 1996. This protection covers the suspension or cancelation of user accounts, including of a sitting or former US president.

72. See, for example, Twitter's "Civic Integrity Misleading Information Policy," Twitter Help Center, accessed February 18, 2023, https://help.twitter.com/en /rules-and-policies/election-integrity-policy. Shortly after acquiring Twitter in October 2022, however, Elon Musk signaled his intent to reform the company's content moderation processes. see Mitchell Clark, "Elon Musk Says Twitter Will Have a 'Content Moderation Council,'" *The Verge*, October 29, 2022. David Kaye, when he was the UN special rapporteur on freedom of

expression, argued that tech companies need to root their screening policies in relevant human rights laws. See his report on "hate speech," UN Doc A/74/486 (October 9, 2019).

73. "Ensuring respect for free expression, through independent judgement," as its mission statement declares. Oversight Board, accessed November 5, 2022, https://www.oversightboard.com/.

74. Aja Romano, "Kicking People Off Social Media Isn't about Free Speech," *Vox*, January 21, 2021. Romano notes that "Twitter has suspended more than 70,000 accounts primarily dedicated to spreading the false right-wing conspiracy theory QAnon." Trump's twitter ban was lifted in November 2022, and his Facebook account reinstated in February 2023.

75. To which matter we return when considering liberty's new and likely future frontiers in chapter 12, on trust.

76. Remarkably, this enduringly apt phrase dates back to one of the Court's earliest internet cases, *Reno v. American Civil Liberties Union* (521 U.S. 844 [1997], at 868).

Chapter 9. Love

1. Associated Press, "Korean Love Story: The Moment an Elderly Husband and Wife Are Reunited After Being Torn Apart by War 60 Years Ago," *South China Post*, October 20, 2015.

2. Thomas Buergenthal, *A Lucky Child* (New York: Little, Brown, 2009).

3. Lonnie Bunch, "Emancipation Evoked Mix of Emotions for Freed Slaves," *Washington Post*, September 7, 2012.

4. For a trip into the peculiar, see Paul Campobasso, "The World's Most Bizarre Relationships and Love Stories (with Non-humans)," *Hubpages*, November 28, 2018.

5. Jessica Pauline Ogilvie, "Scientists Try to Measure Love," *Los Angeles Times*, February 8, 2010.

6. Alain de Botton, *The Course of Love* (London: Penguin, 2016), 4.

7. The quotation comes from Yeats's haunting play *The Land of Heart's Desire* (Chicago: Stone & Kimball, 1894). The words are spoken by an otherworldly "faery child" trying (successfully, as it turns out) to entice a young earthly bride to leave behind her "heavy body of clay, and clinging mortal hope," to join the faery land of her heart's desire.

8. Such is the intricacy of the "the human mating game," as biological anthro-pologist Helen Fischer calls it, that "no other aspect of our behavior is so complex, so subtle, or so pervasive." Fischer, *Anatomy of Love: A Natural History of Mating, Marriage, and Why We Stray* (New York: W. W. Norton, 2017), 1.

9. Oscar Wilde, *The Ballad of Reading Gaol* (1897).

10. Louis de Bernières, *Captain Corelli's Mandolin* (London: Secker & Warburg, 1994; reprinted London: Random House, 1995), 344–45.

11. A. S. Byatt, *Possession* (London: Chatto & Windus, 1990), 195.

12. The original project, the Harvard Study of Adult Behavior (see Harvard Second Generation Study, accessed November 2, 2022, https://www .adultdevelopmentstudy.org/), followed 268 men for more than seventy years

from their adolescence until, for some, well into their nineties. see George Vaillant, "Yes, I Stand by My Words: 'Happiness Equals Love—Full Stop,'" *Positive Psychology News*, July 16, 2009.

13. De Beauvoir, quoted in Wayne Bryant, *Bisexual Characters in Film: From Anaïs to Zee* (New York: Haworth Press, 1997), 143.

14. See Enrique Burunat, "Love Is the Cause of Human Evolution," *Advances in Anthropology* 4, no. 2 (2014): 99–116.

15. See Helen Fisher, *Anatomy of Love* (New York: W. W. Norton, 2017), chapter 3.

16. Victor Karandashev, "A Cultural Perspective on Romantic Love," *Online Readings in Psychology and Culture* 5, no. 4 (2015), https://doi.org/10.9707 /2307-0919.1135.

17. Given the abundant evidence of romance in literature and art across the world and throughout the millennia, it is truly remarkable that this should have been the case within the discipline, but to their credit, as well as shame, they are damned by their own frank admissions. See David Goleman, "After Kinship and Marriage Anthropology Discovers Love," *New York Times*, November 24, 1992; and Charles Lindholm, "Romantic Love and Anthropology," *Romantic Love* 19, no. 1 (2006): 5–21.

18. Rebecca King Pierce in conversation with Dredge Kang, "The New Anthropology of Love," *Hold That Thought*, February 10, 2016, podcast and transcript available in *The Ampersand* (Washington University, Arts and Sciences), https://artsci.wustl.edu/ampersand/new-anthropology-love.

19. Goleman, "After Kinship and Marriage Anthropology Discovers Love."

20. See Pierce in conversation with Kang, "New Anthropology of Love."

21. George Orwell, *1984* (London: Secker & Warburg, 1949), 86.

22. The Afghani ministry, established in 2021, is tasked with enforcing the Taliban's strict interpretation of Islam. See Kathy Gannon, "Taliban Replace Ministry for Women with 'Virtue' Authorities," *Associated Press*, September 19, 2021. In contrast, the reasoning behind Spain's establishment in 2017 of the "Commissioner for the Demographic Challenge" (to give the agency its proper title) was to correct the country's declining birth rate by encouraging people to procreate. See "El Gobierno nombra a Edelmira Barreira nueva comisionada para el reto demográfico," *ABC España*, January 21, 2017.

23. As Orwell says in *1984*: "Not love so much as eroticism was the enemy," 83.

24. "Making love" as a euphemism for sex is, according to the *Oxford English Dictionary*, a relatively recent interpretation (circa 1920s), its original usage (in the Middle Ages) having been to denote courtship rather than intercourse.

25. "Sexuality," writes Dennis Altman, is one of the two "dominant preoccupations of current science and popular debate" (the other being globalization). It is on the connections between the two that his book *Global Sex* (Chicago: University of Chicago Press, 2001), is focused (quote at 1).

26. Shaw, quoted in John Lloyd and John Mitchinson, *If Ignorance Is Bliss, Why Aren't There More Happy People? Smart Quotes for Dumb Times* (New York: Harmony Books, 2008).

27. That is, "the power of sexuality to define who we are as human beings," as Richard Parker puts it, in "Sexuality, Culture, and Society: Shifting Paradigms

in Sexuality Research," *Culture, Health, and Sexuality* 11, no. 3 (2009): 251–66, at 253.

28. Bowers v. Hardwick, 478 U.S. 186 (1986), at 191.

29. Lawrence v. Texas, 539 U.S. 558 (2003).

30. According to *World Population Review* same-sex marriage is now legal in twenty-four countries (including Mexico, albeit only in parts of the country), and in a eleven other countries same-sex civil unions are tolerated. See "Countries Where Gay Marriage Is Legal 2023," World Population Review, accessed February 18, 2023, https://worldpopulationreview.com/country-rankings/countries-where-gay-marriage-is-legal.

31. According to the "Map of Countries That Criminalise LGBT People," Human Dignity Trust, accessed November 1, 2022, https://www.humandignitytrust.org/lgbt-the-law/map-of-criminalisation/.

32. See, respectively, "Alabama Sex Toy Drive-thru Business on the Rise," *CBS News*, December 30, 2010; W. Gardiner Selby, "Colin Jost, on Weekend Update, Says a Texas Law Bars Ownership of More than 6 Dildos," *Politifact*, October 13, 2017, https://www.politifact.com/factchecks/2017/oct/13/colin-jost/colin-jost-weekend-update-texas-dildos-law-6-own-m/.

33. For a global compendium of relevant laws, see the Sexual Rights Initiative (accessed February 18, 2023, https://sexualrightsinitiative.org); and for the US specifically, see Richard Weinmeyer, "The Decriminalization of Sodomy in the United States," *AMA Journal of Ethics* 16, no. 11 (2014): 916–22; and Lily Wakefield, "There Are 16 States in the U.S. That Still Have Sodomy Laws against 'Perverted Sexual Practice'; It's 2020," *Pink News*, January 24, 2020.

34. For a surreal two minutes have a look at the video "Matt and Harmony (RealDoll X Behind the Scenes)," YouTube, accessed November 2, 2022, https://www.youtube.com/watch?v=cNiPmdsLpP4. Introducing Harmony, the "world's first affordable robot with a practical purpose," as Harmony says of herself in the crisp tones of an educated Edinburgh accent, before continuing, "being home use, [pause] or in bedroom use . . . hahaha." Harmony is easy to use, modular and "user-repairable," as her creator Matt McMullen adds. Equally disquietingly entertaining, though fictional (for now, at least), are the novels *Machines Like Me*, by Ian McEwan (London: Random House, 2020), and *Frankissstein*, by Jeanette Winterson (London: Jonathan Cape, 2020).

35. On which, see R. Marie Griffith, *Moral Combat: How Sex Divided American Christians and Fractured American Politics* (New York: Basic Books, 2018).

36. Camille Paglia, *Free Women, Free Men: Sex, Gender, Feminism* (Edinburgh: Canongate, 2018), 36.

37. On the apparent rise and potentially terrible consequences of the latter, see Anna Moore and Coco Khan, "The Fatal, Hateful Rise of Choking During Sex," *The Guardian*, July 25, 2019.

38. Having lived and worked in Australia for more than thirty years, I am still somewhat taken aback by how conservative its political and social agendas are, more like my native Northern Ireland than the carefree image that Australia likes to portray of itself. The legalization of same-sex marriage in Australia in 2017 was a welcome exception to this rule. Same-sex marriage was legalized in the Republic of Ireland in 2015. It was prohibited in Northern Ireland until

January 2020, when it was legalized under the Northern Ireland (Executive Formation etc) Act 2019, finally bringing the province into line with the rest of the United Kingdom, which has permitted same-sex marriage since 2013.

39. Seanad Éireann debates, vol. 242, no. 11, October 20, 2015.

40. Bostock v. Clayton County, Georgia; Altitude Express v. Zarda; and R. G. & G. R. Harris Funeral Homes v. EEOC/Stephens (consolidated under the first-named case), 590 U.S. __ (2020).

41. See Mike DeBonis, "The Push for LGBTQ Civil Rights Stalls in the Senate As Advocates Search for Republican Support," *Washington Post*, June 20, 2021.

42. As argued in written submissions (amici curiae) to the Supreme Court by a coalition of Family Policy Groups and the National Association of Evangelicals, respectively. See "Amici Curiae," in No.17-1618, Gerald Lynn Bostock v. Clayton County, Georgia, The Cert Pool, accessed November 15, 2022, https://certpool.com/dockets/17-1618.

43. Jeffrey Jones, "LGBT Identification in the U.S. Ticks Up to 7.1%," *Gallup News*, February 17, 2022.

44. See "Document Entries," in Bostock v. Clayton County.

45. Léon Treich (ed.), *L'esprit d'Alexandre Dumas* (Paris: Gallimard, 1926), 115 (translation mine). While Treich quotes Dumas as referring to a singular chain ("la chaîne du mariage"), Dumas is otherwise invariably quoted as referring to chains, plural ("les chaînes du mariage"). In a similar vein, Gabriel García Márquez talks of "the arduous calvary of conjugal life," albeit in the cheerier context of leaping over it when one finds love in one's old age. See *Love in a Time of Cholera*, trans. Edith Grossman (London: Penguin, 1989), 420.

46. "In U.S., Record-High Say Gay and Lesbian Relations Morally OK," *Gallup News*, May 20, 2013.

47. Perel, *The State of Affairs: Rethinking Infidelity* (New York: Harper, 2017).

48. Parul Sehgal, "'The State of Affairs' Examines Our Cheating Hearts," *New York Times*, October 24, 2017.

49. See "Oui, une crise cardiaque en plein rapport sexuel est un 'accident du travail,'" *BFM/RMC*, September 13, 2019.

50. See "Worker Injured during Sex Gets Compensation Payout," *NewsComAu*, April 19, 2012. Demonstrating what might be considered extraspecial dedication to her job, the woman involved was employed by the human relations section of a government agency.

51. See George Murdock's seminal work *Social Structure* (London: Macmillan, 1949).

52. Which can be very far indeed. The "most outstanding aspect of [Australian] Aboriginal kinship systems," for example, note Gray, Trompf, and Houston, "is the existence of whole classes of people identified by an Aboriginal person as his or her 'brothers,' 'fathers,' 'sisters,' 'others,' 'husbands,' 'wives,' or the various other classes of affinities." "The Decline and Rise of Aboriginal Families," in Janice Reid and Peggy Trompf (eds.), *The Health of Aboriginal Australia* (Sydney: Harcourt Brace Jovanovich, 1991), 82.

53. As quoted in "George Burns: Biography," Internet Movie Database, accessed November 2, 2022, https://www.imdb.com/name/nm0122675/bio?ref_=nm_ov_bio_sm.

54. Liao, *The Right to Be Loved* (New York: Oxford University Press, 2015).

55. As stressed repeatedly throughout the convention's fifty-four articles.

56. On the definitional difficulties and practical challenges of parental obligations (including the perils to both children and their families), see Asgeir Falch-Eriksen and Elisabeth Backe-Hansen (eds.), *Human Rights in Child Protection: Implications for Professional Practice and Policy* (Cham, Switzerland: Palgrave Macmillan, 2018).

57. An estimated forty-five tons of locks attached to the bridge's railings were removed that year and lock-proof railings installed in their place. Not to be deterred, the love-lock determined have since shifted their attentions to Passerelles Debilly and Léopold-Sédar-Senghor—less romantic bridges, though still subject to the same laws of physics as Pont des Arts.

58. David Hume, *A Treatise of Human Nature* (1739), Book II, Part 3, Section 3, p. 415.

59. Michelle Miller-Day, "Family Communication," *Oxford Research Encyclopedia of Communication*, January 25, 2017, https://doi.org/10.1093/acrefore/9780190228613.013.177.

Chapter 10. Death

1. Yasmine Ryan, "The Tragic Life of a Street Vendor," *Al Jazeera*, January 20, 2011.

2. See Thessa Lageman, "Remembering Mohamed Bouazizi: The Man Who Sparked the Arab Spring," *Al Jazeera*, December 17, 2020, and further references in note 1 above and note 4 below.

3. Ryan, "The Tragic Life of a Street Vendor."

4. Rania Abouzeid, "Bouazizi: The Man Who Set Himself and Tunisia on Fire," *Time*, January 21, 2011.

5. As he felt compelled to do after he led a failed attempt at a military coup in 1970. Suicide in its various forms was a persistent theme throughout Mishima's work. See David Barnett, "The Life and Death of Yukio Mishima: A Tale of Astonishing Elegance and Emotional Brutality" *The Independent*, July 25, 2019.

6. Sherwin Nuland, *How We Die: Reflections on Life's Final Chapter* (New York: Vintage, 1995).

7. The dignity question is further explored through the lens of respect in chapter 11.

8. A "particularly vile," and yet avoidable, cruelty, argues health lawyer Maayan Sudai, in "Not Dying Alone: The Need to Democratize Hospital Visitation Policies during Covid-19," *Medical Law Review* 29, no. 4(2021): 613–38, https://doi.org/10.1093/medlaw/fwab033.

9. Catechism of the Catholic Church.

10. See Oliver Leaman (ed.), *The Qur'an: An Encyclopedia* (London: Routledge, 2005), 177.

11. Kant, quoted in Michael Rosen, *Dignity: Its History and Meaning* (Cambridge, MA: Harvard University Press, 2012), 123.

12. See Frederick White, "Personhood: An Essential Characteristic of the Human Species," *Linacre Quarterly* 80, no. 1 (1993): 74.

13. David Roos, "Human Sacrifice: Why the Aztecs Practised This Gory Ritual," *History*, October 11, 2018.

14. See Muhammad al-Atawneh, "*Shahāda* versus Terror in Contemporary Islamic Legal Thought: The Problem of Suicide Bombers," *Journal of Islamic Law and Culture* 10, no. 1 (2008): 18–29; and Reid Hutchins, "Islam and Suicide Terrorism: Separating Fact from Fiction" *Counter Terrorist Trends and Analyses* 9, no. 11 (2017): 7–11. Although the bombers typically kill themselves as well as others, they and their supporters do not use the term "suicide bomber," as suicide is regarded a grave sin in Islam, preferring instead the term "martyr" or "jihadist."

15. See "State by State," Death Penalty Information Center, accessed November 2, 2022, https://deathpenaltyinfo.org/state-and-federal-info/state-by-state; and Larry Greenemeier, "Cruel and Unusual? Is Capital Punishment by Lethal Injection Quick and Painless?" *Scientific American*, October 27, 2010. The ethical question of having medical practitioners involved in administering the injection and thereby actively contribute to the death of "a patient" is also problematic, albeit that *not* having them present may be equally disturbing; see Amnesty International, *Lethal Injection*, May 18, 2017.

16. "Death Penalty Database: China," Cornell Center on the Death Penalty Worldwide, accessed November 2, 2022, https://deathpenaltyworldwide.org /database/#/results/country?id=16.

17. Furman v. Georgia, 408 U.S. 238 (1972).

18. Gregg v. Georgia, 428 U.S. 153 (1976). *Gregg* was the lead case in a set of five cases heard and decided jointly by the Court, all of which concerned the same legal principle.

19. Roper v. Simmons, 543 U.S. 551 (2005). According to recent annual data collected by Amnesty International, the United States hosted 11 executions in 2021; Iran, at least 314; Egypt, at least 83; Saudi Arabia, 65, and in China, while the government publishes no figures on executions, the number is certainly in the thousands per year. See Amnesty International Global Report, *Death Sentences and Executions 2021* (2022). The United States stands alone among Western nations by retaining capital punishment. Thus, for example, all forty-six Council of Europe member states have ratified the Sixth Protocol to the European Convention on Human Rights, which abolishes the death penalty in peacetime. Before its expulsion from the Council of Europe on March 16, 2022, Russia had signed but not ratified the protocol, though a moratorium on legal executions has been in place in Russia since 2010.

20. As per Protocol I to the Geneva Conventions on the Protection of Victims of International Armed Conflicts (1977), Art. 35.

21. In Rome Statute, Articles 5, 6, 7, and 8.

22. Separate international initiatives exist seeking to ban each of these horrifying weapons. For an overview of and further details on these and other related endeavors, see "About," UN Office for Disarmament Affairs, accessed November 2, 2022, https://www.un.org/disarmament/about/.

23. For an exhaustive tabulation of all reported and suspected instances of such use, see "Timeline of Syrian Chemical Weapons Activity, 2012–22," Arms Control Association, accessed November 2, 2022, https://www.armscontrol .org/factsheets/Timeline-of-Syrian-Chemical-Weapons-Activity.

24. Interestingly, though, psychologist Lenore Walker, one of the first writers to document the phenomenon, used the term to explain why women remain in relationships that are so harmful to them. See her book *The Battered Woman* (New York: HarperCollins, 1979).

25. New York Penal Code, Article 35.

26. Dan Bilefsky, "Wife Who Fired Eleven Shots Is Acquitted of Murder," *New York Times*, October 6, 2011.

27. In Iran, for instance, the death penalty is imposed on wives (including child brides) who kill their abusers; see Mansoureh Mills, "She was a teenage victim of domestic violence and rape. She sought help. This week, Iran executed her," *Time Magazine* October 5, 2018.

28. See, for example, the multijurisdictional study *Women Who Kill in Response to Domestic Violence: How Do Criminal Justice Systems Respond?* Linklaters LLP for Penal Reform International, 2016, https://www.penalreform.org/resource /women-who-kill-in-response-to-domestic-violence/.

29. Case 1 BvR 357/05 (February 15, 2006). Article 1 of Germany's Basic Law (or Constitution) provides: "Human dignity shall be inviolable. To respect and protect it shall be the duty of all state authority."

30. Imperial College COVID-19 Response Team, "Impact of Non-pharmaceutical Interventions (NPIs) to Reduce COVID-19 Mortality and Healthcare Demand," March 16, 2020. See also Jonathan Cooper, "Will Johnson's Coronavirus Response Violate Human Rights Law?" *Open Democracy*, March 16, 2020. As it was, the UK tally of COVID-19-related deaths one year later (in March 2021) was approximately 123,000, out of more than 4 million infections. "COVID-19 Dashboard," Johns Hopkins Coronavirus Resource Center, accessed March 20, 2021, https://coronavirus.jhu.edu/map.html.

31. Sweden's more sustained herd immunity experiment with COVID-19 was heavily criticized for precisely the same reasons of callous disregard for human lives. See Sigurd Bergmann, "Sweden's Experiment with Herd Immunity Is Unethical and Undemocratic and Reveals an Underlying Political Pathology," ABC, October 14, 2020. By March 2021 in Sweden, the tally of COVID-19-related deaths was approximately 13,000, out of some 660,000 infections. "COVID-19 Dashboard."

32. William Shakespeare, *Hamlet*, Act III, Scene I.

33. David Hume, "Of Suicide," written circa 1755, but not published until 1777, posthumously and (initially) anonymously (available at The Open University, accessed November 2, 2022, https://www.open.edu/openlearn/pluginfile.php /623438/mod_resource/content/1/ofsuicide.pdf).

34. Jamie Baker, "Suicide Takes a Major Toll on Those Left Behind," *Laborers' Health and Safety Fund of North America* (November 2017).

35. Reeves was responding to the question "What do you think happens when we die?" put to him by Stephen Colbert during an interview on *The Late Show*, May 11, 2019.

36. "Suicide survivors face grief, questions, challenges," *Harvard Women's Health Watch*, June 8, 2018.

37. See Louise Brådvik, "Suicide Risk and Mental Disorders," *International Journal of Environmental Research and Public Health* 15, no. 9 (2018): 2028.

38. Charles Raison, "Psychiatrist: I Hate Suicide, but I Also Understand It," *CNN*, August 21, 2012.
39. Émile Durkheim, *Suicide: A Study in Sociology* (first published in Paris in 1897), trans. John Spaulding & George Simpson (London: Routledge & Kegan Paul, 1952).
40. According to World Health Organization (WHO) data, Guyana has the highest suicide rate among this age group (58.2 deaths per 100,000 population); of large-population states Russia (19.4 per 100,000) and South Africa (23 per 100,000) have the highest rates, and among OECD countries Finland has the highest rate (18.5 per 100,000). The US rate per 100,000 sits at 17.7, Australia at 12.3, and New Zealand at 13.9, while France, Germany, and the United Kingdom are between 5 and 6. See "Suicide Rate Estimates, Crude, 15–29 and 30–49 Years, Estimates by Country," in "Global Health Observatory Data Repository," updated July 16, 2021, https://apps.who.int/gho/data/node .main.MHSUICIDEAGEGROUPS15293049?lang=en. The suicide rate among young males is strikingly higher than that for females in nearly all countries.
41. On which, see Brian Mishara and David Weisstub, "The Legal Status of Suicide: A Global Review," *International Journal of Law and Psychiatry* 44 (2016): 54–74.
42. See Brådvik, "Suicide Risk and Mental Disorders."
43. Commonwealth v. Carter, No. 15YO0001NE (Mass. Juv. Ct., June 16, 2017).
44. Though originally introduced in 2019, the bill (dubbed "Conrad's Law") has yet to be enacted; see Bill S.2382, An Act Relevant to Preventing Suicide, Commonwealth of Massachusetts, accessed November 3, 2022, https:// malegislature.gov/Bills/191/SD2505. For its latest iteration (Bill SD1302, filed on January 19, 2023) see https://malegislature.gov/Bills/193/SD1302 (accessed February 25, 2023).
45. See Andreas Fontalis et al., "Euthanasia and Assisted Dying: What Is the Current Position and What Are the Key Arguments Informing the Debate?" *Journal of the Royal Society of Medicine* 111, no. 11 (2018): 407–13.
46. For a global review of its legal status, see "Euthanasia and Medical Aid in Dying (MAID) around the World," ProCon.org, updated July 7, 2022, https://euthanasia.procon.org/euthanasia-physician-assisted-suicide-pas-around -the-world/.
47. With its origins in moral philosophy stretching back at least as far as St. Thomas Aquinas, the principle of double effect acknowledges the possibility of separating intention and outcome, as a consequence of which an action taken with moral intent but resulting in morally bad as well as morally good outcomes, may nonetheless still be viewed overall as morally proper. Its application in the medical sense refers to the proper intent behind the treatment and its desired effects potentially mitigating any *supplementary* untoward medical outcomes of the treatment. See Denise Dudzinski, "The Principle of Double Effect in Palliative Care: Euthanasia by Another Name," in Gail Van Norman et al. (eds.), *Clinical Ethics in Anesthesiology* (New York: Cambridge University Press, 2010).
48. On which process, see Bianca Nogrady, *The End: The Human Experience of Death* (Sydney: Random House, 2014), chapters 4 and 5.

49. Roger Magnusson, *Angels of Death: Exploring the Euthanasia Underground* (New Haven, CT: Yale University Press, 2002), 198.
50. For an overview of which, see European Court of Human Rights, *End of Life and the European Convention on Human Rights Factsheet* (April 2021).
51. Luke Hurst and Camille Bello, "Euthanasia in Europe: Where Is Assisted Dying Legal?" *euronews.next*, September 14, 2022.
52. In Europe, Austria, Finland, and Norway also permit passive euthanasia. In Australia, active and passive euthanasia have been legalized everywhere expect in the Australian Capital Territory and the Northern Territory.
53. Vincent Lambert's parents maintained this stance throughout, though most of their other children (Vincent's siblings) and other family members disagreed. Charlie Gard's parents did in the end agree to withdrawal of life support after it became clear that not even exceptional, experimental treatment was feasible. See Dominic Wilkinson and Julian Savulescu, "The Charlie Gard Case," chapter 1 of *Ethics, Conflict, and Medical Treatment for Children* (London: Elsevier, 2018).
54. In addition, in Lambert's case, the UN Committee on the Rights of Persons with Disabilities issued an interim measure (on May 3, 2019) requesting that life support be continued pending the committee's full hearing of the case. Life support was nevertheless withdrawn two months later without any such hearing having taken place. For the legal histories of both cases, see, for Lambert, Dominic Wilkinson and Julian Savulescu, "Current Controversies and Irresolvable Disagreement: The Case of Vincent Lambert and the Role of 'Dissensus,'" *Journal of Medical Ethics* 45 (2019): 631–35; and, for Gard: Wilkinson and Savulescu, "The Charlie Gard Case."
55. Which begs the question to which there is still no definitive answer, When is death? On this remarkably complex matter from a medical perspective, see Alan Shewmon, "Constructing the Death Elephant: A Synthetic Paradigm Shift for the Definition, Criteria, and Tests for Death," *Journal of Medicine and Philosophy* 35 (2010): 256–98.
56. On the many and varied benefits and problems of which, see Deborah Carr and Elizabeth Luth, "Advance Care Planning: Contemporary Issues and Future Directions," *Innovation in Aging* 1, no. 1 (2017): 1–10.

Chapter 11. Respect

1. Barry Flanagan's *San Marco Horse* stands in First Court, Jesus College, Cambridge. It's still there and it's still strikingly beautiful. The lawn, what is more, remains off-limits to all but Fellows of the College and the specially invited.
2. Barack Obama, "Remarks Accepting the Presidential Nomination at the Democratic National Convention in Charlotte, North Carolina," September 6, 2012, American Presidency Project, https://www.presidency.ucsb.edu /documents/remarks-accepting-the-presidential-nomination-the-democratic -national-convention-charlotte. Obama was here echoing John F. Kennedy, who, during his first term as a US senator, declared: "Today, every citizen, regardless of his interest in politics, 'holds office'; every one of us is in a position of responsibility and, in the final analysis, the kind of government we

get depends upon how we fulfill those responsibilities." Kennedy, "Remarks to the American Association of School Administrators Convention in Atlantic City, New Jersey," February 19, 1957.

3. As of August 31, 2022, the total of COVID-19 related outlays of the federal government was $4.6 trillion. "The Federal Response to COVID-19," USASpending.gov, accessed November 4, 2022, https://www.usaspending.gov /disaster/covid-19. See also Adam Gaffney, "America's Extreme Neoliberal Healthcare System Is Putting the Country at Risk," *The Guardian*, March 21, 2020.

4. "Department of Energy Authorizes Additional LNG Exports from Freeport LNG" (media release), US Department of Energy, May 28, 2019.

5. "Ted Cruz Ended His CPAC Speech with the 'Freedom!' Yell from 'Braveheart' and People Are Ruthlessly Mocking Him for It," *Uproxx*, February 26, 2021.

6. "Live free or die" may roll off the tongue nicely, but the precept's most ardent advocates will likely get both if they refuse to wear a mask during a pandemic on the grounds that "it's muzzling yourself, it looks weak . . . especially for men," as Elizabeth Cobbs notes in "Americans Want to Be Free to Be Stupid," *Financial Times*, July 9, 2020.

7. See "World Report 2022: China—Events of 2021," Human Rights Watch, accessed November 4, 2022, at https://www.hrw.org/world-report/2022 /country-chapters/china-and-tibet.

8. Lily Kuo, "China Says UN Criticism of Human Rights Record Is 'Politically Driven,'" *The Guardian*, November 7, 2018.

9. See Lindsay Maizland, "China's Repression of Uyghurs in Xinjiang," *Council on Foreign Relations*, March 1, 2021; and Oliver Young, "Hong Kong Judge Convicts Authors of Children's Books for Sedition," *China Digital Times*, September 9, 2022, respectively. The latter depicted sheep resisting wolves' attempts to take over the village, which the judge, in sentencing the authors to nineteen months in jail, described as "brainwashing."

10. Nike v. Kasky, 539 U.S. 654 (2003).

11. Demands initiated by series of US state attorneys general. See David Hasemyer, "U.S. Supreme Court Refuses to Block Exxon Climate Fraud Investigation," *Inside Climate News*, January 7, 2017. A similar line of argument was used by big tobacco companies in the 1980s and '90s when they sought (also unsuccessfully) to conceal damning reports of their awareness of the health risks of smoking.

12. Masha Gessen, "Mark Zuckerberg Doesn't Know What the First Amendment Is For," *The New Yorker*, October 22, 2019.

13. See the landmark resolution of the UN Human Rights Council 16/18 in 2011, which addresses "combating intolerance, negative stereotyping and stigmatization of, and discrimination, incitement to violence, and violence *against persons* based on religion or belief" (my emphasis).

14. Which under the European Convention on Human Rights, for example, is expressly provided for in Article 9. For an account of the breadth of relevant case law (from the freedoms and restrictions on wearing religious symbols to the freedom not to worship), see "Guide on Article 9 of the European Convention on Human Rights," Council of Europe, August 31, 2022 (update).

15. See Article 19, "UN HRC Resolution 16/18: Consolidating Consensus through Implementation," *Article 19 Briefing*, February 18, 2016, https://www.article19.org/resources/un-hrc-resolution-16-18-consolidating-consensus-through-implementation/.

16. George Kateb, *Human Dignity* (Cambridge, MA: Belknap Press of Harvard University Press, 2011), 10–19.

17. Kateb, 53.

18. Johnathan Powell, *Talking to Terrorists* (London: Vintage, 2014).

19. Powell, at 3; and, regarding the preceding sentence, apologies to William Shakespeare (*Julius Caesar*, Act 3, Scene 2).

20. Powell provides a full account of his perspective on negotiating the Northern Ireland peace process in his book *Great Hatred, Little Room* (London: Bodley Head, 2008).

21. See his essay "Human Rights, Rationality and Sentimentality," in *Truth and Progress: Philosophical Papers* (New York: Cambridge University Press, 1998), 129. "I hope the Russians love their children too," as Sting put it in *Russians* (A&M, 1985), reflecting fears at that time of nuclear war between the West and the Soviet Union, and which words once again resonate in 2023 regarding possible escalation of the war in Ukraine.

22. See Hannes Kuch, "The Rituality of Humiliation: Exploring Symbolic Vulnerability," in Paulus Kaufmann et al. (eds.), *Humiliation, Degradation, Dehumanization* (Dordrecht: Springer, 2011), 37–56.

23. In 2020, the imprisonment rate of Black males in the United States was 5.7 times that of white males, and the imprisonment rate of Black females was 1.7 times the rate of white females, according to Bureau of Justice Statistics, US Department of Justice, "Prisoners in 2020," 23, accessed November 4, 2022, https://bjs.ojp.gov/content/pub/pdf/p20st.pdf. As of June 2021, Aboriginal and Torres Strait Islander (ATSI) prisoners constituted 30 percent of all prisoners in Australia, despite ATSI peoples then making up only 3.8 percent of the total Australian population. See "Prisoners in Australia," Australian Bureau of Statistics, accessed November 4, 2022, https://www.abs.gov.au/statistics/people/crime-and-justice/prisoners-australia/latest-release; and "Estimates of Aboriginal and Torres Strait Islander Australians," ibid., accessed November 4, 2022, https://www.abs.gov.au/statistics/people/aboriginal-and-torres-strait-islander-peoples/estimates-aboriginal-and-torres-strait-islander-australians/latest-release). Further, in the case of Australia, it bears recalling that Indigenous Australians were not recognized as citizens of their country until a referendum in 1967 amending the Constitution permitted them to be so.

24. As demonstrated by Rod Michelmore, "Illicit Financial Flows and Least Developed Countries: A Pro-Poor Approach towards Tax Transparency," unpublished PhD thesis, University of Sydney, 2021.

25. See "Endemic Violence against Women 'Cannot Be Stopped with a Vaccine'—WHO Chief," *UN News*, March 9, 2021. For a condemnatory account of how "pervasive" the problem is in India, see Sudha Ramachandran, "Violence against Women in India Must End. Now," *The Diplomat*, October 5, 2020.

26. See UN Women, *#MeToo: Headlines from a Global Movement* (2020).

27. As argued, for example, by Martha Nussbaum, *Citadels of Pride: Sexual Abuse, Accountability, and Reconciliation* (New York: W. W. Norton, 2021).

28. See "From Where I Stand," *UN Women News*, September 2, 2021, https://www .unwomen.org/en/news/stories/2021/9/from-where-i-stand-william-fernando -rosero.

29. See chapter 5, on wealth, under the heading "Unfreedoms."

30. According to the Congressional Research Service, 8.6 percent of Americans (28 million) have no health care coverage: "U.S. Health Care Coverage and Spending," *In Focus*, April 1, 2022; and chapter 3, on health, under the heading "Healthy Liberty."

31. See chapter 7, on security, under the heading "Anti-terrorism's Freedom Dilemma." See also Ed Pilkington, "'Panic Made Us Vulnerable': How 9/11 Made the US Surveillance—And the Americans Who Fought Back," *The Guardian*, September 4, 2021.

32. Hart Research Associates / Public Opinion Strategies, Study 220699, (NBC News Survey, October 2022), accessed November 5, 2022, https://s3 .documentcloud.org/documents/23171526/220699-nbc-news-october-poll-v3 .pdf. The exact percentages for belief in the other side's existential threat were Republicans, 81 percent, and Democrats, 79 percent; and for preparedness to overlook moral failures, Republicans, 67 percent, and Democrats, 63 percent.

33. "Musk, Trump, and the Demeaning of America," *Robert Reich* (blog), November 7, 2022, https://robertreich.substack.com/p/america-in-the-age-of -the-megalomaniacs. See also chapter 8, on voice, especially under the heading "Voice Control."

34. Jonathan Kirshner, "Gone but Not Forgotten: Trump's Long Shadow and the End of American Credibility," *Foreign Affairs*, March–April 2021.

35. Fintan O'Toole, "Trump Has Unfinished Business. A Republic He Wants to Destroy Still Stands," *Irish Times*, December 26, 2020.

36. Fintan O'Toole, "Donald Trump Has Destroyed the Country He Promised to Make Great Again," *Irish Times*, April 25, 2020.

37. On which point you cannot go past the astonishing example of white evangelicals in the United States. As reported in a 2016 PRRI/Brookings poll, "More than seven in ten (72%) white evangelical Protestants say an elected official can behave ethically even if they have committed transgressions in their personal life—a 42-point jump from 2011, when only 30% of white evangeli- cal Protestants said the same." "Backing Trump, White Evangelicals Flip Flop on Importance of Candidate Character—PRRI/Brookings Survey," PRRI, October 19, 2016, https://www.prri.org/research/prri-brookings-oct-19-poll -politics-election-clinton-double-digit-lead-trump/.

38. Thomas Hobbes, *Leviathan* (1561), Part 2, Chapter 19, p. 150.

39. Svetlana Alexievich, *Secondhand Time: The Last of the Soviets* (New York: Random House, 2016), 9.

40. In an interview with Sean Illing, "A Decade of Revolt," *Vox*, December 26, 2019.

Chapter 12. Trust

1. All details in these paragraphs are drawn from a remarkable memoir of Lien's life written by Bart van Es, *The Cut Out Girl* (New York: Penguin Press, 2019),

in which the original letter and its translation are reproduced on pp. 29–30. Bart van Es is the grandson of the foster parents who took in Lien in 1942.

2. For those who survived, the psychological trauma of the experience was often crippling, for all involved—parents and foster parents, as well as the hidden children themselves. See Bloeme Evers-Emden, "Hiding Jewish Children during World War II: The Psychological Aftermath," *Jewish Political Studies Review* 19, nos. 1–2 (2007): 39–47.

3. Hemingway to Dorothy Connable, February 17, 1953, in Carlos Baker (ed.), *Ernest Hemingway: Selected Letters, 1917–1961* (New York: Scribner, 1981).

4. See Mark Zastrow, "South Korea Is Reporting Intimate Details of COVID-19 Cases: Has It Helped?" *Nature*, March 18, 2020.

5. See Brett Murphy and Letitia Stein's damning investigation, "The Coronavirus Test That Wasn't: How the Federal Health Officials Misled State Scientists and Derailed the Best Chance at Containment," *USA Today*, March 27, 2020; and David Leonhardt, "America's Death Gap," *New York Times*, September 1, 2020.

6. Jean-Jacques Rousseau, *Émile; Or, Concerning Education* (1762), Book II, "The Fox and the Crow: A Fable," Project Gutenberg (2011), https://www.gutenberg .org/files/5427/5427-h/5427-h.htm.

7. For a compilation of cases before or decided by the Court, see European Court of Human Rights, *COVID-19 Health Crisis—Fact Sheet* (July 2021). See also the 2021 case of *Vavřička and Others v. the Czech Republic* (ECHR, Application no. 47621/13 and five others), April 8, 2021, concerning vaccine protocols, discussed in chapter 3, on health, under the heading "The Importance of Information and Argument."

8. Jean-Jacques Rousseau, *The Social Contract* (1762)—one of the most influential political and philosophy texts of all time, which Rousseau described in its preface as a "little thesis" (of some 55,000 words). It was published in the same year as *Émile* (125,000 words in length), which just goes to show how incredibly industrious one can be without electronic aids and distractions.

9. These being the very ingredients or civic virtues, as Philip Pettit reminds us, that constitute the ancient idea of republicanism. Philip Pettit, *Republicanism: A Theory of Freedom and Government* (New York: Oxford University Press, 1999).

10. Benjamin Disraeli, *Vivian Grey* (London: Henry Colburn, 1826), Book VI, Chapter 7. Disraeli was a founding member of the modern British Conservative Party and served twice as prime minister of the United Kingdom.

11. As G. W. F. Hegel put it, "A constitution is not a mere manufacture, but the work of centuries. It is the idea and the consciousness of what is reasonable, in so far as it is developed in a people." *Elements of the Philosophy of Right* (1820), p. 222, para. 274.

12. See Martin Krygier, "Rule of Law," in Michel Rosenfeld and András Sajó (eds.), *The Oxford Handbook of Comparative Constitutional Law* (Oxford: Oxford University Press, 2012).

13. Crowley v. Christensen, 137 U.S. 86 (1890), at 89–90.

14. Her husband, Michael Aris (who died in 1999), was British, as are their two sons, Alexander and Kim.

15. Planned Parenthood of Southeastern Pennsylvania v. Casey, 505 U.S. 833 (1992), at 851–52.
16. This is the so-called Texas Heartbeat Act (2021). For the text, see TX SB8 (2020–21), 87th Legislature, LegiScan, accessed November 6, 2022, at https://legiscan.com/TX/text/SB8/id/2395961.
17. Whole Woman's Health v. Jackson, 594 U.S. __ (2021), decided (5–4) on September 1, 2021. Justice Sonia Sotomayor's impassioned dissent noted, "In effect, the Texas Legislature has deputized the State's citizens as bounty hunters, offering them cash prizes for civilly prosecuting their neighbors' medical procedures." And further, she wrote, "the Act is a breathtaking act of defiance—of the Constitution, of this Court's precedents, and of the rights of women seeking abortions throughout Texas."
18. For discussion of *Dobbs* and its implications for both freedoms and responsibilities, see chapter 3, on health, under the heading "Healthy Liberty."
19. See the earlier discussion under the heading "In 'Trust' We Must Trust."
20. See, for example, Andreas Follesdal, "In Defense of Deference: International Human Rights as Standards of Review," *Journal of Social Philosophy*, November 8, 2021, https://doi.org/10.1111/josp.12449.
21. Section 5(1), the purpose of which was to forestall arguments defending bribery based on claims that it is accepted or even expected in certain overseas cultures or circumstances.
22. The world is "ensnared in a vicious cycle of distrust, fueled by a growing lack of faith in media and government," reports the "2022 Edelman Trust Barometer," which, globally, recorded people's views of both entities as "divisive forces in society" at 48 percent and 46 percent, respectively. See Edelman, accessed November 6, 2022, https://www.edelman.com/trust/2022-trust-barometer.
23. Timothy Snyder, *The Road to Unfreedom: Russia, Europe, and America* (New York: Tim Duggan Books, 2018), 134.
24. For a sardonic look at Putin's life of mendacity, see Andrew Weiss, *Accidental Czar: The Life and Lies of Vladimir Putin* (New York: Roaring Brook Press, 2022).
25. For the full text of the white paper, see "A Next Generation Artificial Intelligence Development Plan," China Copyright and Media, updated August 1, 2017, https://chinacopyrightandmedia.wordpress.com/2017/07/20/a-next-generation-artificial-intelligence-development-plan/.
26. John Lanchester, "Document Number Nine," *London Review of Books* 41, no. 19 (October 10, 2019). Also see "The AI-Surveillance Symbiosis in China: A Big Data China Event," Center for Strategic and International Studies, August 18, 2022, https://www.csis.org/analysis/ai-surveillance-symbiosis-china-big-data-china-event.
27. See Stephen Hutcheon, "'New Secret No. 5656': The Document That Lifts the Lid on Life inside a Chinese Re-education Camp," *ABC News*, November 28, 2019.
28. Thus, for example, in its 131-page response to the UN High Commissioner for Human Rights' report on Xinjiang Uyghur Autonomous Region (published on the same day as the UN report), Beijing glibly asserts both that "respecting and protecting human rights is a basic principle enshrined in the Constitution of

China" and that the "Vocational Education and Training Centres" in Xinjiang are merely administering "voluntary" programs of "de-radicalization" and "psychological correction and behavioural intervention to help trainees change their mindset, re-enter society and re-join their family." See "Fight against Terrorism and Extremism in Xinjiang: Truth and Fact," Information Office of the People's Government of Xinjiang Uyghur Autonomous Region, August 2022, 49–53, Office of the High Commissioner on Human Rights, accessed November 6, 2022, https://www.ohchr.org/sites/default/files /documents/countries/2022-08-31/ANNEX_A.pdf. It is in the blind certainty of the legitimacy of its authority that the righteousness of China's current leadership reveals its darkest levels of malevolent intent to control its citizenry.

29. Helen Davidson, "Chinese Inquiry Exonerates Coronavirus Whistleblower Doctor," *The Guardian*, March 20, 2020.

30. See Andrew Green, "Li Wenliang," obituary, *The Lancet*, February 18, 2020.

31. In 2017 the book *A Country of Big Babies*, by Wu Zhihong, was published and sold for a short time in China before being pulled from the shelves. The book's basic premise, and the matter that attracted the censors' attention, was that Chinese people, having never really grown up, are more supplicants than citizens and depend on the state for direction and control, rather than exercising free-thinking independence.

32. Though there are some signs of the government's growing awareness. See, for example, the "2021 Edelman Trust Barometer" (p. 9), which registered a "precipitous decline" in trust among the population of China throughout 2020. Edelman, accessed November 6, 2022, https://www.edelman.com/sites /g/files/aatuss191/files/2021-01/2021-edelman-trust-barometer.pdf; and Richard Edelman, "Declaring Information Bankruptcy," Edelman, January 12, 2021, https://www.edelman.com/trust/2021-trust-barometer/insights /declaring-information-bankruptcy.

33. See Mark McKenna, "Scott Morrison's Quiet Australians," *The Monthly* (July 2019); and Scott Morrison, address at 2019 Queensland Resources Council annual lunch, transcript (November 1, 2019).

34. It seemed to escape Mr. McCormack—as so much often did—that his label hardly fitted the head of the Australian Defence Force, the deputy governor of the Reserve Bank, and Chair of the Australian Prudential Regulation Authority, all of whom had raised climate change concerns at the time.

35. Morrison continued this line of marketing-slogan invective by characterizing critics of his government's botched handling of COVID-19 vaccine roll-outs throughout 2021 and the inadequacy of adequate quarantine facilities as "hindsight heroes," the irony being that it was precisely Morrison's lack of leadership foresight that his critics were targeting. See "'Hindsight Heroes': Morrison Blasts Vaccine Critics," *New Daily*, September 9, 2021. Morrison's government ended with the general election in May 2022, when his Liberal-National coalition lost to the Labor Party.

36. Nancy Gibbs, "The Danger of Donald Trump's Ignorance," *Time*, October 1, 2019. For data and discussion on Trump's careless disregard for truth and accuracy, including the more than 30,000 lies he told throughout his presidency, see chapter 8, on voice, under the heading "Voice Control."

37. See Karl Mihm, Jacob Apkon, and Sruthi Venkatachalam, "Litigation Tracker: Pending Criminal and Civil Cases against Donald Trump," *Just Security*, September 29, 2022, https://www.justsecurity.org/75032/litigation-tracker -pending-criminal-and-civil-cases-against-donald-trump/.

38. On which, see chapter 11, on respect, under the heading "Disrespect and Irresponsibility."

39. Charles Babington, "Partisan Views Affect Trust in Government," *Pew Trust Magazine*, September 9, 2021. In another report, Pew stresses that the United States is singular in this regard. Michael Dimock and Richard Wike, "America Is Exceptional in the Nature of Its Political Divide," *Pew Research Center*, November 13, 2020.

40. See, for example, Liz Mair, "Things Have Got So Stupid, We're Now Politicizing Food," *The Daily Beast*, November 22, 2018, and Jonathan Haidt, "Why the Past 10 Years of American Life Have Been So Uniquely Stupid," *The Atlantic*, April 11, 2022.

41. Sarah Longwell, "Trump Supporters Explain Why They Believe the Big Lie," *The Atlantic*, April 18, 2022; Jon Greenberg, "Most Republicans Still Falsely Believe Trump's Stolen Election Claims," *Poynter*, June 16, 2022 (collating a number of 2022 poll results).

42. Megan Brenan, "Americans' Trust in Media Dips to Second Lowest on Record," *Gallup*, October 7, 2021.

43. "Remarks by President Biden on the Continued Battle for the Soul of the Nation," White House, September 1, 2022.

44. Doha Madani, "Tennessee Teen Talking about Grandma Who Died of COVID Heckled by Adults at School Board Meeting," *NBC News*, September 10, 2021.

45. Christine Aschwanden, "Why Hatred and 'Othering' of Political Foes Has Spiked to Extreme Levels," *Scientific American*, October 20, 2020.

46. Previously available on twitter account: @realDonaldTrump (October 1, 2019), which account was "permanently" suspended by Twitter Inc. on January 8, 2021.

47. Caitlin Oprysko, "'I Don't Take Responsibility at All': Trump Deflects Blame for Coronavirus Testing Fumble," *Politico*, March 13, 2020.

48. Stuart Russell, *Human Compatible: AI and the Problem of Control* (New York: Penguin, 2019), 231.

49. James Vincent, "Gender and Racial Bias Found in Amazon's Facial Recognition Technology (Again)," *The Verge*, January 25, 2019.

50. Jacob Snow, "Amazon's Face Recognition Falsely Matched 28 Members of Congress with Mugshots," *ACLU*, July 28, 2018, at https://www.aclu.org/blog /privacy-technology/surveillance-technologies/amazons-face-recognition-falsely -matched-28.

51. According to the US Equal Employment Opportunity Commission, more than 83 percent of tech executives and managers are white, and barely 20 percent are women. See "Diversity in High Tech," Equal Employment Opportunity Commission, accessed November 7, 2022, https://www.eeoc.gov /special-report/diversity-high-tech.

52. Sarah Myers West, Meredith Whittaker, and Kate Crawford, "Discriminating Systems: Gender, Race, and the Power of AI," AI Now Institute (2019), 15–19. See also Deborah Raji, "How Our Data Encodes Systemic Racism," *MIT Technology Review*, December 10, 2020; Adrian Johansen, "How Lack of Diversity in Tech Leads to Coding and Algorithm Biases," *Global Comment*, July 14, 2022.

53. Dominic Gates, "Flawed Analysis, Failed Oversight: How Boeing, FAA Certified the Suspect 737MAX Flight Control System," *Seattle Times*, March 17, 2019.

54. Gates, "Flawed Analysis, Failed Oversight."

55. Special Rapporteur on the Promotion and Protection of the Right to Freedom of Opinion and Expression, *Surveillance and Human Rights* (May 28, 2019), UN Doc A/HRC/41/35.

56. Special Rapporteur on the Promotion and Protection of the Right to Freedom of Opinion and Expression, para. 6.

57. Referring to Facebook's role in the scandal, a UK parliamentary committee report in February 2019 commented, "Companies like Facebook should not be allowed to behave like 'digital gangsters' in the online world, considering themselves to be ahead of and above the law." See "Cambridge Analytica and GDPR—1 Year On—A Lot of Words and Some Action," Privacy International, April 30, 2019, https://www.privacyinternational.org/news-analysis /2857/cambridge-analytica-gdpr-1-year-lot-words-and-some-action. Facebook's gangster tactics were again on show two years later when, in the middle of a pandemic, the company blocked a host of strategically targeted Australian Facebook pages, including those providing information on government health services, in an effort to pressure the Australian government to water down a parliamentary bill intended to make social media platforms pay news outlets for using their content. The fact that Facebook's blackmail was largely successful speaks volumes about both the corporation and the Australia government at the time. See Keach Hagey, Mike Cherney, and Jeff Horwitz, "Facebook Deliberately Caused Havoc in Australia to Influence New Law, Whistleblowers Say," *Wall Street Journal*, May 5, 2022.

58. Sanjay Nair, "Trust in Tech Is Wavering and Companies Must Act," Edelman Trust Barometer, April 8, 2019.

59. "2021 Edelman Trust Barometer," 39; Edelman, "Declaring Information Bankruptcy."

60. Even (or perhaps especially) human rights bodies are dumbstruck in the face of such imponderables. See José-Miguel Bello y Villarino and Ramona Vijeyarasa, "International Human Rights, Artificial Intelligence, and the Challenge for the Pondering State: Time to Regulate?" *Nordic Journal of Human Rights* 40, no. 1 (2022): 1–22.

61. See Max Wessel and Nicole Helmer, "A Crisis of Ethics in Technological Innovation," *MIT Sloan Management Review*, March 10, 2020; and chapter 2, under the heading "The Responsibilities of Technology."

62. As the British Academy and the Royal Society advocate in their joint report, *Data Management and Use: Governance in the 21st Century* (June 2017), 7; see

also Ed Wallen, "The Importance of Ethical Leadership in Tech: A Call to Action," *Forbes*, July 27, 2022.

63. A proposal to radically alter the business model of technology companies is one ambitious attempt at providing some such detail, as promoted by the ever-resourceful Center for Human Technology. See its "We Need Zebras (Not Unicorns)," *Insights*, July 21, 2022, https://www.humanetech.com/insights/we-need-zebras-not-unicorns.

64. "It's utopian to think that people can make infallible AI," says philosopher and computer ethics academic Katleen Gabriëls, in *Conscientious AI: Machines Learning Morals* (Brussels: VUB Press, 2021).

65. Of the many versions of the tale, both Plutarch, in *The Parallel Lives* (circa 100 AD), and Henry Fielding, in *A Dialogue between Alexander the Great and Diogenes the Cynic* (1743), portray it thus.

Index

abduction, freedom from, 25–26

abortion and abortion rights: legality of, 12, 277; opposition to, 196; public attitudes toward, 223, 303nn14–15; restrictions on, 73, 185, 277–78, 303n13, 303n15, 342nn16–18

absolute/unconditional freedom, 300n18; of authoritarian states, 258; distinguished from liberty with responsibilities, 6–7, 22, 30–31, 33, 52–53, 59, 80–81, 252–53, 255; of tyrants, 42–44

actions, intentionality of, 44–45, 160–61, 318n3, 318n5, 336n47

Adams, Gerry, 262

advance directives, 248, 337n56

Affordable Care Act, 256

Afghanistan, 31, 166–67, 172, 214, 317n39, 330n22

age restrictions, 56, 151, 164, 212–13, 219

al-Assad, Bashar, 42–43, 235–36

al-Bashir, Omar, 42–43

alcohol use, 37, 56, 72, 73, 79, 90, 95, 142, 164–65, 236, 275

Alexander III (the Great), 292

Alexievich, Svetlana, 267

altruism, 50, 287, 307n58

American Civil Liberties Union, 287

American Revolution, 20, 41, 118, 183, 305n39

Amin, Idi, 42

Amnesty International, 5

Anthropocene, 177, 178, 322n45

antibiotics, 74–75; resistance to, 76

anti-Semitism, 194–95, 202, 269–70, 326n45

antitrust laws, 191

anti-vaccination movements, 73, 76, 77–78, 82–83, 85–86, 87, 253, 305n33, 305n38; "my body, my choice" position, 73, 79–81, 303n16; science-based rebuttals, 83–84

apartheid, 28, 129

apostates, 30, 188

Arab Spring movement, 228–29

Ardern, Jacinda, 105

Arendt, Hannah, 53–54; *Freedom and Politics*, 47, 201

Aristotle, 104

Aron, Arthur, 208

artificial intelligence (AI), 13, 58–60, 155, 286–87; ethics of use, 60–61, 219, 281, 301nn32–34, 346n64

assembly, freedom of, 25–26, 55–56

association, freedom of, 25–26, 55–56

Attlee, Clement, 67–68

Aung San Suu Kyi, 8, 276

Australia, 4, 68, 224, 301n35; aboriginal people, 179, 332n52, 339n23; climate change denialism, 283, 343n34; COVID-19 pandemic, 343n35, 345n57; euthanasia legality, 246, 337n52; free market economy, 121–22; free media, 188; free speech debates, 326n45; gun ownership and gun-related homicides, 173–74, 321n34; inequality of incarceration rates, 264, 339n23; navy, 157–58; same-sex marriages, 221, 331n38; sexuality discrimination, 218; social media, 345n57; suicide rate, 336n40

authoritarianism, 202, 227–28, 266, 282–83

347